Head and Neck Radiology Spot Diagnosis

Ammar Haouimi • Ziaul Haq Choudhuri
Rukhsana Begum • Chelia Boukaaba
Eugene Yu

Head and Neck Radiology Spot Diagnosis

A Casebook

Springer

Ammar Haouimi
Radiology and Medical Imaging
Centre D'imagerie Médicale Aurès
Batna, Algeria

Rukhsana Begum
Radiology and Medical Imaging,
former Chief
Edmundston Regional Hospital
Edmundston, N-B, Canada

Eugene Yu
Princess Margaret Cancer Centre
University of Toronto
Toronto, ON, Canada

Ziaul Haq Choudhuri
Radiology and Medical Imaging,
former Chief
Edmundston Regional Hospital
Edmundston, N-B, Canada

Chelia Boukaaba
Radiology and Medical Imaging
Centre D'imagerie Médicale Aurès
Batna, Algeria

ISBN 978-3-032-14552-9 ISBN 978-3-032-14553-6 (eBook)
https://doi.org/10.1007/978-3-032-14553-6

This Springer imprint is published by the registered company Springer Nature Switzerland AG
The registered company address is: Gewerbestrasse 11, 6330 Cham, Switzerland

Our exceptional mentors and colleagues,
who have guided us through the field of head and neck imaging.
And
Aspiring Head and Neck Radiologists
May this work inspire your curiosity, refine your precision, and fill your heart with compassion as you scan and diagnose every patient.

Foreword

I still remember telling my attendings on the second day of my radiology residency that I wanted to become a Head & Neck Radiologist. They literally started laughing at me and telling this naive first year radiology resident why no one in their "right mind" would enter such a field. They said the anatomy was too complex, the pathology was too difficult, and there were too few educational resources. Well, for all those reasons, I decided to become a Head & Neck Radiologist, and it was one of the best decisions of my life!

Over the past 30 years, the development of new imaging techniques and educational resources has invigorated the field of Head & Neck imaging. Yet, many radiologists are still reluctant to enter this field because of the "aura" of the field being too complex. The head & neck can be complex, but the basic anatomic components and pathologies are the same as elsewhere in the body.

I have always felt that most radiologists know much more about head and neck radiology than they think. One of the major educational gaps has been the lack of a practical case-based book that encourages the reader to explore the field by emphasizing what the radiologist already knows in an understandable and "non-threatening" format.

Fortunately, for all of us, this is exactly what Drs. Haouimi, Choudhuri, Begum, Boukaaba, and Yu have created in this book. This "spotter" format book covers 200 disorders of the extracranial head and neck, which include both common and rare pathologies. The book strongly emphasizes the characteristic findings and the typical clinical presentations which provide the reader to make a "spot" diagnosis, and it aptly named "Head & Neck Radiology Spot Diagnosis"! The scope and breadth of the book's content is comprehensive but not overwhelming so it can be read "cover to cover." The image quality is superb and will be an invaluable educational resource for radiology, otolaryngology, ophthalmology, and neurosurgery trainees at all levels and practicing radiologists. It will also be an outstanding board review for radiologists throughout the world who are considering taking a Head & Neck subspecialization exam.

I want to congratulate the authors for their tireless efforts in creating such an outstanding book. This is an invaluable resource which will be an essential reference that is also fun to read for many years to come. I just wish this book was available when I was a resident and fellow as it would have made my journey in Head & Neck Radiology much easier and more enjoyable!

Suresh K. Mukherji, MD, MBA, FACR

Professor of Radiology,
University of Louisville
and University of Illinois, USA

Profssor of Radiation Oncology (Adjunct),
Robert Wood Johnson Medical School,
Rutgers University
New Brunswick, NJ, USA

Preface

The extracranial head and neck is a region shared among skull base neurosurgeons, ophthalmologists, otorhinolaryngologists, stomatologists, and dental surgeons. Clinical evaluation is often difficult, and endoscopy, while important, can provide only a limited amount of information. Cross-sectional imaging, along with standard X-rays, plays a significant role in the diagnosis of diseases involving this area.

Head and neck radiology is a dynamic field that requires a deep understanding of complex anatomy, pathology, and imaging techniques. This book aims to bridge the gap between theory and practice by presenting key topics in a pictorial and interactive format. Cases are designed to engage readers through self-assessment. Each case begins with high-quality images and clinical history, prompting the reader to evaluate findings and generate a diagnosis or differential. Detailed explanatory notes follow, providing insight into the imaging features, pathophysiology, and clinical relevance of each condition. Differential considerations are highlighted concisely to train the reader in systematic diagnostic reasoning. A short description accompanies each case, including management options, distilling essential information without overwhelming detail. However, this book is not intended to be a replacement for standard textbooks but rather a supplement to them.

Our approach aims to provide clarity while covering the wide spectrum of head and neck disorders. From common to rare entities, the cases span key domains including neoplasms, congenital anomalies, trauma, infections, and vascular conditions. Emphasis is placed on correlation with clinical scenarios, helping readers appreciate the broader context of imaging findings. The interactive design promotes self-paced learning, making it ideal for radiologists, residents, fellows, and other healthcare professionals involved in treating head and neck diseases. By blending visual learning with concise explanations, this book provides an engaging resource to enhance diagnostic accuracy.

We hope it inspires confidence, curiosity, and a deeper appreciation for this complex but fascinating area of radiology.

Batna, Algeria — Ammar Haouimi
Edmundston, NB, Canada — Ziaul Haq Choudhuri
Edmundston, NB, Canada — Rukhsana Begum
Batna, Algeria — Chelia Boukaaba
Toronto, ON, Canada — Eugene Yu

Contents

Authors and Contributors

About the Authors

Ammar Haouimi, MD, DIS, DURP, DUCT, EDUS is a consultant radiologist at Aurès Imaging Center at Batna, Algeria. He got his training from the University of Bordeaux II. He was the head of the Department of Radiology and Imaging at Ohud Hospital and Madinah Maternity and Children Hospital (MMCH), Madinah, Saudi Arabia. Currently, he is one of the editors of the biggest online open-source teaching radiology website "Radiopaedia.org," where he has published more than 2600 cases and contributed to more than 860 articles. He has authored nine books on different Radiology subspecialties, including co-author of *Neuroradiology Spot Diagnosis* (2025), Cambridge Scholars Publishers Editor.

Ziaul Haq Choudhuri, MD, DIS, DUNR, DUMRI, DUEG is a staff neuroradiologist and former chief of the Department of Radiology and Medical Imaging at Edmundston Regional Hospital, NB, Canada. He completed his Neuroradiology training under the mentorship of Prof. Dominique Doyon and Prof. Pierre Lasjaunias at Hôpital Bicêtre, University of Sorbonne (Paris V). He completed his fellowship in Maxillofacial Radiology at the University of Paris Sud. Previously, he served as Senior Consultant at King Fahd Hospital in Medinah, Saudi Arabia. He has extensive teaching experience and has trained many residents both at home and abroad. He is the co-author of *Neuroradiology Spot Diagnosis* (2025), Cambridge Scholars Publishers Editor.

Rukhsana Begum, MD, DIS, DUEG is a staff radiologist and former chief of Radiology and Medical Imaging at Edmundston Regional Hospital, NB, Canada. She specialized from the University of Sorbonne (Paris V) and worked at Hôpital Bicêtre, Hôpital Avicenne, Necker–Enfants Malades, and Hôpital Robert Debré in Paris. She was head of the Department of Radiology and Imaging at Maternity and Children's Hospital, Madinah, Saudi Arabia. She has extensive teaching experience, particularly in Pediatric Neuroradiology. She is the co-author of *Neuroradiology Spot Diagnosis* (2025), Cambridge Scholars Publishers Editor.

Chelia Boukaaba, MD is a consultant radiologist at Aurès Imaging Center at Batna, Algeria. She graduated from the University of Constantine, Algeria. Currently, she is the head of the women's imaging department. She contributed to three books published by Dr. Ammar Haouimi.

Eugene Yu, MD, FRCPC is a neuroradiologist who subspecializes in head and neck imaging at the Princess Margaret Cancer Centre, University Health Network, University of Toronto. He is a Professor in the Departments of Medical Imaging and Otolaryngology Head and Neck Surgery. He obtained his medical school degree, radiology residency, and neuroradiology fellowship at the University of Toronto. He is the former site director for both the Neuroradiology Fellowship and the Radiology Residency Programs at Princess Margaret Cancer Centre, University of Toronto, and former clinical lead of head and neck radiology at the University Health Network. He has published over 100 articles, mostly focused on head and neck radiology, in various peer-reviewed journals. He is the co-author of *Skull Base Cancer Imaging* (2018), Thieme Editor; *Emergency Imaging: Rad Cases* (2014), Thieme Editor; and *Introductory Head and Neck Imaging* (2014), Jaypee Brothers Editor. He has served on the executive board of the North American Skull Base Society. He has been an invited visiting professor at different Universities, including the University of Chicago and Albert Einstein College of Medicine. He served as an Associate Editor of the journal *Head & Neck*. He is a current reviewer for peer review journals like *Radiology*, *Clinical Imaging*, *JAMA Otolaryngology*, *Journal of Neurological Surgery—Skull Base*, and *Neuroradiology*.

Contributors

Reem Adas, MD Department of Medical Imaging, National Guard Hospital, King Abdulaziz Medical City, Jeddah, Saudi Arabia

Amer Alaref, MD Northern Ontario School of Medicine University (NOSMU), Thunder Bay, ON, Canada

Nassim Barchiche, MD Dr Lakhal Imaging Medical Center, Blida, Algeria

Zine-Eddine Boudiaf, MD Aurès Medical Imaging Center, Batna, Algeria

Rabah Bouguelaa, MD, DIS Aurès Medical Imaging Center, Batna, Algeria

Nicolin Hainc, MD, FMH Department of Neuroradiology, University Hospital, Zurich, Switzerland

Chanon Ngamsombat, MD Faculty of Medicine, Siriraj Hospital, Mahidol University, Bangkok, Thailand

Mohamad Fatah Rougui, MD Department of Ophthalmology, Centre Hospitalier Universitaire Batna, Batna, Algeria

Case 1

1

Clinical History

A 5-year-old girl presented with a history of progressive painless swelling of the right fronto-orbital region.

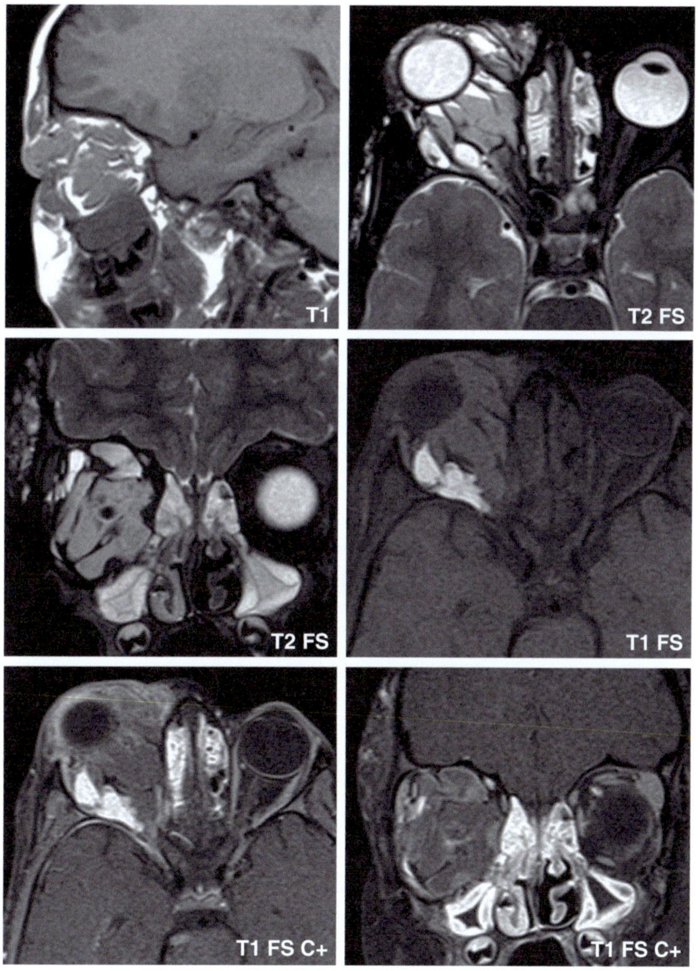

A. Haouimi et al., *Head and Neck Radiology Spot Diagnosis*,
https://doi.org/10.1007/978-3-032-14553-6_1

Findings

A right orbital multiloculated, ill-defined perioptic cystic mass having both intra- and extraconal components. It is causing grade III proptosis with associated locoregional extension and bony remodeling. The lesion appears as an intermediate-to-high signal on T1 and a high signal on T2. Multiple fluid–fluid levels are best seen on T2 fat sat, suggesting hemorrhagic, lymphatic, and proteinaceous contents. Faint enhancement is mainly evidenced at the margins of the cysts.

Diagnosis

Fronto-orbital lymphatic malformation.

Discussion

Orbital lymphatic malformations are rare, benign nontumoral cystic vascular lesions. They are mostly seen in pediatric patients below the age of 2 and may represent up to 1–3% of orbital masses. Histologically, the lesions are unencapsulated and often demonstrate an infiltrative growth pattern, insinuating between the orbital contents. These lesions can be trans-spatial, crossing anatomic boundaries and tissue planes.

The major clinical symptoms are progressive proptosis, ptosis, visual disturbances, and sluggish ocular movements. Although the lesions are benign, they can cause cosmetic deformity and occasionally vision loss secondary to amblyopia or compressive optic neuropathy.

MRI is the investigation of choice and typically shows a cluster of "grape-like" cystic lesions with internal septations. MRI can show the presence of fluid–fluid levels representing the layering of hemoglobin breakdown products from intralesional bleeding, as well as lymphatic and proteinaceous components.

Common Differential Diagnosis

- Capillary hemangioma: intense enhancement.
- Cavernous hemangioma: slow, gradual, irregular enhancement, and delayed washout.
- Orbital venous varix: change of size with Valsalva if not thrombosed.

Management Options

For smaller and asymptomatic lesions, observation should be the most appropriate management. Some physicians prefer to manage cases with corticotherapy, sclerotherapy, or laser therapy, depending on the clinical scenario. Patients with severe cosmetic and visual compromise may need surgical intervention.

References and Further Reading

1. Haouimi A. Fronto-orbital lymphatic malformation. Radiopaedia.org. 2021. https://doi.org/10.53347/rID-86073. Accessed on 20 June 2024.
2. Perry CB, et al. Orbital lymphatic malformation. EyeRounds.org. 2015. http://EyeRounds.org/cases/201-Lymphatic-Malformations.htm. Accessed on 20 June 2024.

Case 2

2

Clinical History

A 55-year-old woman presented with visual floaters and progressive decline in visual acuity over a period of 3 months.

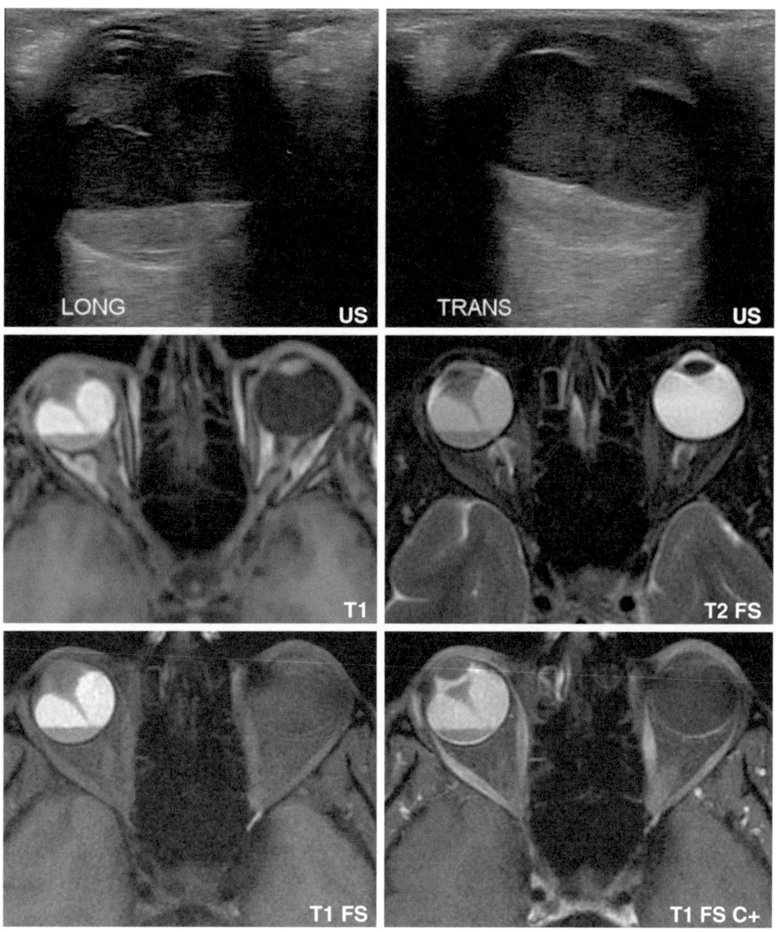

A. Haouimi et al., *Head and Neck Radiology Spot Diagnosis*,
https://doi.org/10.1007/978-3-032-14553-6_2

Findings

Ultrasound reveals a retro-retinal collection with a fluid–fluid level and an interposed canal of Cloquet. MRI shows the intraocular collection with a "V" configuration extending from the ora serrata anteriorly to the optic disc posteriorly. The anterior component represents methemoglobin of high signal while the posterior serum component shows a low signal. No enhancement.

Diagnosis

Retinal detachment.

Discussion

Retinal detachment means separation of the neurosensory layer from the pigmented choroid. Aging, diabetes, and trauma are the common causes. With advancing age, the vitreous shrinks and becomes more liquefied, leading to posterior vitreous detachment (PVD), mostly without any complication. However, when PVD causes a retinal tear, liquified vitreous passes through the torn retina to be collected in the subretinal space, causing separation of the neurosensory layer from the pigmented choroid.

A tiny focal detachment may be asymptomatic but the patients may complain of photopsia, multiple floaters, and visual field defects when a larger area is involved. The mechanism of detachment can be explained by traction, exudation, and rhegmatogenous (secondary to retinal tear). Rhegmatogenous type is by far the most common type.

On imaging, it is typically V-shaped with an anterior insertion to ora serrata. Posteriorly, the detachment converges as it approaches the optic disc. The signal depends on the content of the collection and there is no sign of enhancement.

Common Differential Diagnosis

- Choroidal detachment: lenticular collection, posteriorly diverging from the optic disc.
- Persistent hyperplastic primary vitreous: microphthalmia, leukocoria.
- Retinoblastoma: during infancy, inhomogeneous, T2 low signal, calcification +.

Management Options

Depending on the severity of the tear, surgical intervention, cryopexy, and laser therapy are considered. If diagnosed early, the treatment for retinal detachment works well.

References and Further Reading

1. Gaillard F, El-Feky M. Retinal detachment. Radiopaedia.org. 2024. https://doi.org/10.53347/rID-1975. Accessed on 15 Sept 2024.
2. Haouimi A. Retinal detachment. Radiopaedia.org. 2020. https://doi.org/10.53347/rID-76463. Accessed on 07 Nov 2022.

3 Case 3

Clinical History

A 35-year-old woman with known neurofibromatosis type 1.

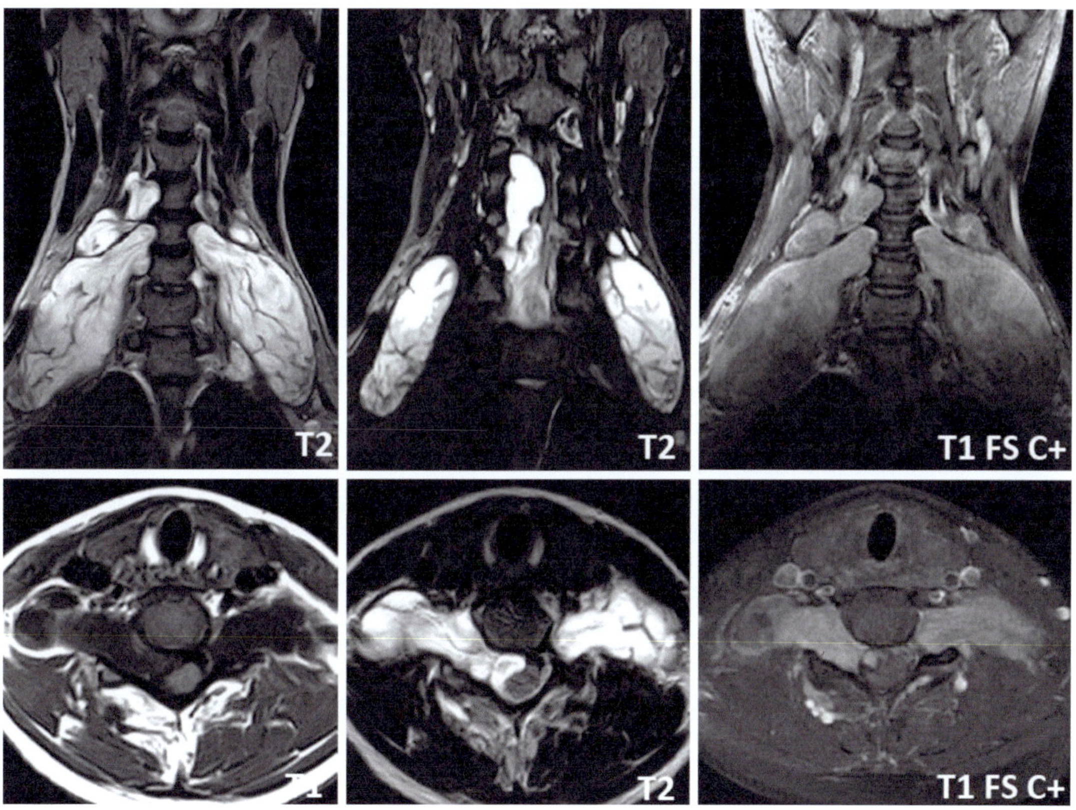

A. Haouimi et al., *Head and Neck Radiology Spot Diagnosis*,
https://doi.org/10.1007/978-3-032-14553-6_3

Findings

Bilateral transforaminal cervical bulging masses along the course of brachial plexus, extending from C3–C4 to C6–C7, are causing extrinsic medullary compression. They are of low signal on T1 and high signal on T2 with intense heterogeneous enhancement resembling "bags of worms."

Diagnosis

Plexiform neurofibromas (PNF).

Discussion

Plexiform neurofibromas are benign, architecturally complex lesions arising from the proliferation of Schwann cells and other components of the peripheral nerve. They are WHO grade 1 lesions, mostly seen in patients with neurofibromatosis type 1 (about 30%). PNFs often have a diffuse growth pattern involving multiple nerve sheaths. The term "plexiform" refers to a complex rope-like or plexiform growth of an interlacing network of nerves and blood vessels.

Up to 10% of cases have malignant potential, leading to a malignant peripheral nerve sheath tumor. They have growth and plateau phases. The lesions tend to grow during puberty and pregnancy due to hormonal changes. The lesions can be both superficial and deep and can arise anywhere in the body except the brain and spinal cord. About half of the cases are seen in the head, neck, face, and larynx. MRI can define the extent and nature of the lesion.

Cosmetic deformity, pain and discomfort, as well as functional impairment (when the lesion compresses the nearby structures) are the main clinical concerns.

Common Differential Diagnosis

- Venous malformations: presence of phleboliths.
- Lymphatic malformations: no enhancement.
- Sarcoma: infiltrative lesions with rapid growth, adenopathy +/−, usually unicentric.

Management Options

Medical treatment with selumetinib is promising. Complete resection is challenging due to the involvement of multiple nerve fibers. Radiotherapy and chemotherapy are used for malignant cases.

References and Further Reading

1. Grover DSB, et al. Imaging diagnosis of plexiform neurofibroma-unravelling the confounding features. Radiol Case Rep. 2021. https://doi.org/10.1016/j.radcr.2021.06.025. PMID: 34386146; PMCID PMC8343807. Accessed on 08 Dec 2024.
2. Haouimi A. Plexiform neurofibromas-neurofibromatosis type 1. Radiopaedia.org. 2020. https://doi.org/10.53347/rID-74336. Accessed on 08 Dec 2024.

Case 4

4

Clinical History

A 17-year-old girl presented with left tinnitus and chronic headache.

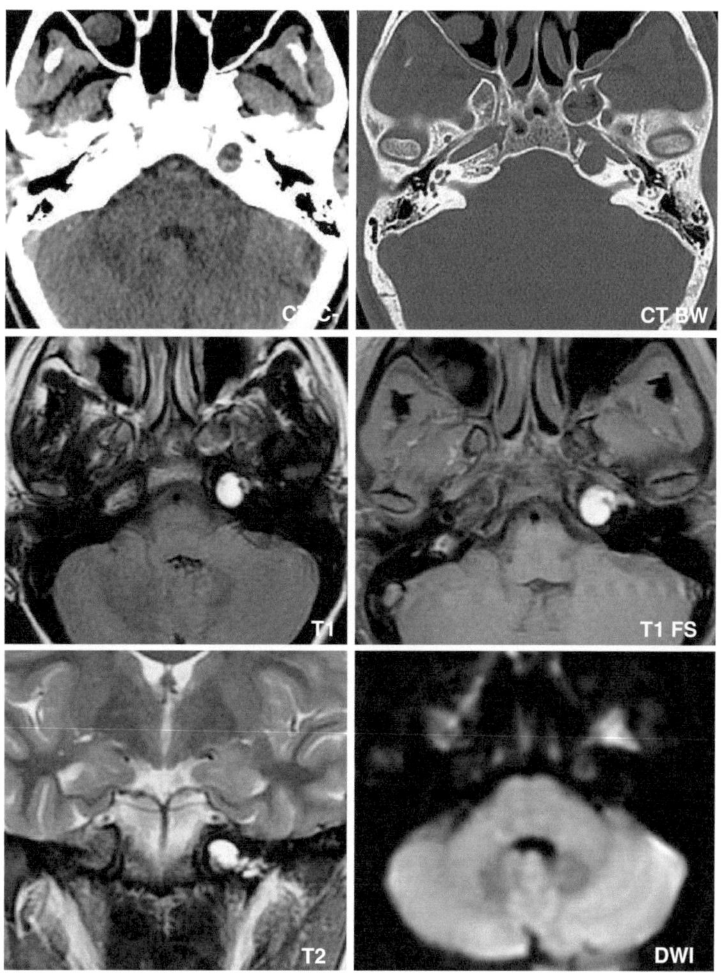

A. Haouimi et al., *Head and Neck Radiology Spot Diagnosis*,
https://doi.org/10.1007/978-3-032-14553-6_4

Findings

CT scan shows a small, well-marginated, expansile lucency involving the left petrous apex with a cortical dehiscence where it marginates the carotid canal. On MRI, the lesion demonstrates homogeneous high signal on T1, T1 fat-sat, and T2 images. No restricted diffusion is seen.

Diagnosis

Petrous apex cholesterol granuloma.

Discussion

Cholesterol granulomas also known as "chocolate cysts" are rare, benign, tumor-like expansile cystic lesions containing chocolate-brown fluid at the tip of the petrous apex. Previously, they were called "congenital epidermoid cysts." The fluid contains cholesterol crystals, hemoglobin breakdown products, including hemosiderin, and multinucleated giant cells surrounded by a fibrous capsule. Obstruction of normal drainage with failure of ventilation and subsequent hemorrhage liberates cholesterol crystals. Cholesterol granulomas develop as a foreign-body response to the cholesterol crystals.

The main etiologies of cholesterol granulomas are chronic infection (CSOM) and trauma. Although the lesions can be asymptomatic, vertigo, tinnitus, and hearing loss may develop due to progressive expansion of the lesion.

On CT, cholesterol granulomas are nonenhancing, well-demarcated, lucent, and expansile with associated cortical thinning and trabecular erosion. On MRI, the lesions appear as hyperintense masses on both T1 and T2. There is no enhancement or restricted diffusion.

Common Differential Diagnosis

- Asymmetric fatty marrow: signal can be suppressed by fat-sat sequence.
- Apical petrositis: low signal on T1.
- ICA aneurysm: heterogeneous signal with expansion of the carotid canal, flow void +.

Management Options

Most of these lesions are asymptomatic and remain either stable or grow very slowly over time. Those patients need imaging follow-up. Surgical drainage may be needed to maintain petrous apex pneumatization in symptomatic cases. Considering the high recurrence rate, percutaneous aspiration and gel foam embolization can also be performed.

References and Further Reading

1. Haouimi A. Cholesterol granuloma-petrous apex. Radiopaedia.org. 2022. https://doi.org/10.53347/rID-97772. Accessed on 26 Aug 2022.
2. Hunt JP, et al. Cholesterol granuloma of the petrous apex. Ear Nose Throat J. 2002. https://pubmed.ncbi.nlm.nih.gov/11987737/. Accessed on 15 July 2023.

Case 5

5

Clinical History

A 75-year-old man presented with a tetraparesis.

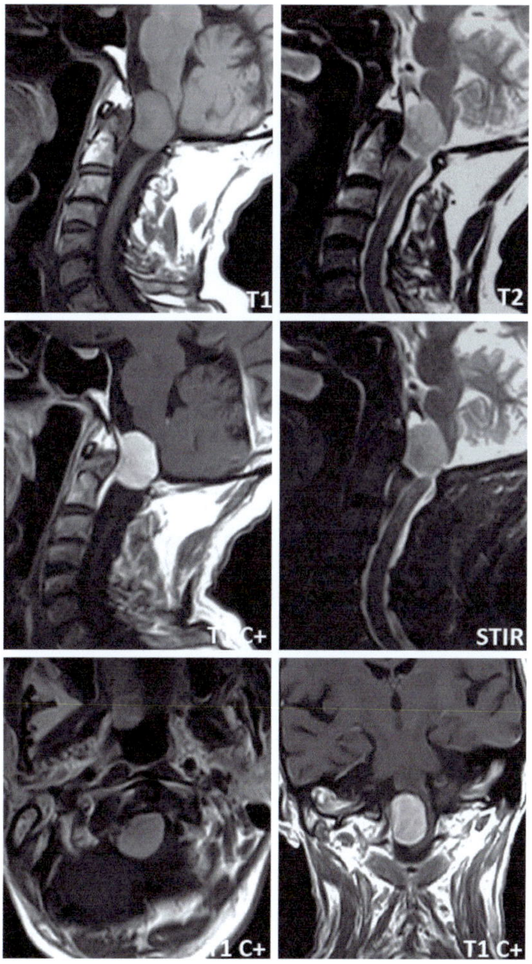

A. Haouimi et al., *Head and Neck Radiology Spot Diagnosis*,
https://doi.org/10.1007/978-3-032-14553-6_5

Findings

A broad, dural-based, extra-axial, well-defined mass located anteriorly at the foramen magnum, lateralized to the right. Extrinsic medullary compression causes displacement of the bulbomedullary junction to the left. The lesion appears isointense to the spinal cord on T1, hyperintense on T2 with vivid homogeneous enhancement showing "dural tail sign."

Diagnosis

Foramen magnum meningioma.

Discussion

Foramen magnum meningiomas (FMM) can develop at the skull base cranio-cervical junction. In general, meningiomas represent up to 25% of all intracranial tumors, and among them, FMM constitute up to 3%. The vast majority of meningiomas are benign, WHO grade 1 tumors. The lesions develop from the proliferation of arachnoid meningoepithelial cells. Because of their unique location, FMM are considered one of the most challenging meningiomas.

Symptoms develop slowly over years and are often misdiagnosed. The lesions are discovered late because of their slow growth and indolent development. The anatomic proximity of FMM to the cerebellar tonsils, medulla oblongata, lower cranial nerves, rostral spinal cord, and upper cervical nerves leads to highly variable symptomatology.

On MRI, the lesion appears as isosignal on T1 and slightly high signal on T2 with marked enhancement and positive "dural tail sign." On plain CT, FMM appear as high-density enhancing lesion. Bone algorithm CT can define the bony anatomy, identify calcification and hyperostosis, and allow surgical planning for bone resection. An optimal surgical planning always requires both CT and MR imaging to assess bone and soft tissues appropriately.

Common Differential Diagnosis

- Skull base schwannoma: "no dural tail sign."
- Skull base dural metastasis: known primary, heterogeneous, no hyperostosis, rapid growth.
- Chordoma: high T2 midline heterogeneous lesion, destructive.

Management Options

Surgery is the mainstay of treatment. Other options are radiotherapy and radiosurgery.

References and Further Reading

1. Bir SC, Maiti TK, Nanda A. Foramen magnum meningiomas. Handb Clin Neurol. 2020. https://doi.org/10.1016/B978-0-12-822198-3.00038-0. Accessed on 07 Dec 2024.
2. Haouimi A. Meningioma – foramen magnum. Radiopaedia.org. 2022. https://doi.org/10.53347/rID-98382. Accessed on 07 Dec 2024.

Case 6

6

Clinical History

An 85-year-old diabetic man presents with persistent right periauricular earache (worse with manipulation), local redness and swelling with thick, purulent, foul-smelling otorrhea.

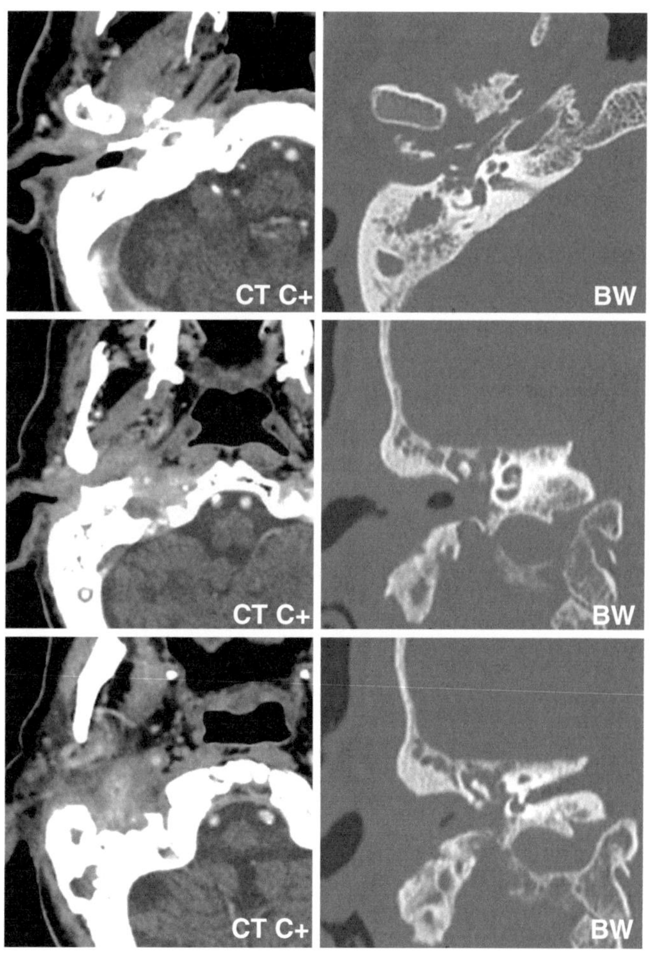

A. Haouimi et al., *Head and Neck Radiology Spot Diagnosis*,
https://doi.org/10.1007/978-3-032-14553-6_6

Findings

Soft tissue filling of the right middle ear and mastoid air cells. Enhancement and swelling of the EAC. Osteolytic changes of the tympanic bone, styloid process, and clivus (images not shown). Inflammatory and edematous changes involving neighboring soft tissues with enhancement, including the carotid sheath and the wall of the ICA with narrowing of the lumen. Associated sigmoid sinus thrombosis extending to internal jugular vein at jugular foramen.

Diagnosis

Malignant otitis externa with internal carotid arteritis and sigmoid sinus thrombosis.

Discussion

The terms malignant otitis externa and malignant otitis media are used interchangeably. Use of the term malignant otitis externa is more appropriate as the infection originates in the external auditory canal before extending to the neighboring structures. The infections are mostly bacterial, caused by *Pseudomonas aeruginosa* and occasionally by *Candida* or *Aspergillus*. Diabetics, immunosuppressed, cancer, and elderly patients are more vulnerable to this condition. Though the lesions are nonneoplastic, the term "malignant" is used due to their highly aggressive nature and can be potentially life threatening. Proteases and other toxins produced by *Pseudomonas* cause osteomyelitis of adjacent bony structures and the soft tissue involvement can lead to multiple cranial nerve neuropathies as well as involvement of intracranial structures.

Clinically, patients initially present with otalgia aggravated by manipulation and persistent foul-smelling otorrhea. Conductive hearing deficit, cranial neuropathies, and trismus can arise. Symptoms like fever, malaise, and weight loss are seen only in advanced cases.

Common Differential Diagnosis

- EAC squamous cell carcinoma: lymphadenopathy +, destructive, irregular wall thickening.
- EAC cholesteatoma: no enhancement, intramural bony flakes +/−.
- EAC keratosis obturans: enlarged canal diameter, no bony erosion.

Management Options

Empiric IV antibiotherapy is the mainstay of treatment. Local debridement to remove debris and necrotic tissue.

References and Further Reading

1. Guan H. Necrotising otitis externa. Radiopaedia.org. 2022. https://doi.org/10.53347/rID-149334. Accessed on 25 Jan 2025.
2. Walizai T, et al. Necrotising otitis externa. Radiopaedia.org. 2024. https://doi.org/10.53347/rID-19937. Accessed on 25 Jan 2025.

Case 7

7

Clinical History

A 30-year-old woman presented with a painless right orbital swelling since childhood.

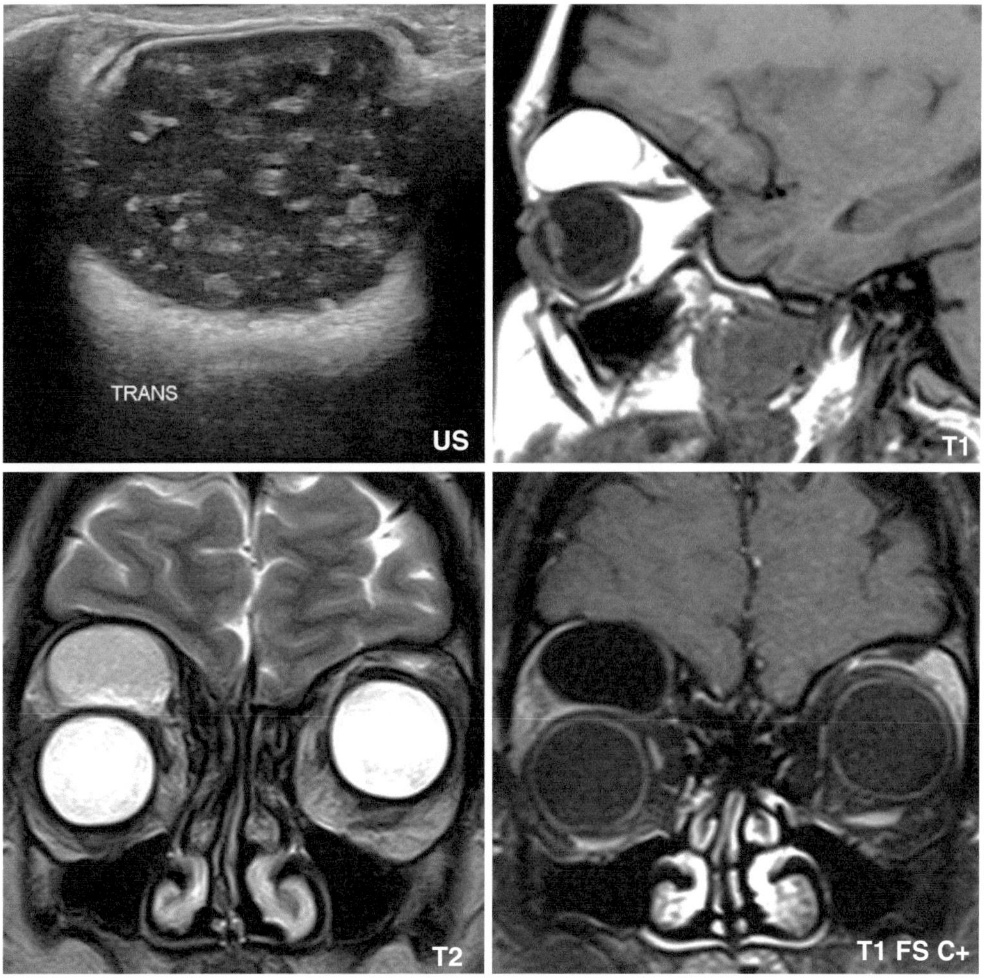

A. Haouimi et al., *Head and Neck Radiology Spot Diagnosis*,
https://doi.org/10.1007/978-3-032-14553-6_7

Findings

Ultrasound shows a hypoechoic intraorbital lesion containing numerous tiny echogenic foci with a "sack of marbles appearance." On MRI, this supraocular extraconal lesion appears well defined, showing high signal on both T1 and T2, attenuated signal with T1 fat saturation, and no enhancement. Downward displacement of ocular globe and superior rectus muscle.

Diagnosis

Orbital dermoid cyst.

Discussion

Dermoids are benign developmental choristoma representing up to 5% of orbital masses. They are derived from dermal and epidermal tissues trapped in the cranial fusion lines during closure of the neural tube in embryogenesis. The lesions contain dermal elements and skin appendages such as hair follicles and sebaceous and sweat glands. Malignant transformation is rare. Clinically, patients present with a slow-growing, painless swelling. A sudden increase in size indicates rupture and may be associated with signs of locoregional inflammation.

The intralesional echogenic foci on ultrasound correspond to aggregations of multiple tiny fatty tissue globules and produce the "sack of marbles sign." On MRI, the lesions are typically heterogeneous, composed of soft tissue, fluid, and fatty tissue (sebum). These extraconal lesions show smooth margins without any enhancement. Occasionally, calcifications may be present. Presence of fatty tissue on MRI is quasi-pathognomonic.

Common Differential Diagnosis

- Idiopathic pseudotumor: acute painful onset.
- Lacrimal cancer: infiltrative lesion involving adjacent bone and fatty tissue.
- Frontal mucocele: CSF intensity lesion on all sequences.

Management Options

Surgical resection. Anti-inflammatory drugs to reduce postrupture inflammation.

References and Further Reading

1. Bansal R, et al. Orbital dermoidcyst. Indian J Ophthalmol. 2022. https://doi.org/10.4103/ijo.IJO_145_22. Accessed on 05 June 2022.
2. Haouimi A. Orbital dermoid cyst-sack of marbles sign. Radiopaedia.org. 2020. https://doi.org/10.53347/rID-83352. Accessed on 04 Sept 2022.
3. Pham NS, et al. Dermoid cyst of the orbit and frontal sinus: a case report. Skull Base. 2010. https://doi.org/10.1055/s-0030-1247631. Accessed on 02 May 2023.

Case 8

8

Clinical History

A 10-year-old boy presented with partial epilepsy.

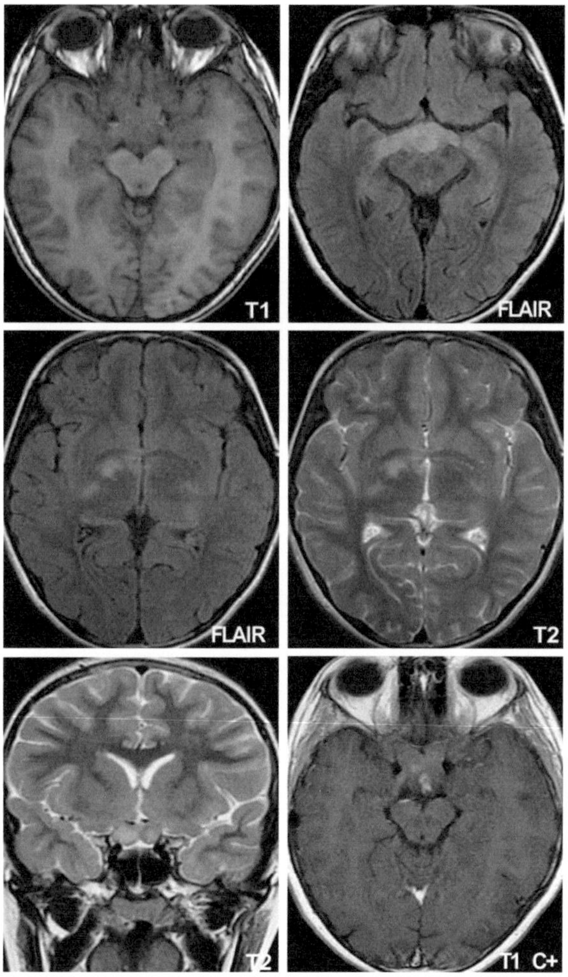

A. Haouimi et al., *Head and Neck Radiology Spot Diagnosis*,
https://doi.org/10.1007/978-3-032-14553-6_8

Findings

Markedly thickened optic chiasm as well as pre- and postchiasmatic segments of the optic nerves. On MRI, these structures are isointense to gray matter on T1, hyperintense on T2 and FLAIR, and show mild enhancement. No intraorbital optic nerve abnormality.

Diagnosis

Optic pathway glioma (OPG).

Discussion

OPGs are benign tumors categorized as pilocytic astrocytoma. They account for up to 15% of supratentorial tumors in children in the setting of neurofibromatosis type 1. However, isolated adult cases can also be seen and those are often aggressive. OPG arises from the precortical optic pathways and can involve any segment of visual pathway, including the hypothalamus.

The clinical symptoms depend on the specific area of involvement. Symptomatic cases often present with vision loss, painless proptosis, nystagmus, and signs of increased intracranial pressure and epilepsy in Dodge type 3 lesions. Patients can also complain of hypothalamopituitary dysfunction, such as precocious puberty and signs of hormonal imbalance. CT scan may also show an enlarged optic canal. MRI is the modality of choice and reveals a fusiform enlargement of the affected optic nerve with T1 iso- or hypointense signal. On T2, the lesions are centrally hyperintense with a thin peripheral low signal representing the dura. The enhancement is variable. MRI can better show the relationship to neighboring structures such as the hypothalamus and infundibulum. Larger lesions are mostly heterogeneous and can have both cystic and solid components.

Common Differential Diagnosis

- Optic nerve sheath meningioma: no chiasmatic involvement, calcification.
- Optic neuritis: acute onset, enhancement +.
- Sarcoidosis: systemic, predilection for lacrimal gland, orbital inflammation.

Management Options

Chemotherapy is the first line of treatment. Resistant cases may need radiotherapy.

References and Further Reading

1. Gaillard F, Smith D. Optic pathway glioma. Radiopaedia.org. 2025. https://doi.org/10.53347/rID-6665. Accessed on 15 July 2025.
2. Haouimi A. Optic pathway glioma. Radiopaedia.org. 2019. https://doi.org/10.53347/rID-67734. Accessed on 01 Sept 2022.
3. Huang M, et al. Optic nerve glioma. Stat Pearls Publishing; 2024. https://www.ncbi.nlm.nih.gov/books/NBK557878/. Accessed on 19 June 2025.

Case 9

Clinical History

A 30-year-old man presented with acute onset of unilateral left orbital pain and blurred vision.

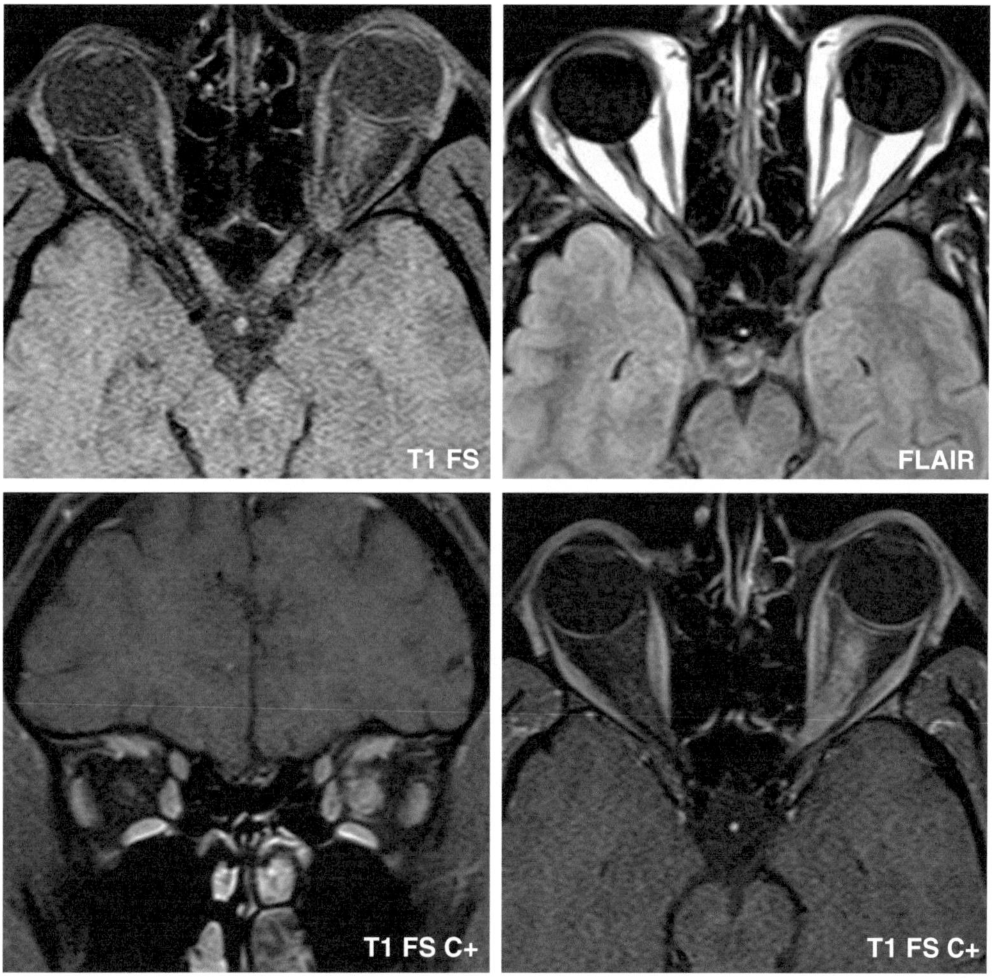

A. Haouimi et al., *Head and Neck Radiology Spot Diagnosis*,
https://doi.org/10.1007/978-3-032-14553-6_9

Findings

Thickening of the left retrobulbar optic nerve. It appears isointense on T1 and hyperintense on FLAIR. Homogeneous enhancement of the optic nerve and perineural sheath on postcontrast images.

Diagnosis

Optic neuritis.

Discussion

Optic neuritis is an inflammatory condition causing demyelination of the optic nerve. An autoimmune mechanism has been described to explain the etiology of optic nerve demyelination. Viral infections are believed to precipitate autoimmune reactions. Optic neuritis also has a causal relationship between HLA-DRB1and HLA-B27 antigen. The risk factors are multiple sclerosis (MS), neuromyelitis optica, and high-altitude dwellers.

Optic neuritis is commonly seen in the setting of multiple sclerosis but can also present as an isolated clinical syndrome in which it is unilateral and involves only a short segment. Patients often present with acute onset of orbital tenderness worsening with ocular movement, dyschromatopsia, followed by visual impairment within a few days of onset.

MRI shows a swollen retrobulbar segment of the optic nerve. The optic nerve appears isosignal on T1 and high signal on T2 with enhancement in early stage (up to 3 weeks following onset of symptoms) before starting to atrophy.

Common Differential Diagnosis

- Multiple sclerosis: additional brain and spinal cord lesions.
- Optic nerve sheath meningioma: painless, MRI "tram track sign," and "doughnut sign" +.
- Neuromyelitis optica: associated longitudinally extensive spinal cord lesions.

Management Options

Most cases are self-limiting. Patients are treated with corticosteroids to reduce recovery time. Intravenous immunoglobulin and plasma exchange are reserved for nonresponsive cases.

References and Further Reading

1. Bennett JL. Optic neuritis. Continuum (Minneap, Minn). 2019. https://doi.org/10.1212/CON.0000000000000768. Accessed on 15 July 2025.
2. Gaillard F, Baba Y. Optic neuritis. Radiopaedia.org. 2025. https://doi.org/10.53347/rID-29943. Accessed on 01 Sept 2025.
3. Haouimi A. Optic neuritis with perineuritis. Radiopaedia.org. 2021. https://doi.org/10.53347/rID-94805. Accessed on 10 Dec 2022.

Case 10

10

Clinical History

A 75-year-old woman presented with a left-sided exophthalmos.

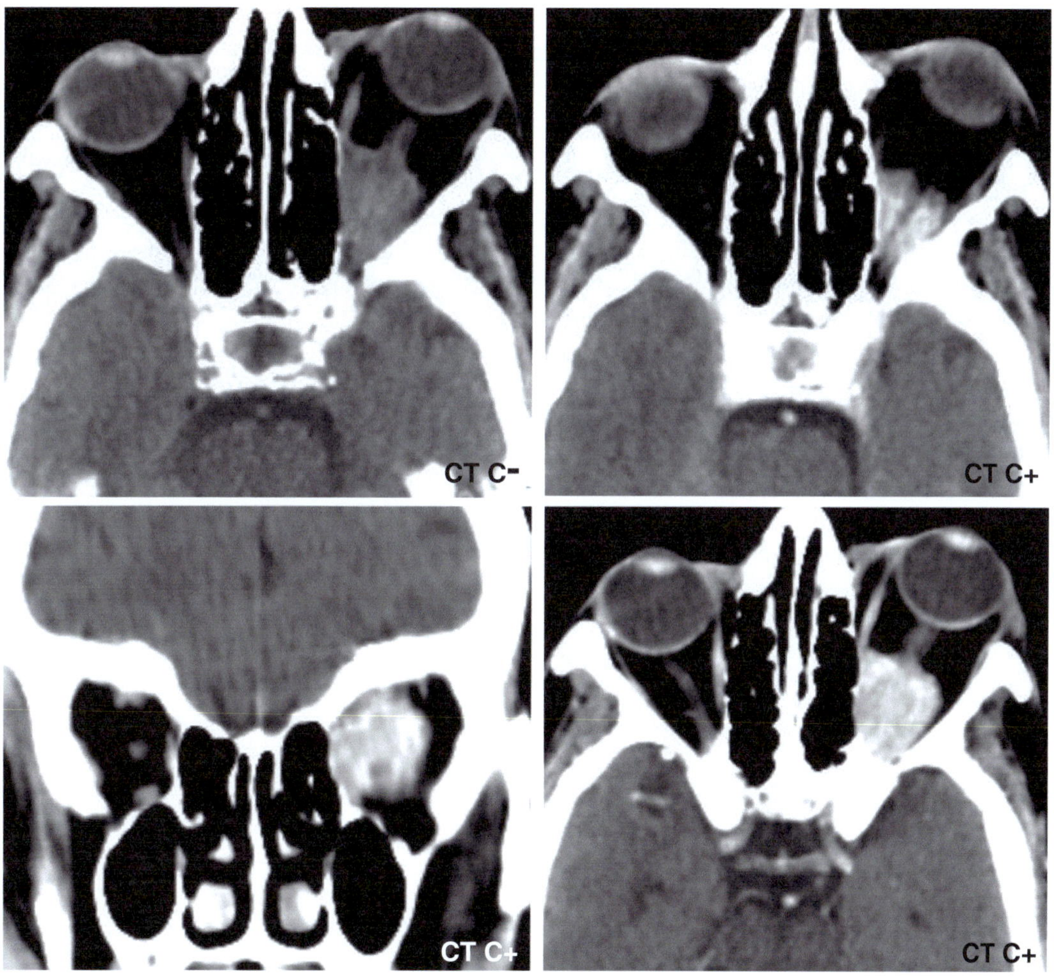

A. Haouimi et al., *Head and Neck Radiology Spot Diagnosis*,
https://doi.org/10.1007/978-3-032-14553-6_10

Findings

An intraconal mass encasing the left optic nerve, isodense to the nerve on the unenhanced image with intense homogeneous enhancement. The lesion creates a "tram track" appearance on enhanced axial images and a "nonenhancing dot sign" on enhanced coronal reconstruction. The lesion extends to the optic canal with ipsilateral axial proptosis grade III.

Diagnosis

Optic nerve sheath meningioma (ONSM).

Discussion

Optic nerve sheath meningiomas are uncommon benign tumors and are the second most common primary optic nerve tumor. They represent an overall 1–2% of all meningiomas. ONSMs are almost always unilateral except in patients with NF2. They originate from meningothelial cells of the meninges neighboring the optic nerve. Though they rarely invade the optic nerve, the lesions are unencapsulated and remain tightly adherent to perineural pia.

Clinically, patients present with slow-growing painless proptosis with or without diplopia and monocular vision loss. The diagnosis is confirmed with neuroimaging. Biopsy is not necessary in the typical clinical context with characteristic neuroimaging findings.

CT shows isodense, enhancing, perioptic soft tissue tubular lesions involving the nerve sheath. Calcifications may have a "tram track" appearance and may be present in up to 50% of cases. MRI shows a homogeneously enhancing isointense thickened nerve sheath on both T1 and T2. The tubular thickening of the nerve sheath encasing the optic nerve often produces a characteristic MRI "tram track sign" on axial images and a "doughnut sign" on coronal images.

Common Differential Diagnosis

- Optic nerve glioma: fusiform lesion of the optic nerve, no calcification.
- Optic neuritis: enhancement of the optic nerve, often associated with multiple sclerosis.
- Orbital pseudotumor: history, mostly involves extraocular muscles and retro-orbital fat.

Management Options

Stereotactic radiotherapy provides the best chance for vision preservation. Surgical excision with preservation of vision is practically impossible.

References and Further Reading

1. Haouimi A. Optic nerve sheath meningioma-axial exophthalmos grade 3. Radiopaedia.org. 2019. https://doi.org/10.53347/rID-72137. Accessed on 03 Sept 2022.
2. Gaillard F, Yadegarfar M. Optic nerve sheath meningioma. Radiopaedia.org. 2024. https://doi.org/10.53347/rID-9624. Accessed on 01 Sept 2022.

Case 11

11

Clinical History

A 1-year-old girl with a congenital mass in left paranasal region.

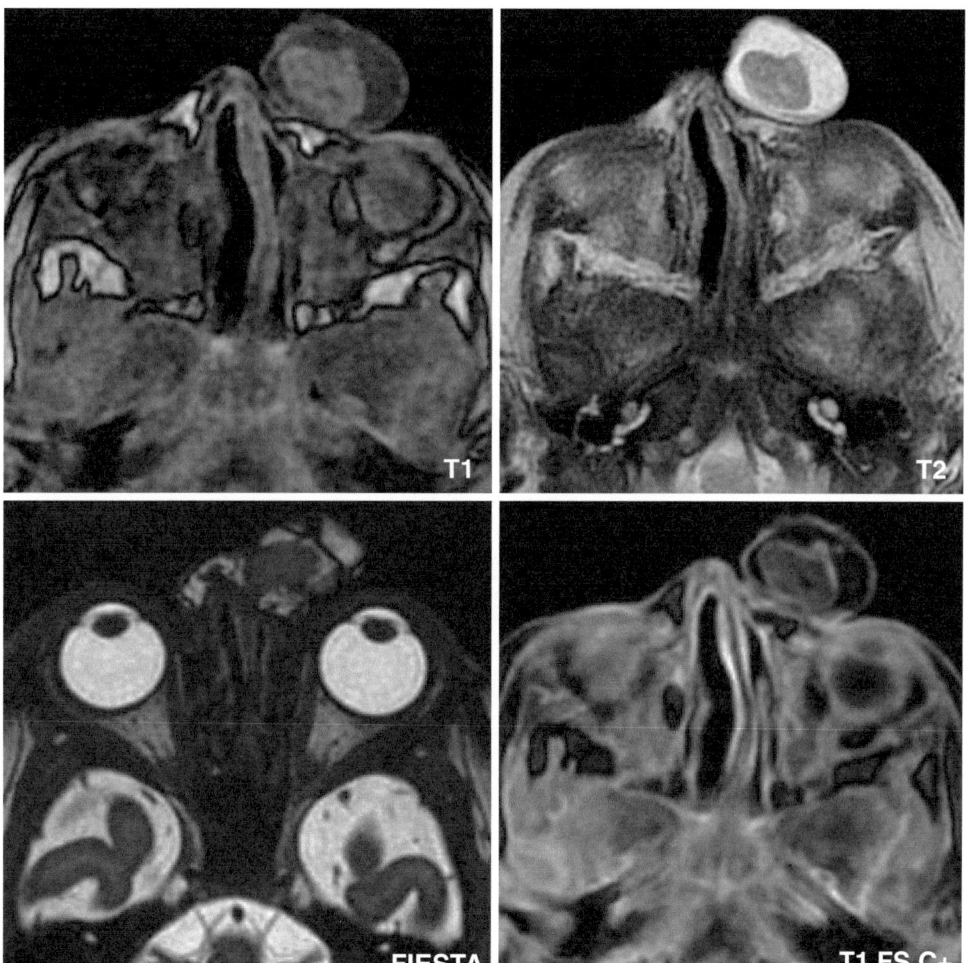

A. Haouimi et al., *Head and Neck Radiology Spot Diagnosis*,
https://doi.org/10.1007/978-3-032-14553-6_11

Findings

A left off-midline lesion at the root of the nose showing central isosignal (to the brain tissue) on both T1 and T2 with peripheral low signal on T1 and high signal on T2 (CSF-like signal). Intense peripheral enhancement of the solid component. No communication with intracranial structures or subarachnoid space.

Diagnosis

Nasal glioma.

Discussion

Nasal gliomas, also known as nasal glial heterotopia, are rare congenital lesions with no malignant potential. Histologically, they are composed of dysplastic glial tissue. They represent sequestered dysplastic neurogenic tissue isolated from the subarachnoid space. It is thought to be due to premature fusion of potential anterior skull base spaces before the regression of the dural diverticulum. They occur sporadically without any gender or familial predilection and without any other brain abnormalities.

The lesions can be intraoral or extranasal. Clinically, extranasal lesions (approximately two-thirds of cases) are paramedian masses at the level of the glabella, covered with red skin. These lesions do not increase in size while crying or Valsalva. Intranasal lesions are seen medial to the middle turbinate and often present as firm submucosal lesions extending toward the nostril inferiorly. The main complaints of intranasal lesions are nasal obstruction, epistaxis, epiphora, and rhinorrhea.

MRI is the investigation of choice, and lesions appear isointense on all sequences. Occasionally, an intracranial obliterated fibrous stalk can be visualized on high-resolution MRI.

Common Differential Diagnosis

- Encephalocele: connection with CSF space and brain tissue, increases while crying.
- Solitary sinonasal polyp: usually not seen in infants, more translucent than glioma.
- Epidermoid: low signal intensity, not isointense.

Management Options

Early surgical excision is necessary to minimize craniofacial distortion. Extranasal cases need stalk resection, whereas intranasal cases need to be resected endoscopically.

References and Further Reading

1. Haouimi A. Nasal glial heterotopia. Radiopaedia.org. 2022. https://doi.org/10.53347/rID-98794. Accessed on 22 Nov 2022.
2. Midyett FA, Mukherji SK. Nasal glioma. In: Skull base imaging. Cham: Springer. https://doi.org/10.1007/978-3-030-46447-9_20.
3. Radswiki T, El-Feky M. Nasal glioma. Radiopaedia.org. 2022. https://doi.org/10.53347/rID-12965. Accessed on 07 Nov 2022.

Case 12

12

Clinical History

A 50-year-old woman known for Graves' disease presented with bilateral painless neck swelling.

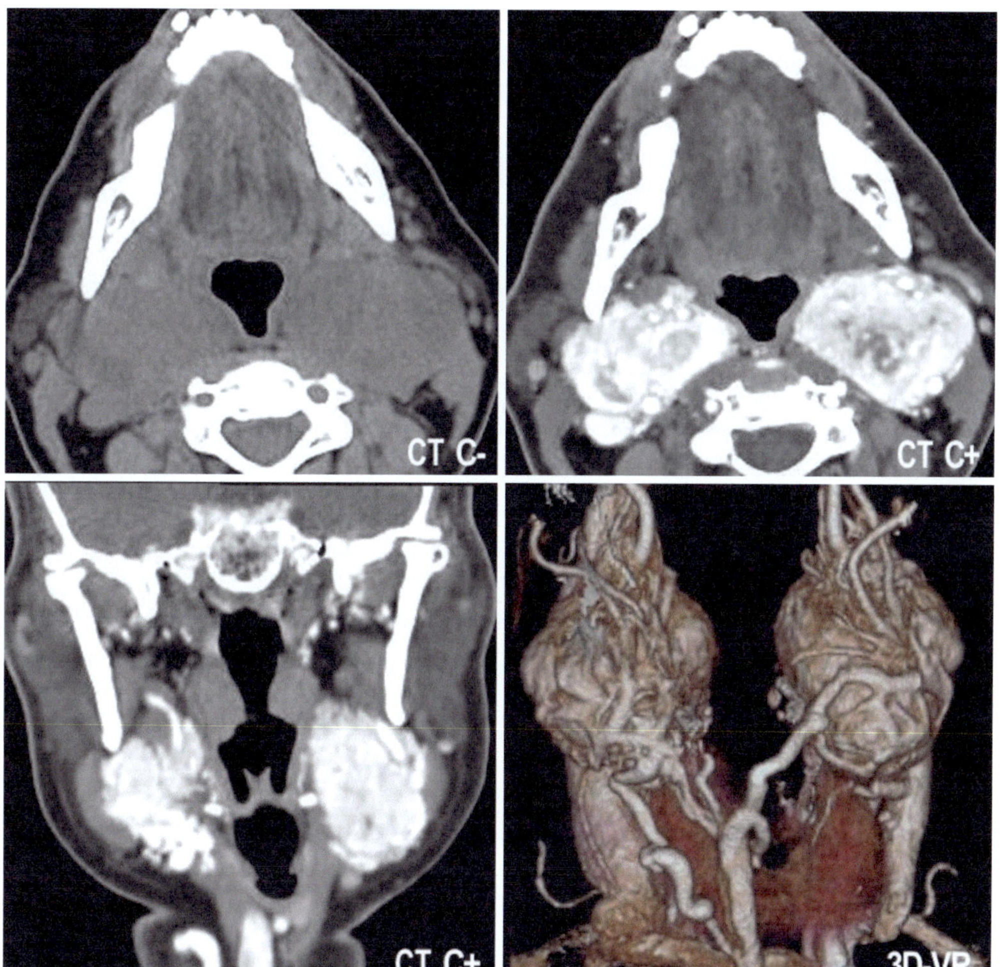

A. Haouimi et al., *Head and Neck Radiology Spot Diagnosis*,
https://doi.org/10.1007/978-3-032-14553-6_12

Findings

Bilateral well-defined carotid space masses, isodense to muscle with vivid enhancement on CT. Splaying of the internal and external carotid arteries showing typical "lyre sign."

Diagnosis

Bilateral carotid body paraganglioma (CBP).

Discussion

CBPs arise from clusters of neuroendocrine cells and are mostly seen between the third and sixth decades of life. About 10% of the cases are bilateral. They have rare malignant potential.

Most of the carotid body paragangliomas remain asymptomatic. Patients usually present with a slow-growing, painless, pulsatile lateral neck mass near the angle of the mandible, anterior to the sternocleidomastoid muscle, at the level of hyoid bone. Larger lesions can cause dysphagia, odynophagia, hoarseness of voice, and other lower cranial nerve deficits due to proximity to the lower four cranial nerves. Increase in size leads to splaying and encasement of the internal and external carotid arteries without narrowing the vascular lumen. Symptoms such as hypertension, sweating, and headache can be seen in a few patients due to vasoactive catecholamines produced by CBP.

On plain CT, the lesion is isodense to soft tissue. Splaying of the internal and external carotid arteries is better appreciated on enhanced CT due to marked enhancement of the lesion. On MRI, larger lesions may show a "salt-and-pepper appearance" on both T1 and T2. When carotid body paraganglioma is suspected, the radiologist must look for second lesion such as glomus jugulare and glomus vagale.

Common Differential Diagnosis

- Schwannoma: displaces the carotid space anteriorly; splaying of the ICA and ECA is rare.
- Lymphoma: multiple bilateral lymph nodes, mild homogeneous enhancement.
- Castleman disease: homogeneous enhancement, not in carotid space.

Management Options

Treatment options include observation, radiation therapy, and surgery.

References and Further Reading

1. Haouimi A. Bilateral carotid body tumour. Radiopaedia.org. 2022. https://doi.org/10.53347/rID-149310. Accessed on 25 Aug 2022.
2. Hosalkar RM, et al. Carotid body paraganglioma. Ann Maxillo fac Surg. 2019. https://doi.org/10.4103/ams.ams_183_18. Accessed on 12 Apr 2024.
3. Ikram A, Rehman A. Paraganglioma. Stat Pearls Publishing; 2025. https://www.ncbi.nlm.nih.gov/books/NBK549834/. Accessed on 19 Aug 2025.

Case 13

13

Clinical History

A 30-year-old man presented with a low-growing, hard, painless mandibular mass.

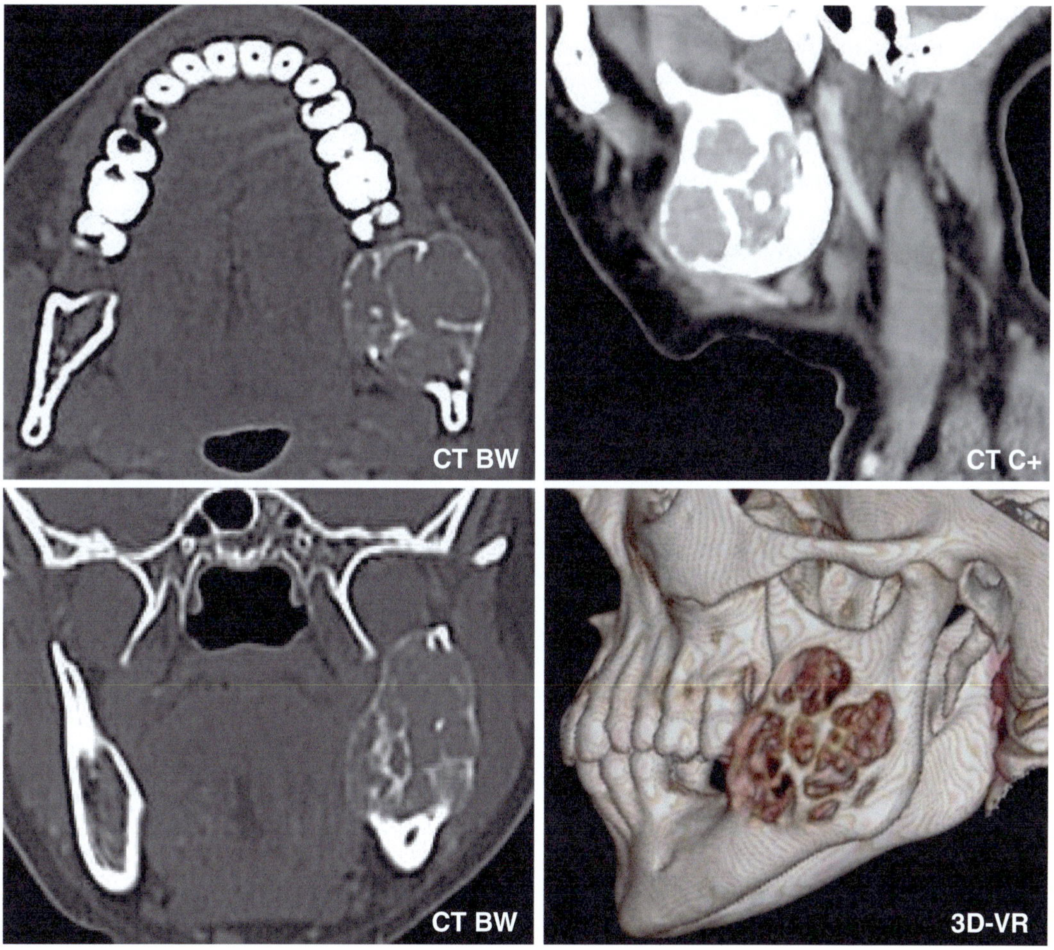

A. Haouimi et al., *Head and Neck Radiology Spot Diagnosis*,
https://doi.org/10.1007/978-3-032-14553-6_13

Findings

A multilocular, expansile "soap-bubble" lesion of the left mandibular angle with solid enhancing components. Unerupted third molar tooth (#38) with areas of cortical thinning. No locoregional soft tissue or lymph node involvement.

Diagnosis

Ameloblastoma.

Discussion

Ameloblastomas are benign odontogenic lesions with remote malignant potential. These are locally aggressive tumors arising from odontogenic epithelium with a high rate of recurrence. The exact etiology is not known. A possible genetic mutation activating a specific signaling pathway (mitogen-activated protein kinases [MAPK]) may play a role in its pathogenesis. About 20% of cases are associated with dentigerous cyst.

Clinically, patients may be asymptomatic, and it may take years to be symptomatic, until they notice facial swelling and asymmetry. They typically present as a slow-growing, painless mass near the angle of the mandible. Loose dentition and delayed healing after tooth extraction may occur. Occasionally, the patients may complain of a change in bite and lesions are detected by the dentist on routine dental panoramic radiographic films.

On CT, ameloblastomas often show bony expansion and dental root resorption. The multiloculated radiolucent lesions giving a typical "soap-bubble" appearance. They may also be associated with unerupted teeth.

Common Differential Diagnosis

- Periapical abscess: clinically painful, no bone expansion.
- Fibrous dysplasia: ground-glass matrix.
- Aneurysmal bone cyst: fluid–fluid level, no enhancing mural nodule.

Management Options

The treatment is surgical excision for smaller lesions and "en bloc" removal for bigger lesions. Curettage is discouraged. Radiotherapy and chemotherapy are contraindicated.

References and Further Reading

1. Haouimi A. Ameloblastoma-mandible. Radiopaedia.org. 2023. https://doi.org/10.53347/rID-99357. Accessed on 25 Aug 2022.
2. Hisatomi M, et al. Diagnostic value of dynamic contrast-enhanced MRI for unilocular cystic-type ameloblastomas with homogeneously bright high signal intensity on T2-weighted or STIR MR images. Oral Oncol. 2011. https://doi.org/10.1016/j.oraloncology.2010.11.009. Accessed on 21 July 2025.
3. Palanisamy JC, et al. Ameloblastoma. Stat Pearls Publishing; 2023. https://www.ncbi.nlm.nih.gov/books/NBK545165/. Accessed on 24 July 2024.

Case 14

14

Clinical History

A 50-year-old man presented with a painless swelling of the right parotid region.

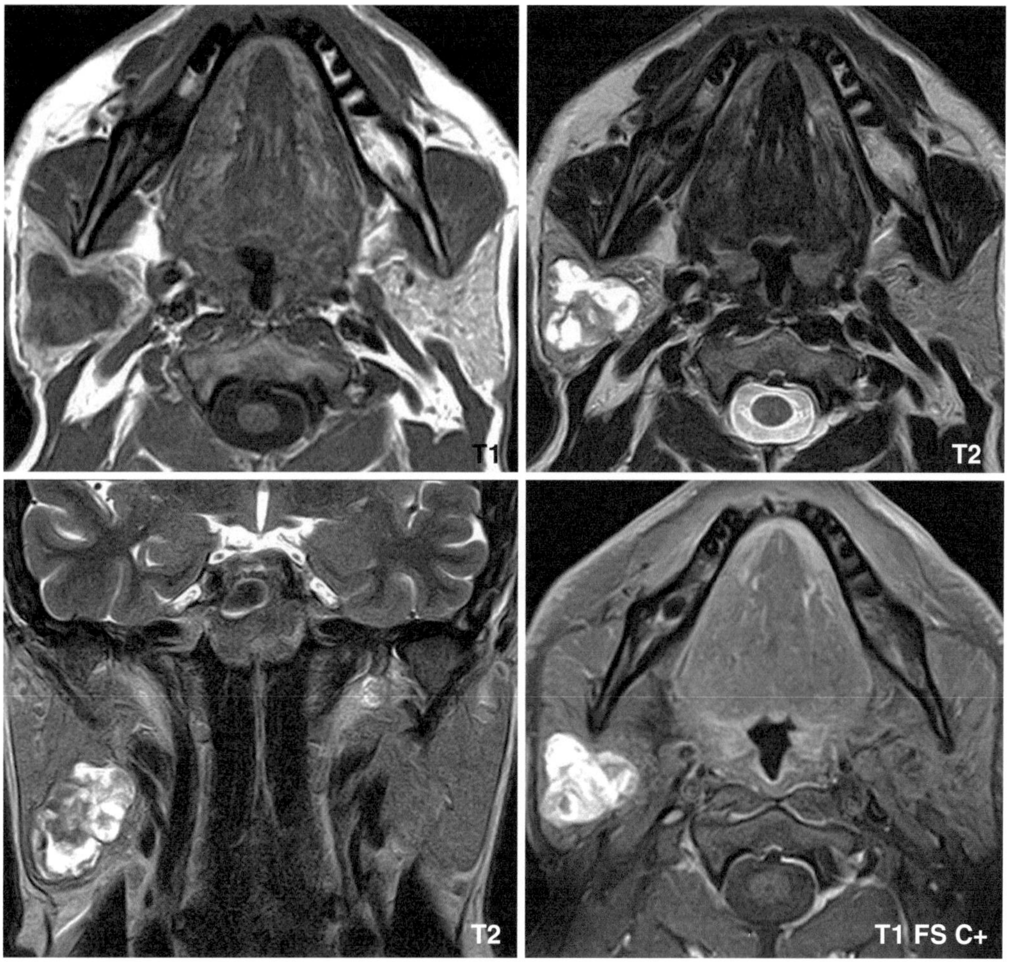

A. Haouimi et al., *Head and Neck Radiology Spot Diagnosis*,
https://doi.org/10.1007/978-3-032-14553-6_14

Findings

A well-defined, lobulated right parotid mass involving both superficial and deep parotid lobes. It is of low signal on T1 and heterogeneous high signal on T2 with a faint, hypointense peripheral demarcating capsule. Intense, nonhomogeneous enhancement following IV contrast.

Diagnosis

Pleomorphic adenoma of the parotid gland.

Discussion

Pleomorphic adenomas or benign mixed parotid tumors are slow-growing, well-defined lesions with a 15% chance of malignant transformation if left untreated. They are the most common parotid space tumors of unknown origin. Most of the cases originate in the superficial lobe. The deep lobe can occasionally be involved. Histologically, they originate from the distal ductal system, having epithelial, myoepithelial, and stromal components. Larger lesions may contain solid, cystic, and dystrophic calcifications.

Clinically, patients present with slowly progressing painless parotid swelling without signs of any facial nerve involvement.

CT shows lobulated intraglandular homo- or heterogeneous (presence of necrosis and calcification) soft tissue hypodensity. On MRI, the lesions are of low signal on T1 and high signal on T2. A rim of peripheral low signal on T2 represents the surrounding fibrous capsule. The parenchymal signal may be homo- or heterogeneous, depending on tissue composition, and the solid component usually enhances.

Common Differential Diagnosis

- Warthin's tumor: no calcification.
- Parotid carcinoma: infiltrative lesion, nodal involvement, and perineural spread +/−.
- Parotid nodal metastasis: known periauricular skin cancer, melanoma, or known remote malignancy.

Management Options

The treatment is surgical. Tumor spillage during the surgical procedure may lead to recurrence. Open surgical biopsy should not be performed to avoid such possibility. Radiotherapy is reserved for recurrent and residual lesions with questionable benefit.

References and Further Reading

1. Bokhari MR, Greene J. Pleomorphic adenoma. Stat Pearls Publishing; 2025. https://www.ncbi.nlm.nih.gov/books/NBK430829/. Accessed on 13 July 2025.
2. Haouimi A. Pleomorphic adenoma-parotid. Radiopaedia.org. 2022. https://doi.org/10.53347/rID-97061. Accessed on 26 Aug 2023.
3. Kato H, et al. Pleomorphic adenoma of salivary glands: common and uncommon CT and MR imaging features. Jpn J Radiol. 2018. https://doi.org/10.1007/s11604-018-0747-y. Accessed on 18 July 2025.

Case 15

15

Clinical History

A 35-year-old man presented with a painless pulsatile left cervical swelling.

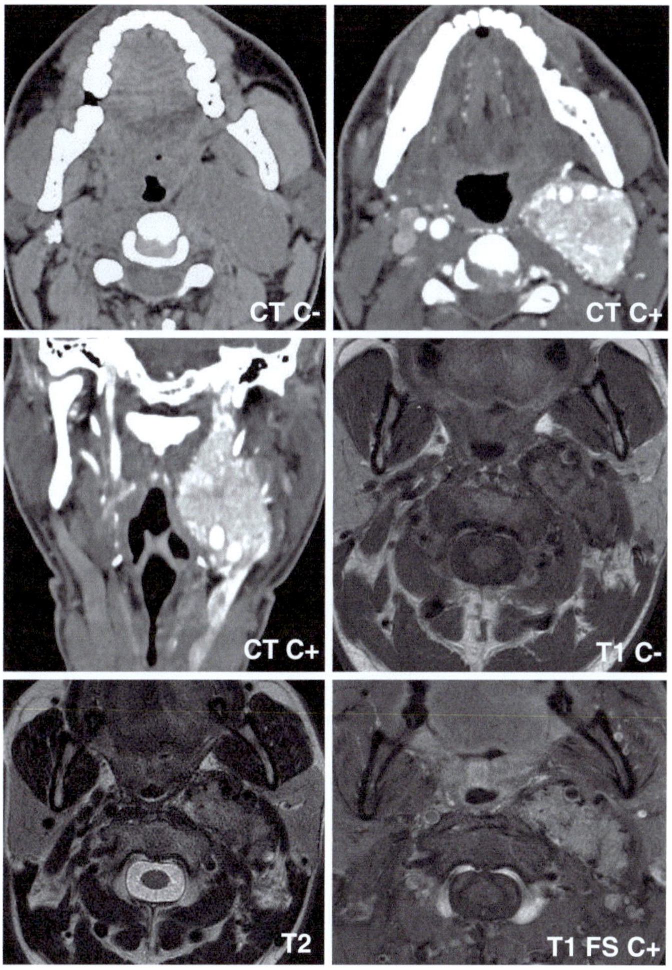

A. Haouimi et al., *Head and Neck Radiology Spot Diagnosis*,
https://doi.org/10.1007/978-3-032-14553-6_15

Findings

An ovoid lesion of the left carotid space, isodense to muscles with vivid enhancement, displacing the internal and external carotid arteries anteriorly on CT. It causes a mass effect on adjacent parapharyngeal space. On MRI, this enhancing mass appears well encapsulated. It shows an intermediate signal on T1, an intermediate-to-high signal on T2 with multiple flow voids creating a "salt-and-pepper appearance."

Diagnosis

Glomus vagale paraganglioma.

Discussion

Vagal paragangliomas are rare and benign tumors representing up to 5% of head and neck paragangliomas. They arise predominantly from the nodose ganglion in the carotid sheath.

Clinically, patients often present with a painless, pulsatile lateral neck mass. Symptoms can be associated with hoarseness and lower cranial nerve neuropathy.

Vagal paragangliomas appear as a well-defined, intense, homogeneously enhancing masses on CT. MRI is the modality of choice. A typical "salt-and-pepper" appearance on T1 can be seen. This sign is not however specific for vagal paraganglioma. Catheter angiography reveals a vascular tumor with large feeding arteries, intense tumor stain, and early draining veins.

Common Differential Diagnosis

- Carotid body tumor: widening of carotid bifurcation, "lyre sign."
- Glomus jugulare paraganglioma: epicenter within the jugular foramen.
- Vagal schwannoma: less vascular, cystic foci, no tumor blush on angiography.

Management Options

Treatment options include observation, surgical excision, and radiotherapy. Preoperative endovascular embolization may be used to reduce tumor vascularity.

References and Further Reading

1. Bhatt S, et al. Glomus vagal tumour, can it be diagnosed only on sonography. J Ultrasound. 2017. https://doi.org/10.1007/s40477-016-0237-y. Accessed on Sept 2024.
2. Haouimi A. Glomus vagal tumour. Radiopaedia.org. 2019. https://doi.org/10.53347/rID-67994. Accessed on 30 Aug 2022.
3. Ikram A, Rehman A. Paraganglioma. StatPearls Publishing; 2025. https://www.ncbi.nlm.nih.gov/books/NBK549834/. Accessed on 24 Sept 2025.

Case 16

Clinical History

A 4-year-old child. Incidental finding during ENT examination.

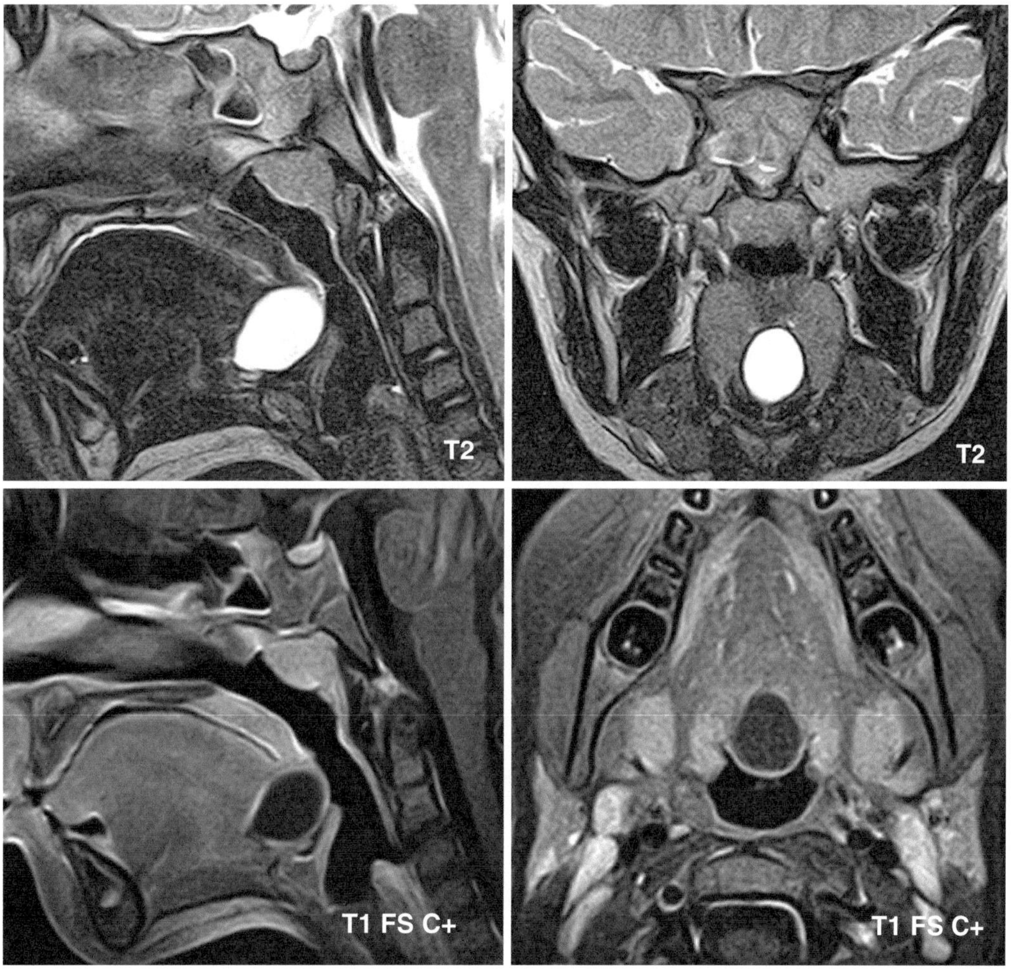

A. Haouimi et al., *Head and Neck Radiology Spot Diagnosis*,
https://doi.org/10.1007/978-3-032-14553-6_16

Findings

A well-defined midline suprahyoid cystic lesion at the tongue base showing homogeneous high signal content on T2 with very smooth thin peripheral rim enhancement.

Diagnosis

Lingual thyroglossal duct cyst.

Discussion

Thyroglossal duct cyst (TGDC) is a congenital epithelial cyst arising from the persistence of the thyroglossal duct, the embryologic tract of thyroid descent. The duct typically should disappear after the descent of the thyroid from the foramen cecum. These cysts can be found at any level along the tract, from the hyoid bone to the strap muscles.

Clinically, patients complain of a painless, smooth, and fluctuant midline mass, usually located below the hyoid bone. The lesion moves upward with swelling or tongue protrusion due to its attachment to the foramen cecum. When they get infected, the lesions may show a tender and erythematous midline mass.

Ultrasound is the imaging modality of choice. On ultrasound, the lesions appear as well-defined, anechoic, or hypoechoic cystic lesions with possible internal debris when they get infected. A smooth, thin-walled, low-attenuation lesion in the midline, sometimes showing rim enhancement when infected, is seen on CT. Lesions are hypointense on T1 (unless proteinaceous or complicated by hemorrhage), hyperintense on T2, with a thin wall and no solid enhancement, unless complicated. Diagnosis is confirmed by imaging correlation with clinical findings. Rapidly progressing lesions with focal enhancement and calcification may suggest malignancy.

Common Differential Diagnosis

- Ectopic lingual thyroid: solid lesion with intense enhancement.
- Mixed laryngocele: off-midline, not embedded in the strap muscles.
- Epidermoid cyst: superficial to the strap muscles, may show restricted diffusion.

Management Options

Complete surgical resection of the cyst as well as the duct up to the foramen cecum is often recommended. Recurrence is rare after complete resection. However, simple excision of the cyst is often associated with high recurrence rates.

References and Further Reading

1. Haouimi A. Lingual thyroglossal duct cyst. Radiopaedia.org. 2022. https://doi.org/10.53347/rID-96109. Accessed on 31 Aug 2023.
2. Li W, et al. Presentation, management, and outcome of lingual thyroglossal duct cyst in pediatric and adult populations. J Craniofac Surg. 2019. https://doi.org/10.1097/SCS.0000000000005522. Accessed on 15 Aug 2025.

17 Case 17

Clinical History

A 40-year-old woman presented with a flaccid paralysis of the left upper extremity.

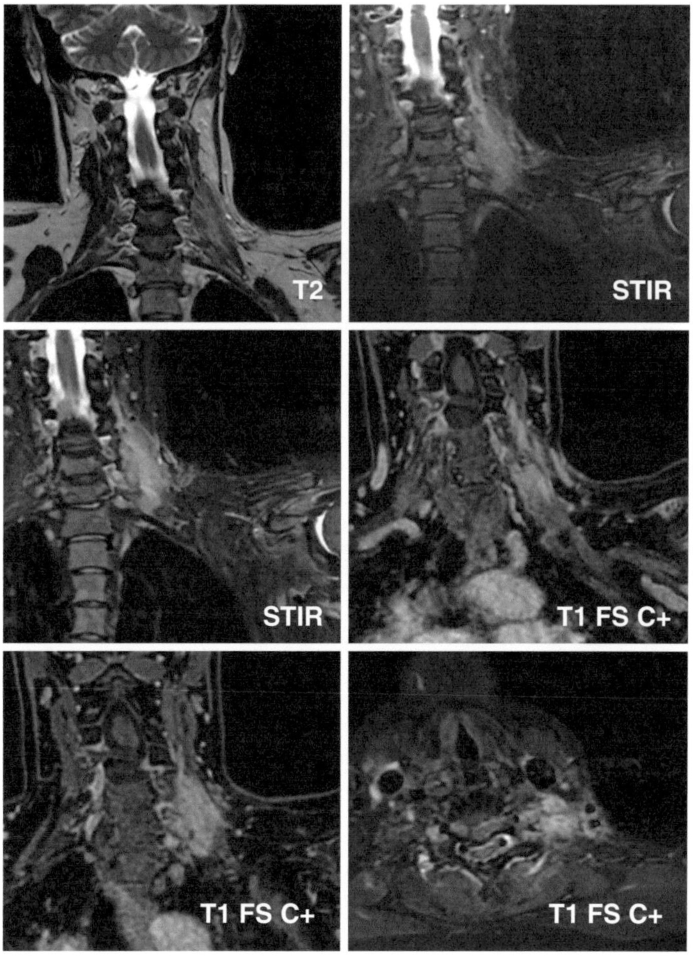

A. Haouimi et al., *Head and Neck Radiology Spot Diagnosis*,
https://doi.org/10.1007/978-3-032-14553-6_17

Findings

Diffuse fusiform thickening of left extraforaminal C3 to T1 nerve roots with intense enhancement. Significant soft tissue edema including neighboring scalene and rotator cuff muscles. The edema extends to the trunks of brachial plexus.

Diagnosis

Brachial plexitis.

Discussion

Brachial plexitis, also known as Personage–Turner syndrome or neuralgic amyotrophy, is an acute brachial plexus inflammation that can arise secondary to multiple etiologic factors. Recent viral upper respiratory tract infection and vaccination may predispose to this condition. Neoplastic compression and genetic factors have also been hypothesized.

The clinical presentations include acute sharp, burning, or stabbing pain in the shoulder and upper extremity, followed by muscular weakness of arm and shoulder. The condition may further lead to flaccid paralysis. The sensory symptoms vary from numbness to complete loss of sensation. MRI is the investigation of choice. MRI shows the neural elements as low signal on T1 and high signal on T2 with thickening and enlargement of the affected segment of brachial plexus. In the acute stage, there is edema of adjacent muscles, which may undergo atrophic and fatty infiltration in 4–6 weeks' time.

Common Differential Diagnosis

- Pancoast tumor: gradual onset, compressive lesion at lung apex.
- Disc herniation: not of acute onset (except traumatic type), with pain in dermatomal distribution.
- Rotator cuff tear: history of trauma, pain localized to shoulder, and normal brachial plexus.
- Lyme disease: history of tick bite, associated with erythema migrans rash.

Management Options

The treatment is conservative. Physiotherapy to prevent complications and restore functionality. Multidisciplinary management optimizes the outcome.

References and Further Reading

1. Ortiz Torres M, Gudlavalleti A, Mesfin FB. Brachial plexitis. Stat Pearls Publishing; 2024. https://www.ncbi.nlm.nih.gov/books/NBK448114/. Accessed on 20 July 2025.
2. Upadhyaya V, et al. Status of magnetic resonance neurography in evaluating patients with brachial plexopathy. Neurol India. 2019. https://doi.org/10.4103/0028-3886.250730. Accessed on 15 May 2025.

Case 18

18

Clinical History

A 20-year-old man presented with a painless supra-labial hemifacial swelling on the left side.

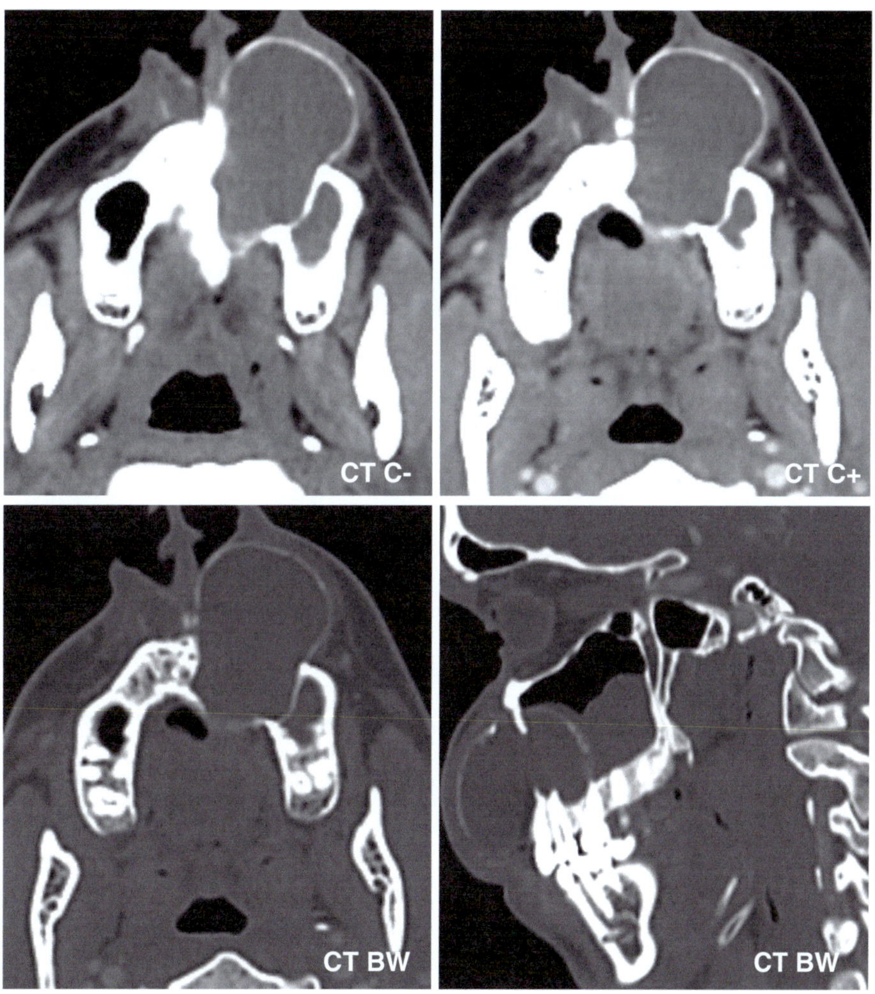

A. Haouimi et al., *Head and Neck Radiology Spot Diagnosis*,
https://doi.org/10.1007/978-3-032-14553-6_18

Findings

A smooth homogeneous hypodense expansile cystic lesion of the left maxilla with scalloped well-corticated borders without cortical breach. The lesion appears to arise from alveolar process with premolar tooth as epicenter. No obvious contrast enhancement. Associated retention cyst of left maxillary sinus.

Diagnosis

Odontogenic keratocyst.

Discussion

Odontogenic keratocysts are benign, locally aggressive developmental lesions arising in the maxilla or mandible. The lesions are believed to originate from remnants of dental lamina and are often solitary. Multiple lesions may be a component of basal cell nevus also known as Gorlin syndrome. Most of the lesions are epicentered in the mandibular ramus while maxillary involvement accounts for approximately 10% of cases. The cysts contain straw-colored fluid or purulent and cheese-like contents.

Clinically, no obvious signs and symptoms even if the lesion is large. Occasionally, patients present with symptoms like local pain and swelling, purulent discharge, and loose teeth. Continued expansion may lead to facial deformity and tilting of teeth.

Radiographically, odontogenic keratocysts are uni- or multiloculated radiolucent, well-demarcated lesions with scalloped or rounded margins. On CT, the cysts appear hypodense. The density varies with viscosity of the contents. Mandibular lesions grow along the length of the bone with minimal buccolingual expansion, whereas the maxillary lesions may cause expansion into the maxillary sinus. Presence of cortical breach suggests possible soft tissue involvement. Due to rich cholesterol and keratin content, the cysts appear as high signal on T1 and heterogeneously high signal on T2 with restricted diffusion. They may show peripheral enhancement (not nodular).

Common Differential Diagnosis

- Ameloblastoma: multilocular, “soap-bubble” appearance, enhancing internal components.
- Radicular cyst: arising from apex of the tooth, no scalloping.
- Basal cell nevus (Gorlin syndrome): multiple lesions.

Management Options

Aggressive curettage and enucleation. The lesions have high recurrence rate and need follow-up.

References and Further Reading

1. Alwakeel A, et al. Odontogenic keratocyst presented as multi-locular radiolucency in mandibular canine and premolar region: a case report. Cureus. 2023. https://doi.org/10.7759/cureus.39291. Accessed on 20 June 2025.
2. Haouimi A. Odontogenic keratocyst-maxilla. Radiopaedia.org. 2022. https://doi.org/10.53347/rID-80186. Accessed on 01 Sept 2023.

Case 19

19

Clinical History

A 15-year-old immunosuppressed girl presented with a recurrent purulent discharge from the ventral aspect of the tongue. No previous history of surgery.

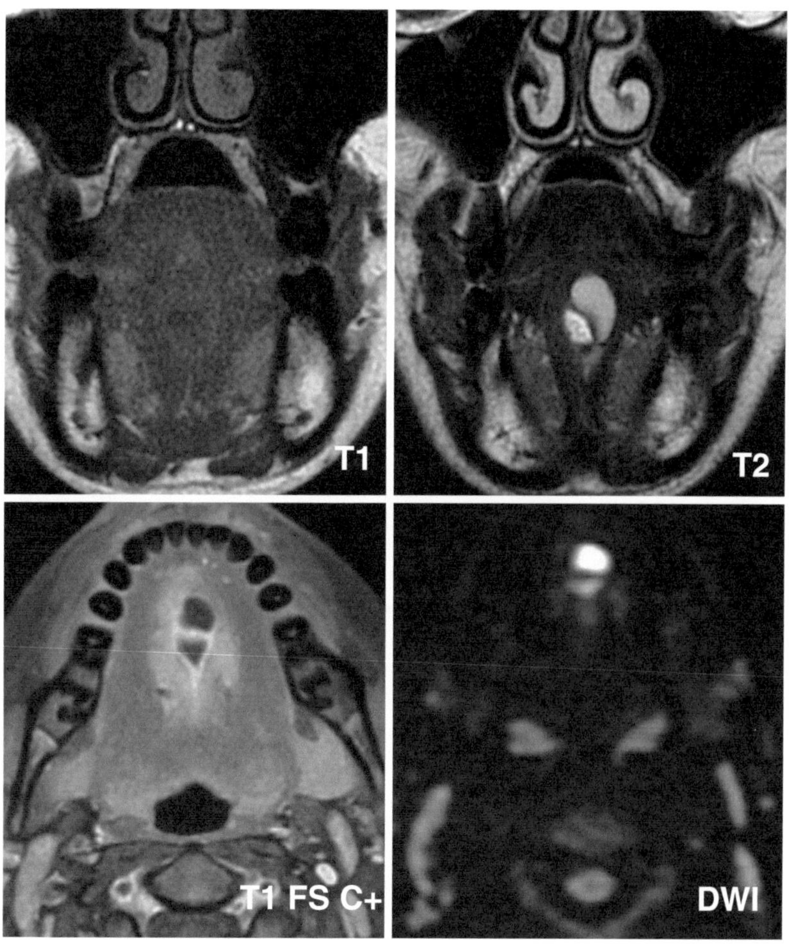

A. Haouimi et al., *Head and Neck Radiology Spot Diagnosis*,
https://doi.org/10.1007/978-3-032-14553-6_19

Findings

Midline intralingual loculated lesion appearing hypointense on T1, hyperintense on T2 with restricted diffusion. Displacement of the genioglossus muscles laterally with smooth and regular peripheral rim enhancement. Enhancement of the genioglossi muscles as well as both submandibular glands.

Diagnosis

Lingual abscess.

Discussion

The tongue is relatively immune to infection due to natural protective barriers, including the compact lingual musculature, the squamous lining, continuous cleaning by saliva, and a rich vascular and lymphatic supply. Lingual abscess is an unusual condition but can be life threatening. Most tongue abscesses are unilateral and seen in the anterior two-thirds. Abscesses of the tongue base most often originate from infected lingual tonsils, infected thyroglossal duct cysts, and from locoregional extensions of radicular infections from the dentition.

Clinically, patients present with fever, painful tongue swelling, and difficulty in talking. In the absence of adequate and timely management, it can lead to complications such as phlegmonous glossitis and development of fatal mediastinitis.

CT scan shows intraglossal uni- or multiloculated low-density area with peripheral ring enhancement. On MRI, the typical tongue abscess appears as T1 hypointensity and T2 hyperintensity surrounded by an enhancing T1 hyperintense rim. Occasionally, an abscess may also present as a pseudotumor-like lesion that enhances diffusely or peripherally.

Common Differential Diagnosis

- Ludwig's angina: cellulitis of the floor of mouth, trans-spatial inflammation, tongue displaced upward.
- Tongue cancer: solid +/− thick irregular enhancement.
- Postradiation necrosis: known clinical history.

Management Options

Treatment of tongue abscess is surgical drainage, rinsing of the oral cavity with antiseptic solutions, followed by aggressive intravenous antibacterial and anti-inflammatory treatment. The other important key to successful management, particularly for the posterior lingual abscess, is airway maintenance.

References and Further Reading

1. Haouimi A. Lingual abscess. Radiopaedia.org. 2021. https://doi.org/10.53347/rID-78864. Accessed on 04 Sept 2022.
2. Ozturk M, et al. Tongue abscesses: MR imaging findings. AJNR Am J Neuroradiol. 2006. PMID: 16775284; PMCID: PMC8133947. Accessed on 13 June 2025.

Case 20

20

Clinical History

A 45-year-old woman presented with a painful right upper neck swelling.

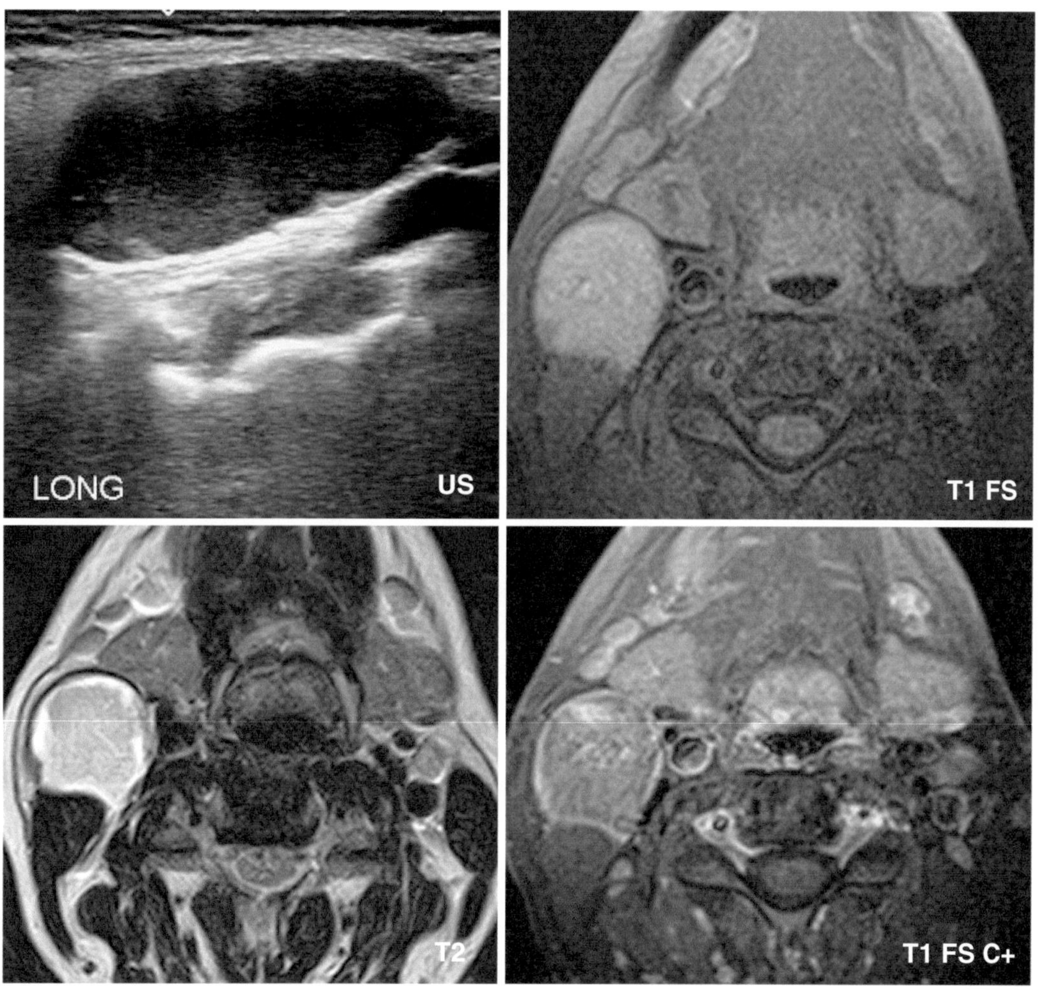

A. Haouimi et al., *Head and Neck Radiology Spot Diagnosis*,
https://doi.org/10.1007/978-3-032-14553-6_20

Findings

A homogeneous hypoechoic cystic lesion with internal debris seen on ultrasound. MRI shows a well demarcated, slightly lobulated lesion anterior to th border of sternocleidomastoid and posterior to the submandibular gland, lateral to the carotid sheath. It appears hyperintense on T1 fatsat and T2 with smooth, thick, and regular peripheral enhancement, “dirty cyst.”

Diagnosis

Infected second branchial cleft cyst.

Discussion

Branchial cleft cysts are congenital anomalies with remote malignant potential. They arise due to the failure of obliteration of an embryological cervical sinus. Most of the second branchial cleft cysts are found in submandibular space. The anomalies may present as cysts, sinus tract, and or fistula.

Though congenital, they may not be obvious or symptomatic until later. Clinically, they appear as painless fluctuant lateral neck mass at the mandibular angle, anterior to sternocleidomastoid muscle and lateral to the carotid space but posterior to the submandibular gland.

The ultrasound appearance of the second branchial cleft cyst is variable depending on the contents. Most are sharply defined and anechoic with posterior acoustic enhancement. On CT, they appear as well-defined thin-walled cystic lesions. The projection of the thin cystic wall between the carotid arteries just above the bifurcation, producing a “notch sign” is highly suggestive. When the cystic wall is lined by ciliated columnar epithelium, the cystic content can be mucoid and may appear slightly hyperintense on T1 as in this case. On T2, the lesion is of high signal with no contrast enhancement in noncomplicated cysts.

Common Differential Diagnosis

- Cystic malignant adenopathy: thick irregular enhancement; FNA is helpful.
- Thymic cyst: at infrahyoid level, located in the lateral visceral space.
- Vagal schwannoma: carotid space lesion.

Management Options

To avoid the risk of repeated infection and further enlargement, elective surgical excision is recommended. However, emergency surgical intervention may be required if there is airway compromise or abscess formation.

References and Further Reading

1. Haouimi A. Infected second branchial cleft cyst. Radiopaedia.org. 2024. https://doi.org/10.53347/rID-67657. Accessed on 20 July 2025.
2. Coste AH, et al. Branchial cleft cyst. Stat Pearls Publishing; 2022. Accessed on 12 Apr 2024.

Case 21

21

Clinical History

Incidental finding in a 60-year-old woman.

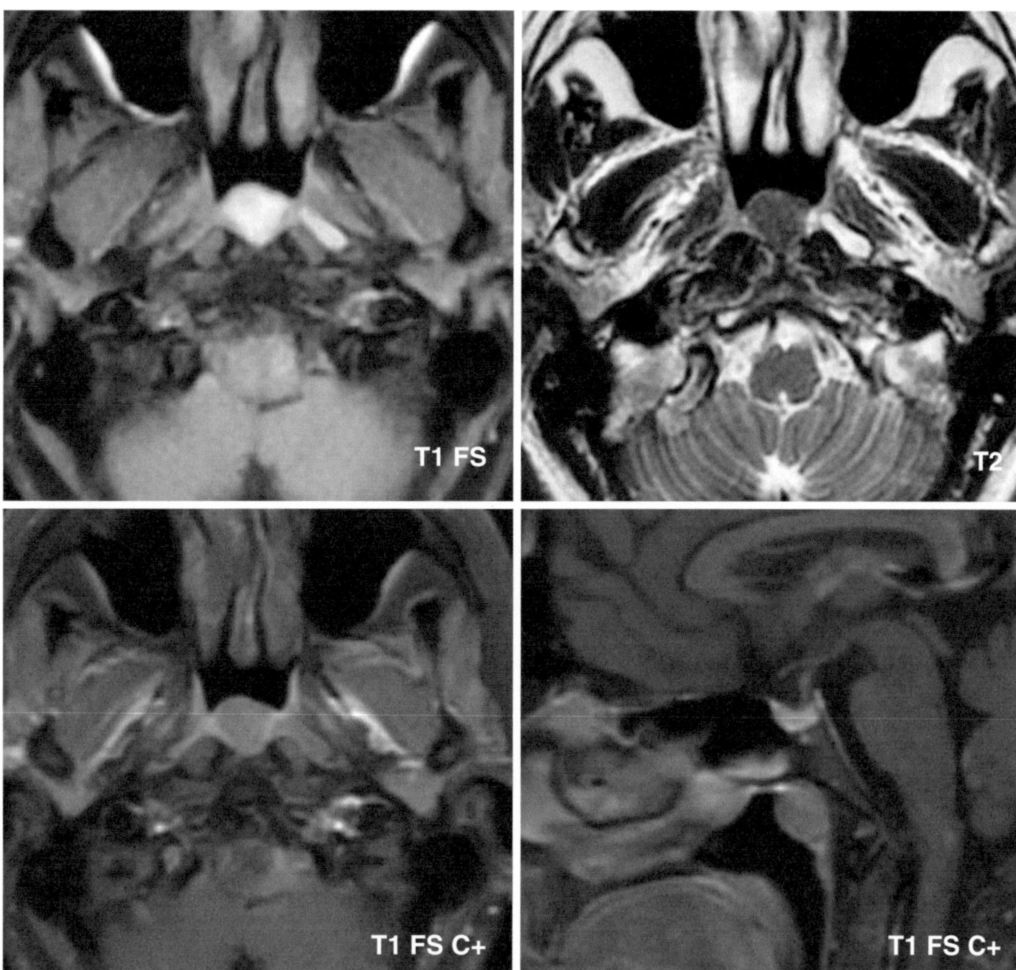

A. Haouimi et al., *Head and Neck Radiology Spot Diagnosis*,
https://doi.org/10.1007/978-3-032-14553-6_21

Findings

A well-defined midline cystic lesion of the posterior nasopharyngeal wall interposed between longus colli muscles. It is of high signal on T1 (high protein content) and slightly hypointense on T2. No enhancement following contrast. Normal adjacent bone and soft tissue signal.

Diagnosis

Tornwaldt cyst.

Discussion

Tornwaldt cysts are benign congenital midline nasopharyngeal cysts seen at pharyngeal mucosal space, anterior to the prevertebral muscles. The cysts arise from notochordal remnants, possibly due to inflammation or mechanical obstruction of the embryological pharyngeal bursa. They are often round or ovoid in shape. The size ranges from a few millimeters up to 3 cm.

Tornwaldt cysts are almost always asymptomatic. Occasionally, halitosis or periodic foul-tasting unpleasant fluid discharge into the mouth can occur if infected. When such symptoms occur, it is called Tornwaldt disease.

Tornwaldt cysts are an incidental imaging finding and are rarely of any clinical significance. On CT, these midline cysts are of low density with or without thin rim of peripheral enhancement. The MRI signal is variable on T1, depending on protein concentration and homogeneously high signal on T2 with normal surrounding soft tissue.

Common Differential Diagnosis

- Nasopharyngeal carcinoma: ill-defined and infiltrative, mostly off-midline.
- Benign mixed tumor: enhancing lesion.
- Retention cyst: often multiple.

Management Options

Tornwaldt cysts are incidental "do not touch" lesions with no clinical significance. Chronic infected cases are treated surgically by either excision or marsupialization.

References and Further Reading

1. Alshuhayb Z, et al. Tornwaldt nasopharyngeal cyst. Int J Surg Case Rep. 2020. https://doi.org/10.1016/j.ijscr.2020.09.105. Accessed on 12 Apr 2024.
2. Cetinkaya EA. Thornwaldt cyst. J Craniofac Surg. 2018. https://doi.org/10.1097/SCS.0000000000004559. Accessed on 05 Jan 2025.
3. Haouimi A. Tornwaldt cyst. Radiopaedia.org. 2019. https://doi.org/10.53347/rID-71909. Accessed on 02 Sept 2022.

Case 22

22

Clinical History

A 50-year-old woman presented with bilateral parotid enlargement, treated as chronic parotitis.

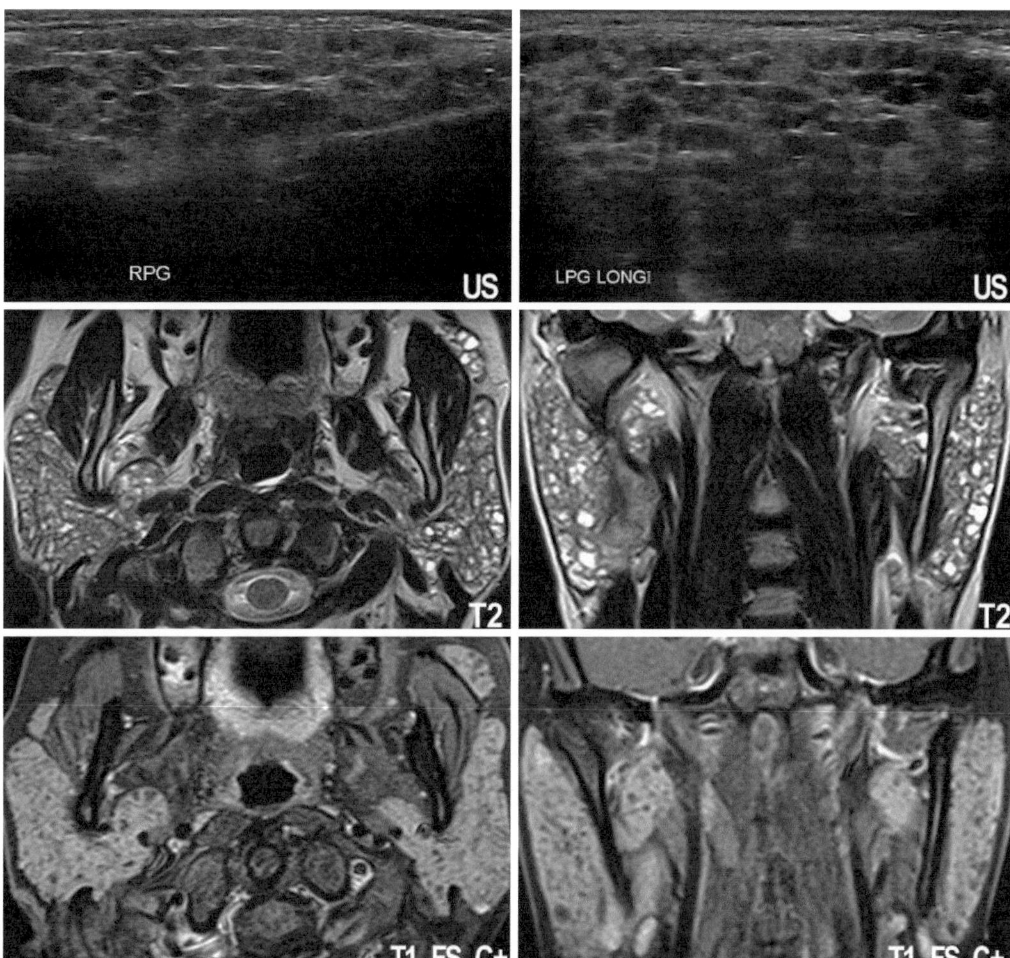

A. Haouimi et al., *Head and Neck Radiology Spot Diagnosis*,
https://doi.org/10.1007/978-3-032-14553-6_22

Findings

Ultrasound shows multiple diffuse bilateral miliary patterns of parotid glands with tiny anechoic microcysts giving a "leopard skin" appearance. MRI shows bilateral intraparenchymal high-signal areas, with a "honeycomb appearance" involving both superficial and deep lobes with mild diffuse enhancement of both parotids.

Diagnosis

Sjögren syndrome.

Discussion

Sjögren syndrome, also known as sicca syndrome, is the second most common multisystem autoimmune disease of unknown origin, following rheumatoid arthritis. This chronic systemic exocrinopathy primarily affects the parotid and lacrimal glands. It is thought to result from a combination of genetic and environmental triggers, such as exposure to certain viruses (like EBV or hepatitis C) and bacteria.

Clinically, patients typically experience repeated episodes of painful parotid swelling. The hallmark symptoms include dryness of the mouth, skin, and eyes, a condition known as keratitis sicca. Those patients carry a higher risk of developing non-Hodgkin lymphoma.

Ultrasound can be normal or can show a diffuse miliary pattern of tiny, echogenic microcysts, giving both parotids a "leopard skin" appearance. CT can reveal bilaterally enlarged parotids with multifocal tiny solid and cystic lesions, along with intraglandular calcifications. No enlarged lymphadenopathy. Enlarged parotid glands show a "honeycombing" pattern on T2 due to microcysts on MRI. Postcontrast fat-suppressed images provide better visualization of heterogeneous intraparenchymal nodular enhancement, as well as the fibrous component.

Common Differential Diagnosis

- Chronic parotitis: unilateral involvement.
- Warthin tumor: mostly at parotid tail, characteristic parenchymal heterogeneity.
- Sarcoidosis: systemic, mixed solid and cystic components, cervical lymphadenopathy.

Management Options

Isolated cases are treated symptomatically by moisture-replacing therapy. However, in case of systemic involvement, immunotherapy is often recommended.

References and Further Reading

1. Haouimi A. Sjögren syndrome. Radiopaedia.org. 2024. https://doi.org/10.53347/rID-67792. Accessed on 07 Nov 2022.
2. Wang KY, Wintermark M, Penta M. Imaging characteristics of Sjögren's syndrome. Clin Imaging. 2022. https://doi.org/10.1016/j.clinimag.2022.08.022. Epub 2022 Sep 16. Accessed on 21 July 2025.

Case 23

Clinical History

A 65-year-old woman with type 2 diabetes mellitus presented with chronic headache.

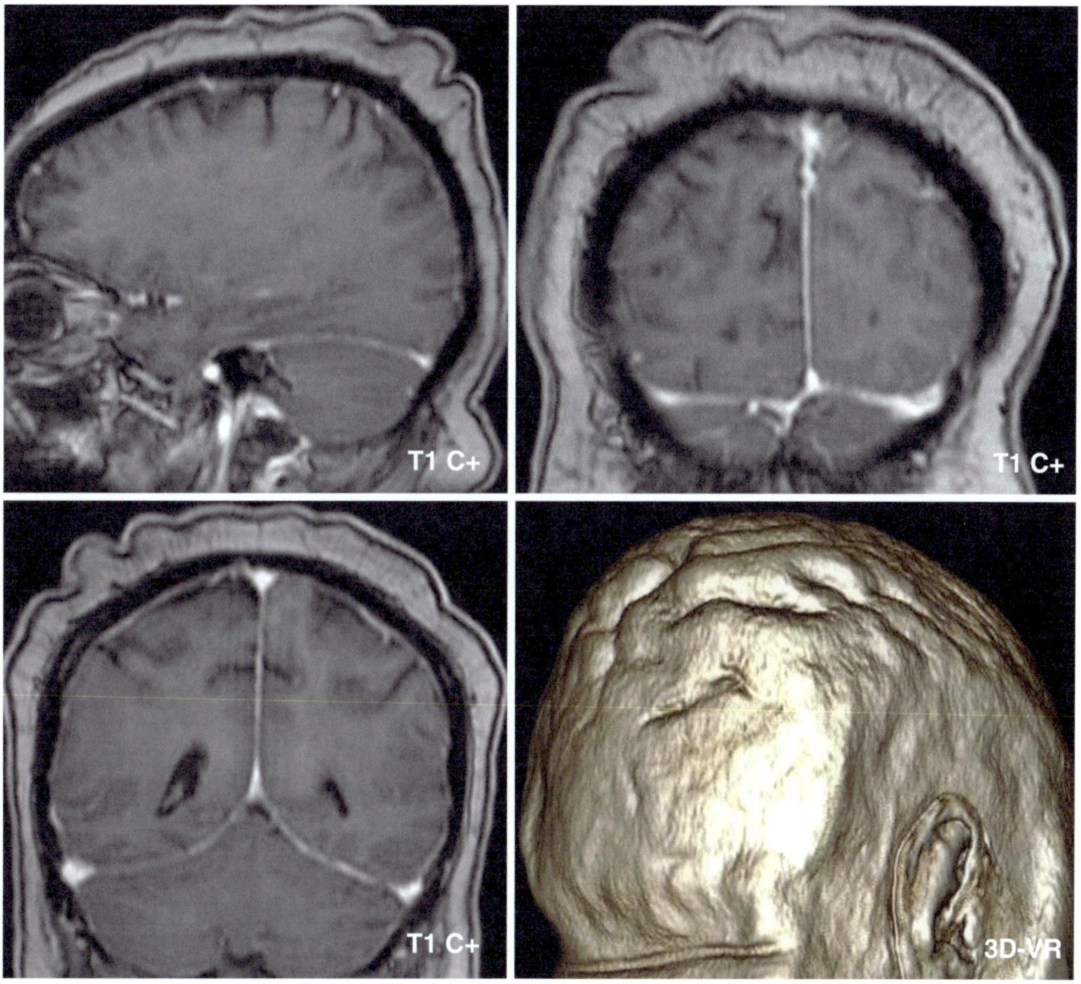

A. Haouimi et al., *Head and Neck Radiology Spot Diagnosis*,
https://doi.org/10.1007/978-3-032-14553-6_23

Findings

Diffusely thickened scalp with prominent ridges and furrows without any brain abnormality. Anteroposterior direction of skin folds more marked at right occipital region.

Diagnosis

Cutis verticis gyrata (CVG), also known as "bulldog scalp syndrome."

Discussion

Cutis verticis gyrata is a rare medical condition with male predominance, with a reported male-to-female ratio of 5:1. Cutis verticis gyrata can be primary or secondary to underlying conditions such as neuropsychiatric disorders, acromegaly, ocular abnormalities, or inflammatory conditions. The etiology of primary CVG is not known but increased peripheral use of testosterone has been hypothesized. The male predominance may also suggest an X-linked inheritance. In this rare condition, the visible scalp resembles cerebral gyri and sulci due to the convoluted skin folds with deep furrows. Occasionally, it can be complicated by the development of melanoma within a melanocytic nevus.

CVG is a progressive condition and cosmetically troublesome. It usually starts to develop after puberty, and can be both uni- or bilateral. The number of folds can vary but they are typically soft and spongy with occipitotemporal predominance. The diagnosis is clinical. Most of the cases are asymptomatic. Accumulation of secretions may cause itching, ulcerations, and bad odor.

Common Differential Diagnosis

- Acromegaly: associated pituitary abnormalities.
- Ehlers–Danlos syndrome: multiple ovoid scalp calcifications, better seen on CT.
- Pachydermoperiostosis (PDP): involvement of bones, not scalp.

Management Options

The management of primary CVG includes good scalp hygiene to keep the areas between the folds clean. Surgical intervention is performed for psychological or cosmetic reasons. In secondary cases, the focus is to treat the primary causes.

References and Further Reading

1. Adôrno IF, et al. Primary essential cutis vertices gyrata. Radiol Bras. 2019. https://doi.org/10.1590/0100-3984.2017.0218. PMID: 31435095; PMCID: PMC6696756. Accessed on 20 June 2025.
2. Haouimi A. Cutis verticis gyrata. Radiopaedia.org. 2021. https://doi.org/10.53347/rID-87909. Accessed on 22 July 2022.
3. Shareef S, et al. Cutis vertices gyrata. Stat Pearls Publishing; 2023. https://www.ncbi.nlm.nih.gov/books/NBK539812/. Accessed on 20 June 2025.

Case 24

24

Clinical History

A 55-year-old man presented with chronic headache, anosmia, and nasal obstruction.

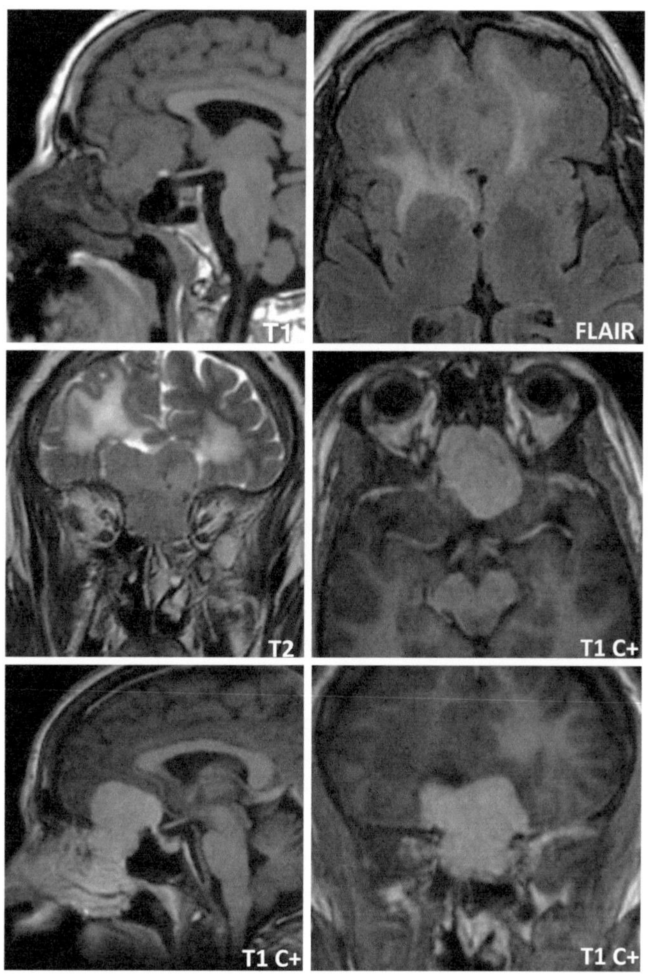

A. Haouimi et al., *Head and Neck Radiology Spot Diagnosis*,
https://doi.org/10.1007/978-3-032-14553-6_24

Findings

A soft tissue mass at the roof of the nasal cavity, epicentered on the cribriform plate of the ethmoid bone, having both intra- and extracranial components. It appears isointense to muscles on T1, T2, and FLAIR with a moderate perilesional edema and extrinsic compression of the adjacent brain parenchyma. Intense homogeneous enhancement following contrast. No "dural tail sign," hemoglobin breakdown products, or calcification.

Diagnosis

Esthesioneuroblastoma (ENB).

Discussion

Esthesioneuroblastomas or olfactory neuroblastomas are rare malignant neuroectodermal tumors of neural crest origin with cribriform plate epicenter. The incidence seems to have increased in the last decade. Olfactory neuroblastomas represent up to 6% of nasal cavity and paranasal sinus cancers. Patients may experience nasal stuffiness, anosmia, epistaxis, and rhinorrhea. On CT, the lesions show enlargement of nasal fossa along with bony remodeling. Speckled intratumoral calcifications are better seen on nonenhanced scan. On MRI, the lesions appear heterogeneously isointense on both T1 and T2 with moderate to intense enhancement. Up to one-fourth of the cases can extend into the intracranial cavity with marginal cysts. Any dumbbell-shaped lesion with "waisting" at cribriform plate and intracranial marginal cysts must be considered as ENB until proven otherwise.

Common Differential Diagnosis

- Olfactory groove meningioma: mostly intracranial, hyperostosis, calcification +.
- Nasopharyngeal carcinoma: epicenter more posteriorly at the nasopharynx.
- Juvenile nasopharyngeal angiofibroma: male adolescents, sphenopalatine epicenter.

Management Options

Combined endoscopic craniofacial resection and radiotherapy is the method of management. Chemotherapy is usually reserved for larger lesions.

References and Further Reading

1. Dublin AB, Bobinski M. Imaging characteristics of olfactory neuroblastoma (esthesioneuroblastoma). J Neurol Surg B Skull Base. 2016. https://doi.org/10.1055/s-0035-1564053. Epub 2015 Sep 14. PMID: 26949582; PMCID: PMC4777621. Accessed on 15 June 2025.
2. Haouimi A. Esthesioneuroblastoma. Radiopaedia.org. 2024. https://radiopaedia.org/cases/199700. Accessed on 19 Jan 2025.
3. Limaiem F, et al. Esthesioneuroblastoma. Stat Pearls Publishing; 2023. https://www.ncbi.nlm.nih.gov/books/NBK539694/. Accessed on 18 May 2024.

Case 25

25

Clinical History

A 25-year-old man presented with a reduced right visual acuity.

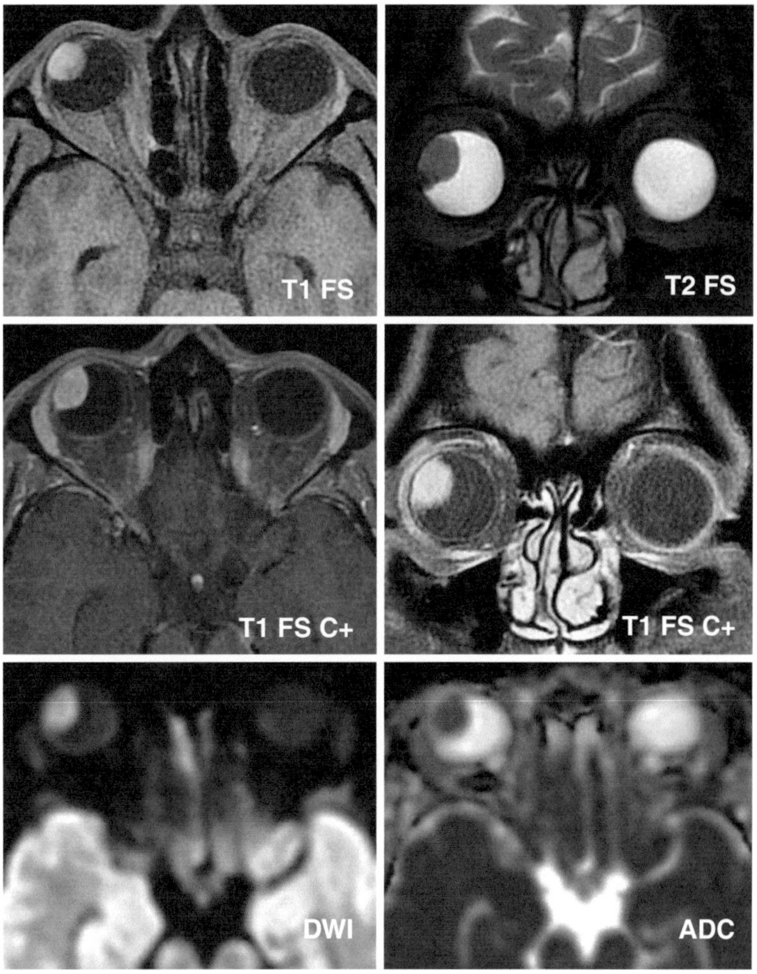

A. Haouimi et al., *Head and Neck Radiology Spot Diagnosis*,
https://doi.org/10.1007/978-3-032-14553-6_25

Findings

A homogeneous right intraocular ovoid lesion showing T1 high signal and T2 low signal in the temporal quadrant. It shows restricted diffusion and moderate homogeneous enhancement. Invasion of the iris, ciliary body, and posterior chamber. No extraocular extension nor to the surface of the optic nerve head.

Diagnosis

Choroidal melanoma.

Discussion

Choroidal melanomas are the most common eye cancer in adults, having an inherited component. Caucasians are more predisposed to this condition. Lesions are believed to develop from previously existing melanocytic nevi or from melanocytes within the choroid. On ophthalmologic examination, the lesions are seen as a "dome-shaped" mass of variable pigmentation. As the lesion grows bigger, there is secondary accumulation of lipofuscin pigments and drusen in the overlying retinal pigment epithelium.

The condition often goes unrecognized until the development of symptoms. The clinical symptoms include visual disturbance, blurred vision, and scotoma. There may be associated signs of retinal detachment or vitreous hemorrhage, like floaters.

Diagnosis is clinical. MRI is needed to evaluate the locoregional involvement. On MRI, the choroidal melanomas show broad choroidal base having high signal on T1 and slightly of low signal on T2. Mixed pigmentation would be suggested by heterogeneous signal intensities.

Common Differential Diagnosis

- Retinoblastoma: mostly in infants, isosignal on both T1 and T2, calcification +.
- Metastasis: known primary, low signal on T1.
- Choroidal detachment: extend beyond the ora serrata.

Management Options

Small melanomas are monitored to assess the size. Medium and large lesions are treated with radiation and/or surgery. The prognosis is poor with locoregional and extraocular extension.

References and Further Reading

1. Haouimi A. Choroidal melanoma. Radiopaedia.org. 2022. https://doi.org/10.53347/rID-96381. Accessed on 09 Nov 2023.
2. Jha P, Yap J. Primary uveal malignant melanoma. Radiopaedia.org. 2025. https://doi.org/10.53347/rID-8552. Accessed on 21 June 2025.
3. Jiblawi A, et al. MRI diagnosis of choroidal melanoma. Cureus. 2021. https://doi.org/10.7759/cureus.16628. PMID: 34458039; PMCID: PMC8385474. Accessed on 12 Mar 2023.

Case 26

26

Clinical History

A 12-year-old girl presented with a painless left proptosis.

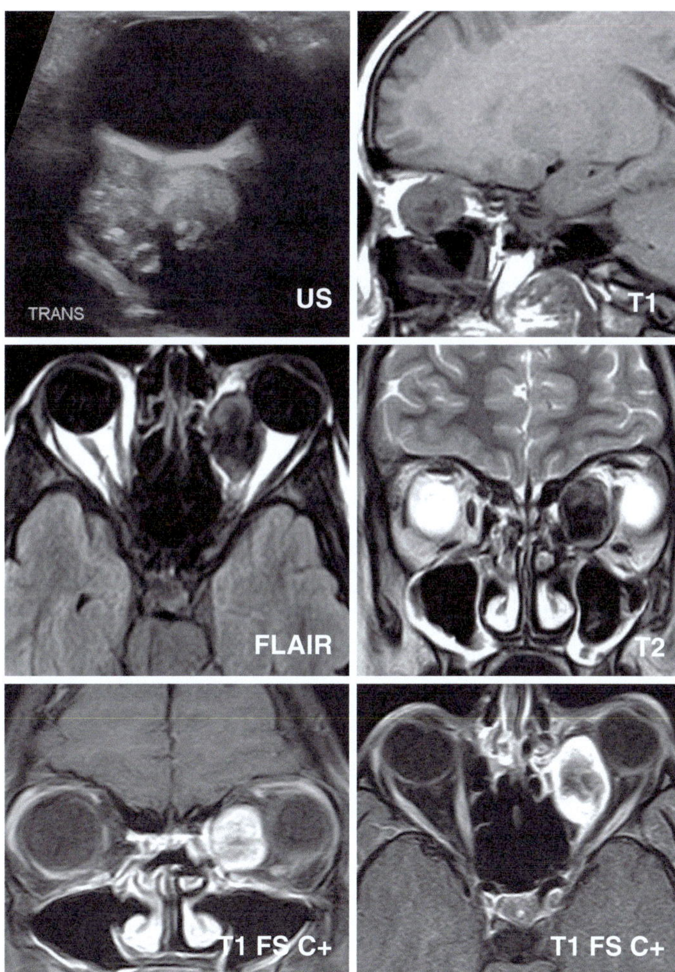

A. Haouimi et al., *Head and Neck Radiology Spot Diagnosis*,
https://doi.org/10.1007/978-3-032-14553-6_26

Findings

Ultrasound shows a left orbital retro-ocular hyperechoic lesion containing hyperechoic foci with posterior acoustic shadowing, suggesting calcific components. MRI shows grade 1 proptosis and a well-defined intraconal oval lesion compressing and displacing the optic nerve laterally and medial rectus muscle medially. The lesion appears isointense to the cortical gray matter peripherally on T1, T2, and FLAIR with central hypointense area (calcifications). Intense homogeneous enhancement of the peripheral solid component.

Diagnosis

Cavernous hemangioma.

Discussion

Cavernous hemangiomas are benign hamartomatous lesions in adults and are the most common vascular lesion of orbit. About 80% of the cases are intraconal. They have a slight female predilection. The growth rate is very slow and may even stop after a certain period. However, a rapid growth may be observed during pregnancy. Pathologically, these well-delineated lesions consist of large dilated venous channels with a fibrous capsule. The patients may present with slowly progressive painless proptosis and diplopia. On ultrasound, the lesions appear as a well-defined, homogeneous, hyperechoic mass. Color Doppler ultrasound shows large low-flow vascular spaces. On CT, the lesions appear isodense with patchy dynamic enhancement. Intralesional calcifications represent phleboliths. MRI shows a well-demarcated intraorbital mass iso-/hypointense to muscle on T1 and hyperintense on T2. Enhancement is heterogeneous at the beginning and then becomes homogeneous and intense over time, which is characteristic.

Common Differential Diagnosis

- Optic nerve meningioma: fusiform lesions, “tramtrack” and “doughnut sign” calcifications +/−.
- Orbital varix: inhomogeneous enhancement, size change with Valsalva.
- Orbital schwannoma: no calcification.

Management Options

Smaller lesions need follow-up and symptomatic treatment. However, larger lesions often need surgical resection with an excellent prognosis.

References and Further Reading

1. Haouimi A. Orbital cavernous haemangioma. Radiopaedia.org. 2022. https://doi.org/10.53347/rID-98488. Accessed on 10 Nov 2022.
2. Xian J, et al. Evaluation of MR imaging findings differentiating cavernous haemangiomas from schwannomas in the orbit. Eur Radiol. 2010. https://doi.org/10.1007/s00330-010-1774-y. Accessed on 10 Nov 2022.

Case 27

27

Clinical History

A 40-year-old woman presented with a right proptosis.

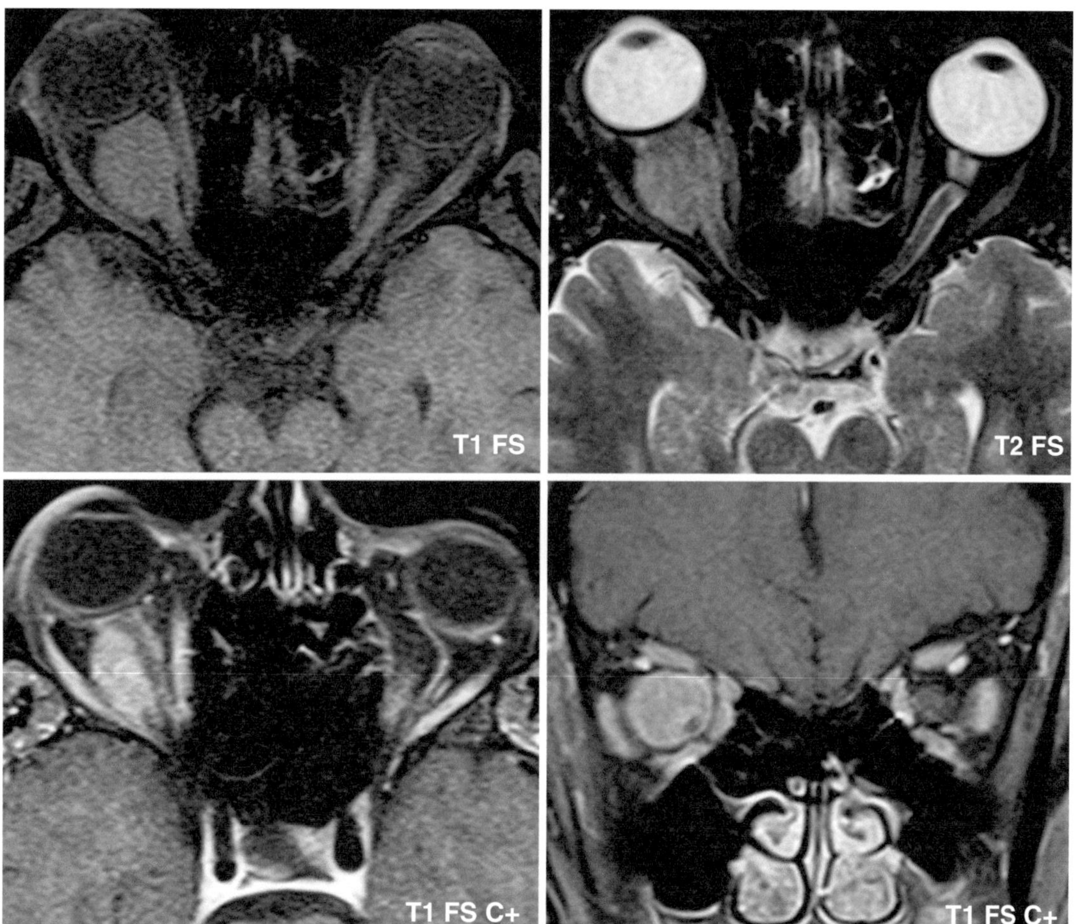

A. Haouimi et al., *Head and Neck Radiology Spot Diagnosis*,
https://doi.org/10.1007/978-3-032-14553-6_27

Findings

A well-circumscribed fusiform right intraorbital, retro-ocular lesion with mild proptosis. It shows homogeneous isosignal to cortical gray matter on T1 and T2 with intense enhancement, encircling the optic nerve, showing positive "tram track sign" and "doughnut sign."

Diagnosis

Optic nerve sheath meningioma (ONSM).

Discussion

ONSM represent about 2% of all orbital tumors and only 1% of all meningiomas. They are benign lesions arising from arachnoid "cap cells." It is a different entity from spheno-orbital meningiomas extending through the orbital apex. The lesions usually involve the intraorbital and intracanalicular portions of the optic nerve sheath. Though benign and slowly progressive, their location is critical. It directly affects the anterior visual pathway and can lead to severe visual loss. Clinically, patients may present with progressive unilateral vision loss, transient visual obscuration, and diplopia. The lesions can calcify and can be seen on nonenhanced CT. CT can also show hyperostosis and anatomical bony changes secondary to tumor. On MRI, the lesions can have a tubular, globular, or fusiform contour. Lesions are isointense to gray matter on both T1 and T2. Intense enhancement of the lesions produces a characteristic "tram-track sign" on axial images. The enhanced tissue corresponds to ONSM encircling the nonenhancing optic nerve. This is seen as a "doughnut" or "nonenhancing dot" sign on coronal images.

Common Differential Diagnosis

- Cavernous hemangioma: oval lesion with extrinsic compression on optic nerve.
- Orbital varix: inhomogeneous enhancement, size change with Valsalva.
- Optic nerve glioma: thickened optic nerve, nerve may enhance.

Management Options

Stable lesions with no or minimal visual impairment are monitored. In symptomatic cases, radiotherapy is the management of choice. Surgical intervention needs to be considered for lesions with intracranial extension.

References and Further Reading

1. Haouimi A. Optic nerve sheath meningioma. Radiopaedia.org. 2021. https://doi.org/10.53347/rID-81629. Accessed on 10 Nov 2022.
2. Patel BC, De Jesus O, Margolin E. Optic nerve sheath meningioma. Stat Pearls Publishing; 2025. https://www.ncbi.nlm.nih.gov/books/NBK430868/. Accessed on 20 Sept 2025.

Case 28

28

Clinical History

A 16-month-old baby boy presented with a spongy compressible soft tissue mass in the right cervicofacial region, which increases in size while crying.

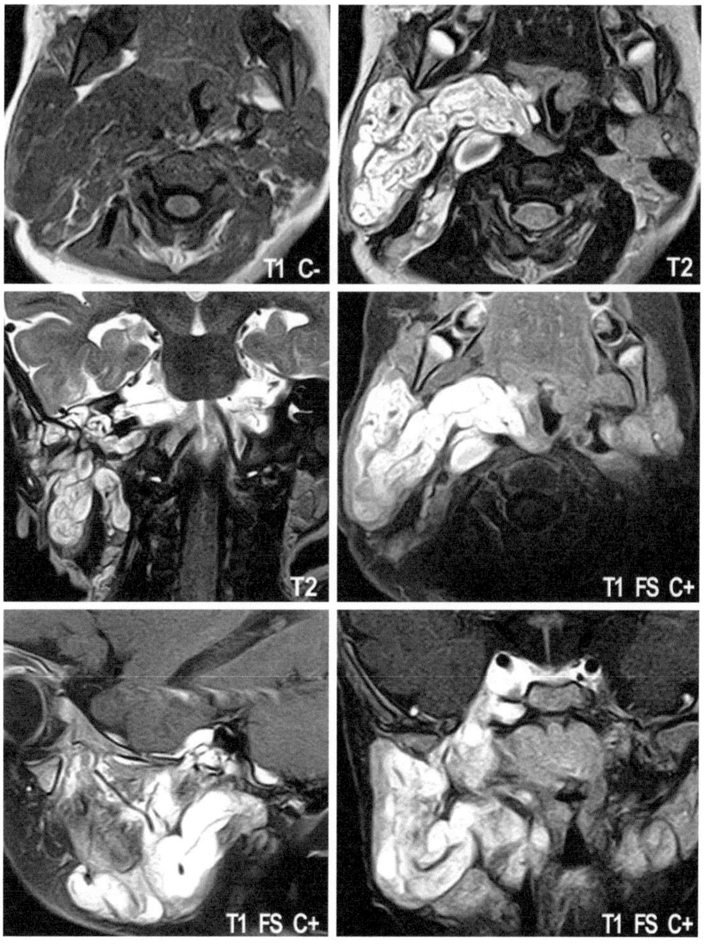

A. Haouimi et al., *Head and Neck Radiology Spot Diagnosis*,
https://doi.org/10.1007/978-3-032-14553-6_28

Findings

A large cervicofacial soft tissue mass centered in the right parotid space. Numerous intralesional serpiginous vascular structures of low signal on T1 and high signal on T2 with vivid enhancement representing dilated vascular lakes. Low-signal-intensity intralesional dots representing phleboliths.

Diagnosis

Venous vascular malformations (VVM).

Discussion

VVMs are the most common slow-flow vascular lesions of the neck, composed of endothelial-lined sinusoids and demonstrating continuous growth. Pathologically, the venous vascular malformations are thinly encapsulated, poorly circumscribed, multilobulated, heterogeneous lesions with venous dilatations. Lesions are trans-spatial and thought to arise from congenital defects during morphogenesis.

These venous vascular malformations are prone to bleeding and frequent invasion of adjacent structures. Any lobulated Valsalva-related soft tissue compressive spongy lesion with phleboliths should always be considered as VVM until proven otherwise.

The Doppler ultrasound can demonstrate this low-flow vascular lesion. Plain CT shows isodense mass with phleboliths and heterogeneous enhancement. These enhancing lesions typically appear as low signal on T1 and high signal on T2 with the presence of low-intensity intralesional dots representing phleboliths.

Common Differential Diagnosis

- Hemangioma: high flow signal voids.
- Lymphatic malformation: negative Doppler signal, no phleboliths.
- Ranula: no septation, no enhancement, no phleboliths.

Management Options

Management options include percutaneous embolization, sclerotherapy, and laser photocoagulation. Surgical options may be considered based on the location and extent of the lesion.

References and Further Reading

1. Beata D, et al. Venous vascular malformations and compressive neuropathy. Interdiscip Neurosurg. 2019. https://doi.org/10.1016/j.inat.2019.01.010.
2. Güneyli S, et al. Imaging findings of vascular lesions in the head and neck. Diagn Interv Radiol. 2014. https://doi.org/10.5152/dir.2014.14004. Accessed on 10 Sept 2025.
3. Haouimi A. Slow flow vascular malformation. Radiopaedia.org. 2022. https://doi.org/10.53347/rID-153644. Accessed on 01 Dec 2022.

Case 29

29

Clinical History

A 10-year-old girl presented with a painless purple swelling along the left lateral border of the tongue.

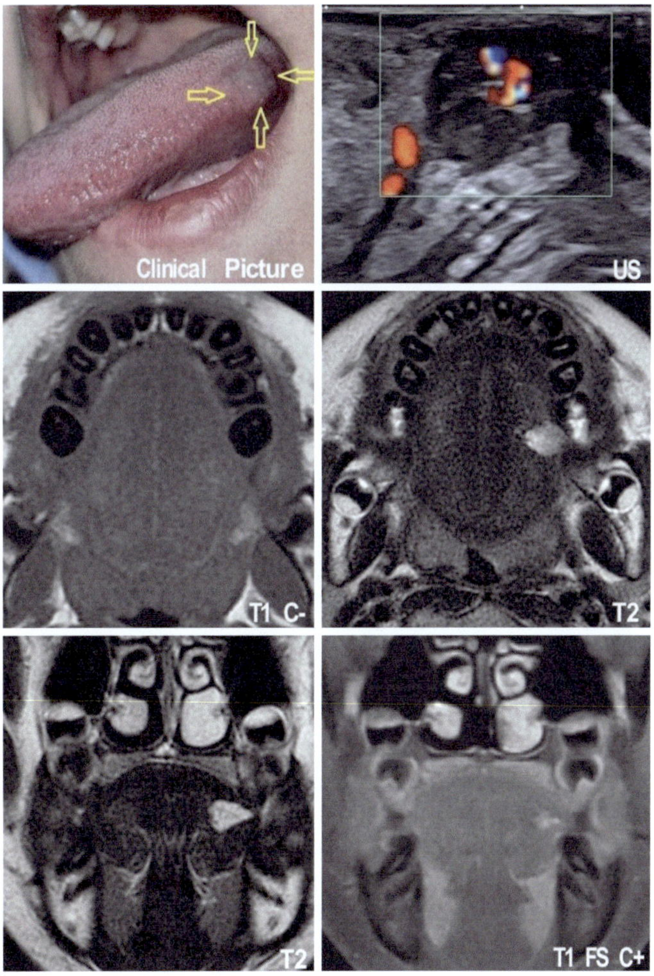

A. Haouimi et al., *Head and Neck Radiology Spot Diagnosis*,
https://doi.org/10.1007/978-3-032-14553-6_29

Findings

A "dome-shaped" purple lesion seen along left lingual margin. The lesion appears well defined and slightly hypoechoic with internal vascularity on ultrasound color Doppler images. On MRI, the lesion is isointense on T1 (almost invisible) and high signal on T2 with a tiny central enhancement.

Diagnosis

Lingual hemangioma.

Discussion

Lingual hemangiomas are benign lesions due to proliferation of endothelial cells. The etiology is poorly understood. Genetic mutations, embolic phenomenon, and hormones may play a significant role in their development. Infection and repeated trauma may also trigger the lesion. Pathologically, the hemangiomas are believed to develop through a combination of both angiogenesis and vasculogenesis. In the natural history, the lesions show initial endothelial proliferation, rapid growth, and finally a spontaneous involution.

The diagnosis is clinical. Color Doppler ultrasound shows a well-defined, slightly hypoechoic lesion with internal vascularity. A contrast-enhanced MRI is the imaging modality of choice and is considered superior to CT. Due to a high risk of bleeding, biopsy of the tongue is often avoided.

Common Differential Diagnosis

- Benign tongue ulcer: clinically straightforward, not dome shaped.
- Lingual lipoma: extremely rare, slow-growing, painless yellowish lesion, high signal on T1.
- Squamous cell carcinoma: mostly in adults, associated lymphadenopathy.

Management Options

Most lingual hemangiomas will involute over time and do not require treatment. Persistence into adulthood or interference with speech and swallowing may prompt the need for medical and/or surgical attention. Most symptomatic cases are treated with beta-blockers. Occasionally, larger lesions may need surgical resection with preoperative embolization. Sclerotherapy with direct puncture can be used for superficial lesions.

References and Further Reading

1. Haouimi A. Tongue haemangioma. Radiopaedia.org. 2021. https://doi.org/10.53347/rID-86631. Accessed on 08 June 2023.
2. Kamala KA, et al. Cavernous hemangioma of the tongue: a rare case report. Contemp Clin Dent. 2014. https://doi.org/10.4103/0976-237X.128680. Accessed on 08 June 2025.
3. Kripal K, et al. Cavernous hemangioma of the tongue. Case Rep Dent. 2013. https://doi.org/10.1155/2013/898692.

Case 30

30

Clinical History

A 3-year-old girl presented with a painless right neck doughy mass, increasing in size since birth.

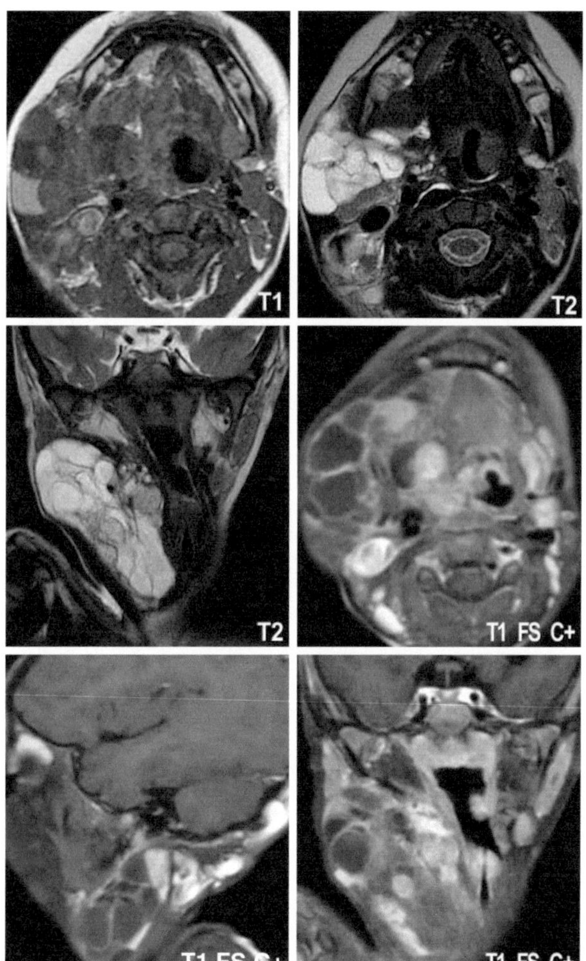

A. Haouimi et al., *Head and Neck Radiology Spot Diagnosis*,
https://doi.org/10.1007/978-3-032-14553-6_30

Findings

A right cervical multilocular cystic trans-spatial mass with internal septa, centered on the retro and submandibular regions. It appears hypointense on T1, with a high signal component (protein content) and high signal on T2. Peripheral rim enhancement and enhancement of the internal septa. There is a mass effect on the adjacent airway, causing oropharyngeal luminal narrowing.

Diagnosis

Cystic lymphangioma.

Discussion

Cystic lymphangiomas, also known as cystic hygromas, are benign trans-spatial lesions that arise due to abnormal development of lymphatic sacs. There is no malignant potential. Acquired cases can arise secondary to trauma, inflammation, or lymphatic obstruction. The lesions can be uni- or multilocular and tend to insinuate into neighboring structures.

They represent up to 5% of benign congenital cervical masses, and their clinical revelation is generally in the first 2 years of life. Lesions are mostly discovered incidentally. Parents may notice a doughy compressible painless soft tissue cervical mass commonly in the posterior cervical or submandibular space.

On ultrasound, the lesions are anechoic with septa of variable thickness or hypo-/hyperechoic because of infections, hemorrhage, high lipid content, etc. On CT, the lesions are usually multiloculated and cystic. The relationship with vascular structures and surrounding organs is outlined after contrast. On MRI, the insinuating lesions are homogeneously hypointense on T1 and hyperintense on T2 with hypointense septa. Septal enhancement makes the multiloculated appearance more obvious.

Common Differential Diagnosis

- Second branchial cleft cyst: mostly unilocular and at the level of mandibular angle.
- Thyroglossal duct cyst: midline unilocular cysts embedded in strap muscles.
- Multiple nodal metastases: clinical history, central necrosis, thick and irregular wall.

Management Options

Cystic lymphangiomas are "do not touch" lesions. Options like sclerotherapy, radiofrequency ablation, laser treatment, and surgical resection are reserved only in selected cases depending on size and symptoms.

References and Further Reading

1. Auerbach N, et al. Stat Pearls Publishing. 2025. https://www.ncbi.nlm.nih.gov/books/NBK560672/. Accessed on 12 July 2025.
2. Haouimi A. Cervical cystic lymphangioma. Radiopaedia.org. 2021. https://doi.org/10.53347/rID-87834. Accessed on 02 Dec 2022.

Case 31

31

Clinical History

A 35-year-old man presented with an acute loss of vision in the right eye and anosmia. Fundoscopy revealed right papilledema. History of similar symptoms in the left eye 4 years prior.

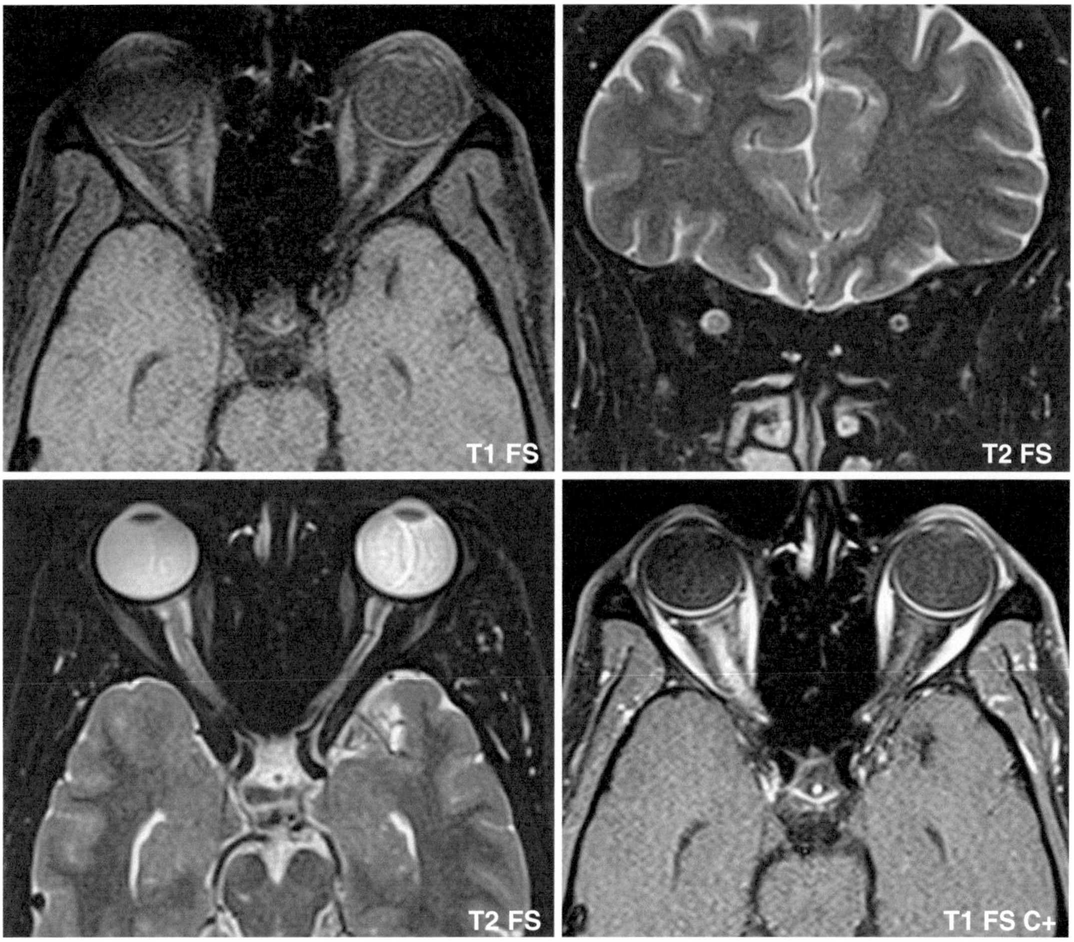

A. Haouimi et al., *Head and Neck Radiology Spot Diagnosis*,
https://doi.org/10.1007/978-3-032-14553-6_31

Findings

Swelling with high T2 signal intensity and contrast enhancement of the intraorbital segment of the right optic nerve. Atrophied left optic nerve. Normal brain and spinal cord.

Diagnosis

Pseudo-Foster Kennedy syndrome.

Discussion

True Foster Kennedy syndrome refers to a syndrome of visual loss due to compressive optic atrophy in one eye and papilledema in the contralateral eye arising from increased intracranial pressure. The cause is due to the presence of an intracranial space-occupying mass that compresses the ipsilateral optic nerve, resulting in optic atrophy. The lesion also increases intracranial pressure and causes papilledema in the contralateral eye. Meningiomas are the most frequent type of tumors found in the brain of patients with FKS. When similar clinical findings are seen without any detectable intracranial lesion, it is referred to as Pseudo-Foster Kennedy syndrome. Pseudo-Foster Kennedy Syndrome is also characterized by unilateral optic atrophy with contralateral optic disc edema. The etiology is poorly understood but is thought to be related to bilateral sequential anterior ischemic optic neuropathy (both arteritic and nonarteritic). The risk factors include hypertension, diabetes, smoking, and giant cell arteritis in the elderly. Benign intracranial hypertension and B12 deficiency may play a significant role.

MRI shows swelling with high T2 signal intensity and contrast enhancement of the intraorbital segment of the affected optic nerve and atrophy of the opposite nerve. Imaging is indicated for atypical cases and to rule out intracranial lesion.

Common Differential Diagnosis

- True Foster Kennedy syndrome: presence of an intracranial mass such as an olfactory groove meningioma.
- Multiple sclerosis: clinical history: multiphasic, multiple brain and spinal cord lesions.
- Neuromyelitis optica: extensive cord involvement and positive anti-AQP4 antibody.

Management Options

Primary prevention including control of vasculopathic risk factors. Spontaneous recovery occurs within a few weeks in primary Pseudo-Foster Kennedy syndrome. Corticosteroids, B12, and other appropriate agents are useful in secondary cases.

References and Further Reading

1. Haouimi A. Pseudo-Foster Kennedy syndrome. Radiopaedia.org. 2018. https://doi.org/10.53347/rID-65137. Accessed on 12 June 2024.
2. Micieli JA, et al. Pseudo-Foster Kennedy syndrome due to idiopathic intracranial hypertension. Can J Ophthalmol. 2014. https://doi.org/10.1016/j.jcjo.2014.05.002. Accessed on 12 June 2024.

Case 32

32

Clinical History

A 30-year-old asthmatic woman presented with nasal obstruction. Prior history of repeated surgery for nasal polyposis and aspirin intolerance.

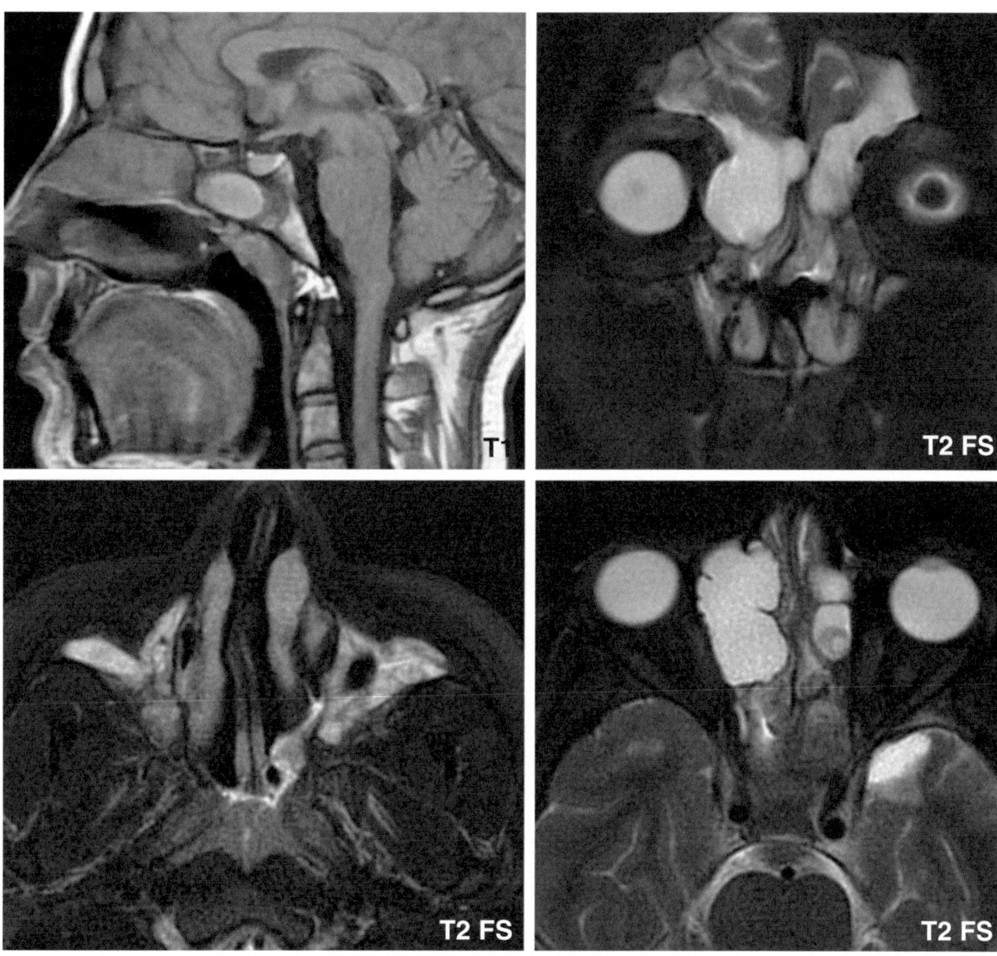

A. Haouimi et al., *Head and Neck Radiology Spot Diagnosis*,
https://doi.org/10.1007/978-3-032-14553-6_32

Findings

Extensive mucosal thickening with almost complete soft tissue opacification of the paranasal sinuses. The intrasinusal soft tissue appears as intermediate signal on T1 and high signal on T2. Areas of high signal within the left ethmoid air cells and sphenoid sinus on T1 showing low signal on T2 (protein-rich content or fungal infection). Bilateral ethmoid mucoceles.

Diagnosis

Widal syndrome.

Discussion

Widal syndrome, also known as aspirin-exacerbated respiratory disease (AERD), is an underrecognized entity not very infrequent in asthma clinics. The frequency is about 8.5% among asthmatics. It could be of genetic origin. It arises secondary to dysregulation of the arachidonic acid metabolic pathway and the cause of this dysregulation is poorly understood. There is a close relation of the syndrome with increased cysteinyl leukotrienes.

Patients often have an allergic or atopic background. The clinical triad known as Samter's triad is characterized by association of nasal polyposis, bronchial asthma, and aspirin intolerance. Rhinitis is most commonly the first symptom. The disorder typically progresses to asthma, then nasal polyposis, with aspirin sensitivity coming last. Hyposmia or anosmia is also found in more than 90% of patients due to involvement of olfactory receptors. The diagnosis is clinical.

Common Differential Diagnosis

- Kartagener syndrome: situs inversus.
- Nasal polyposis: absence of clinical triad.
- Sinonasal malignancy: locoregional invasion, absence of clinical triad.

Management Options

Treatment includes anti-asthmatic drugs. Surgical management of polyposis, if not controlled medically. There is recent interest in treatment with monoclonal antibodies.

References and Further Reading

1. Haouimi A. Widal syndrome. Radiopaedia.org. 2019. https://doi.org/10.53347/rID-69821. Accessed on 03 Dec 2022.
2. Leimgruber A. La triade de Widal (asthme-polypose nasale-intolérance à l'aspirine). Rev Med Suisse. 2005. Accessed on 13 May 2024.
3. Tudorache V, et al. Sindromul Widal este totdeauna o maladie severă. Pneumologia. 2006. Accessed on Apr 2025.

Case 33

33

Clinical History

A 50-year-old man presented with a nasal obstruction.

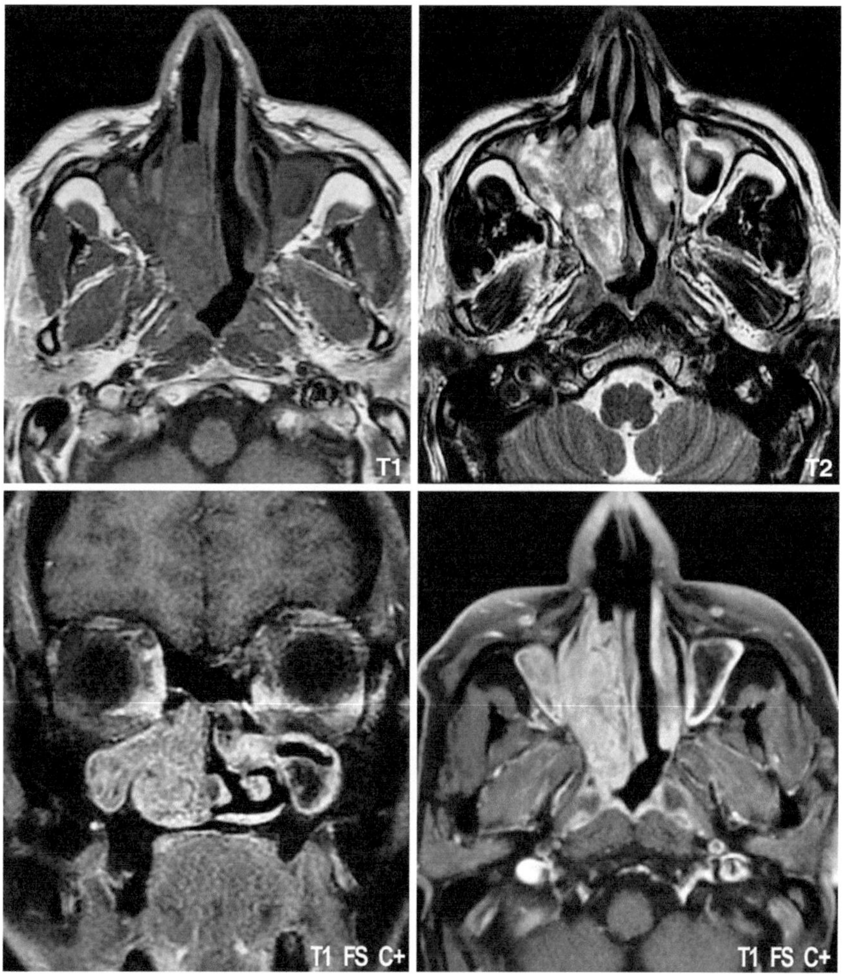

A. Haouimi et al., *Head and Neck Radiology Spot Diagnosis*,
https://doi.org/10.1007/978-3-032-14553-6_33

Findings

Soft tissue mass arising from the lateral wall of the right nasal cavity, enlarging the ostiomeatal complex and extending into the ipsilateral maxillary antrum and choana. The mass is isosignal to muscle on T1, heterogeneous high signal on T2 with alternating lines of high- and low-signal intensity giving a characteristic "convoluted cerebriform pattern" on postcontrast images. Small retracted maxillary sinuses with mucosal thickening.

Diagnosis

Inverted papilloma.

Discussion

Inverted papillomas, also known as endophytic papillomas, are locally aggressive, rare tumors with 5%–10% of malignant potential (squamous cell carcinoma). They mostly affect middle-aged men.

The etiology is poorly understood. A strong association with human papillomavirus has been reported in up to 40% of cases. Association of allergy and chronic sinusitis has also been suggested as a possible cause. The lesions mostly arise from nasal fossa mucosa and neighboring middle meatus, and have a tendency of extending to involve the adjacent sinuses and orbit.

An expanding lesion leads to obstructive ipsilateral sinusitis secondary to ostiomeatal obstruction. Pathologically, these are epithelial tumors of the nasal mucosa. Endoscopic examination often fails to reveal the full extent of the lesion.

On imaging, the lesions present as enhancing lesions with a convoluted cerebriform texture with bony remodeling and obstructive type of sinus opacification. The lesions often enter the ipsilateral maxillary sinus through an enlarged infundibulum. Pre-surgical coronal sinus CT or MRI must be performed, considering high risk of recurrence following incomplete surgical resection.

Common Differential Diagnosis

- Antro-choanal polyp: no enhancement.
- Juvenile angiofibroma: epicenter at sphenopalatine foramen, younger male patients.
- Squamous cell carcinoma: epicenter at maxillary antrum, bony destruction.

Management Options

Treatment for inverted papilloma must be aggressive. Surgery is the mainstay of treatment.

References and Further Reading

1. Haouimi A. Inverted papilloma. Radiopaedia.org. 2021. https://doi.org/10.53347/rID-95388. Accessed on 14 Dec 2022.
2. Chawla A, et al. Imaging features of sinonasal inverted papilloma: a pictorial review. Curr Probl Diagn Radiol. 2016. https://doi.org/10.1067/j.cpradiol.2015.10.004. Accessed on 14 Aug 2025.

Case 34

34

Clinical History

A 70-year-old man presented with chronic headache.

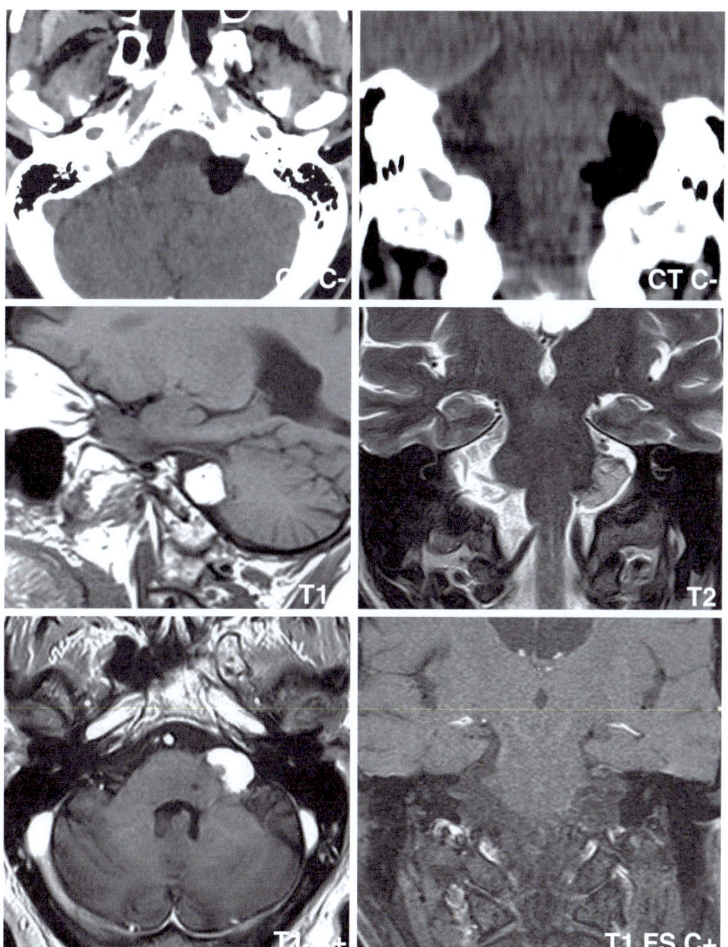

A. Haouimi et al., *Head and Neck Radiology Spot Diagnosis*,
https://doi.org/10.1007/978-3-032-14553-6_34

Findings

A left cerebellopontine angle CT low-density lesion causing slight mass effect on adjacent brain parenchyma. It appears as high signal on T1 and T2 without enhancement. Complete suppression of the signal on fat saturation sequence.

Diagnosis

CPA lipoma.

Discussion

Lipomas are congenital malformations rather than neoplastic. They arise from abnormal differentiation of the mesodermal layer, leading to development of adipose tissue in the central nervous system. They typically grow slowly and do not usually increase in size.

Lesions are mostly asymptomatic. Larger-sized CPA lipomas may cause sensorineural hearing loss due to compression on the vestibulocochlear nerve and facial numbness, and facial weakness can arise due to involvement of the trigeminal and facial nerves, respectively. Cerebellar compression can cause ataxia. It can also cause dizziness, tinnitus, and vertigo.

The lesions appear as a low-density extra-axial mass on CT without contrast enhancement. MRI is the investigation of choice. MRI shows high signal on both T1 and T2 without any intracanalicular extension or enhancement. The intralesional signals will be suppressed by applying fat-suppression sequences.

Common Differential Diagnosis

- CPA epidermoid cyst: restricted diffusion.
- CPA acoustic neuroma: "ice-cream cone" lesion, enhancement, intra-canalicular extension.
- CPA meningioma: enhancement, "dural tail sign," usually no intracanalicular extension.

Management Options

The treatment for a cerebellopontine angle (CPA) lipoma depends on the patient's symptoms and the tumor characteristics.

References and Further Reading

1. Brodsky JR, et al. Lipoma of the cerebellopontine angle. Am J Otolaryngol. 2006; https://doi.org/10.1016/j.amjoto.2005.11.002. Accessed Apr 2022.
2. Haouimi A. Cerebellopontine angle lipoma. "Radiopaedia.org". 2021. https://doi.org/10.53347/rID-93062. Accessed Dec 7 2024.
3. Kanaya T, et al. Acoustic neurinoma with synchronous ipsilateral cerebellopontine angle lipoma: a case report and review of the literature. Diagnostics (Basel). 2022; https://doi.org/10.3390/diagnostics12010120. Accessed 2 June 2024. PMID: 35054286; PMCID: PMC8775160.

Case 35

35

Clinical History

A 60-year-old man came to the oncology clinic after being diagnosed with a laryngeal mass. He has had a tracheostomy at another institution.

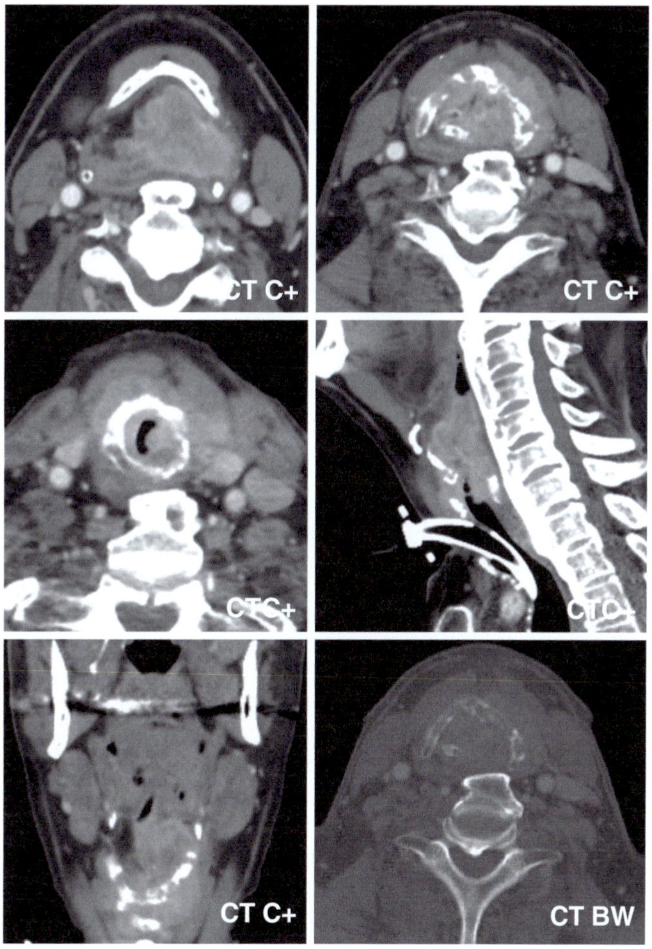

A. Haouimi et al., *Head and Neck Radiology Spot Diagnosis*,
https://doi.org/10.1007/978-3-032-14553-6_35

Findings

A large, enhancing, infiltrative mass occupying the supraglottic, glottic, and infraglottic larynx seen on enhanced CT. Infiltration of the laryngeal cartilage with extra-laryngeal extension, as well as a few enlarged lymph nodes. The sagittal MPR depicts the complete obliteration of the airway and tracheostomy tube to ensure airway patency below the tumor.

Diagnosis

Trans-glottic squamous cell carcinoma of the larynx.

Discussion

Most laryngeal tumors originate from the mucosa, and the commonest type is squamous cell carcinoma with a male predominance. Genetic, environmental, and infectious factors (such as HPV and EPV) play a major role in their development. Smoking and alcohol/opium use are common risk factors. Glottic location accounts for more than half of the cases. About one-third of the lesions are seen at supra-glottic locations. Subglottic involvement is rare <10%).

Direct laryngoscopy with biopsy is the gold standard for diagnosis. Imaging has a major role in determining the extent of the lesion for staging. Tumors confined to the larynx are classified as T1 and T2. Vocal cord fixation or cartilage invasion indicates T3. Extra-laryngeal spread is classified as T4. CT scans often show heterogeneous masses with irregular margins. Soft tissue contrast is better seen on MRI and allows identification of submucosal extension and invasion of pre- and para-glottic fat planes.

Common Differential Diagnosis

- Laryngeal polyp or nodule: smooth, well-defined, noninvasive.
- Laryngeal chondrosarcoma: “rings and arc” calcifications, epicentered on cartilage.
- Tuberculosis: no cartilage invasion, association of extra-laryngeal involvement.
- GPA: subglottic stenosis, inflammation without obvious mass.

Management Options

Advanced trans-glottic T4 cases are usually treated with radiotherapy and chemotherapy. Surgical options may be considered for localized lesions without cervical lymphadenopathy or metastasis.

References and Further Reading

1. Liberale C, et al. Risk factors and oncogenesis. Int J Mol Sci. 2023; https://doi.org/10.3390/ijms241612913. Accessed 24 June 2025.
2. Sahu A, et al. Staging and management of larynx and hypopharynx cancer. Indian J Med Paediatr Oncol. 2023; https://doi.org/10.1055/s-0042-1759504. Accessed 13 Apr 2024.

36

Case 36

Clinical History

A 40-year-old woman presented with a painless right lateral suprahyoid neck swelling.

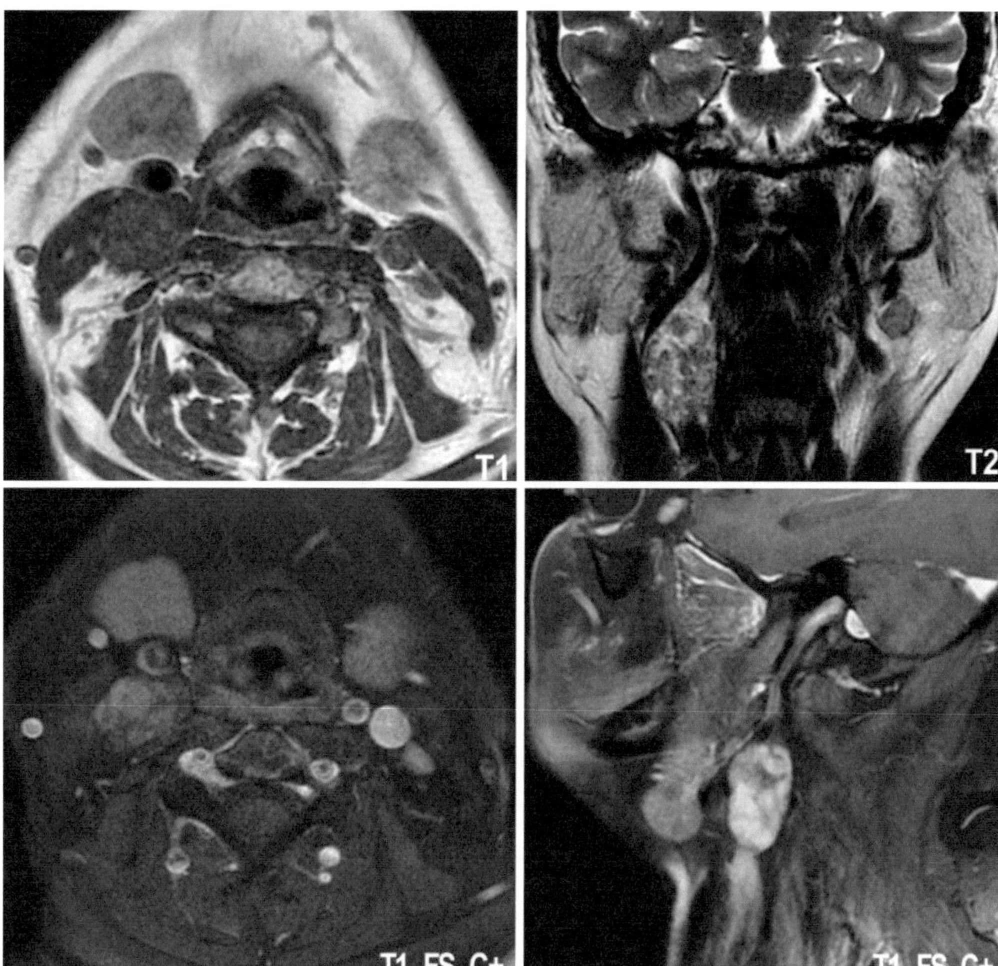

A. Haouimi et al., *Head and Neck Radiology Spot Diagnosis*,
https://doi.org/10.1007/978-3-032-14553-6_36

Findings

Well-encapsulated right carotid space soft tissue mass located between the carotid bifurcation anteriorly and internal jugular vein laterally. It shows an intermediate signal on T1, heterogeneous high signal on T2 with moderate and heterogeneous enhancement. The lesion separates the internal carotid artery and internal jugular vein, displacing the ICA anteromedially.

Diagnosis

Vagal schwannoma.

Discussion

Vagal schwannomas are rare, encapsulated oval or fusiform benign carotid space lesions with remote malignant potential. Bilateral cases are often associated with NF2. They can occur in any location but mostly arise in the suprahyoid neck in the carotid space. Most of the cases manifest between the third and sixth decades.

Clinically, they present as a painless, slow-growing lateral neck mass. Initially, the lesions can be a cosmetic concern. Larger lesions can be palpated along the medial border of the sternocleidomastoid muscle and may cause symptoms such as dysphagia, dysphonia, sleep apnea, and Horner syndrome.

On ultrasound, the vagal schwannomas appear as a nonvascular, well-defined, round, or elliptical mass containing internal echoes. On CT, they are isodense to adjacent muscles, showing uniform enhancement. On MRI, the lesions show low signal on T1 and heterogeneously high signal on T2 without any sign of flow voids. The central low intensity on enhanced T1 represents cystic changes. Multiple tiny, circular, low-intensity areas surrounded by a background of mild hyperintensity on T2, may show a fascicular appearance on axial images. MRI better delineates the relationship between the schwannoma and its nerve of origin than CT.

Common Differential Diagnosis

- Carotid body tumor: "lyre sign."
- Hypervascular lymphadenopathy: usually multiple and bilateral.
- Pseudoaneurysm: pulsatile lesion having connection with vascular lumen.

Management Options

Only symptomatic slow-growing tumors need surgical enucleation. There is a risk of severe transient bradycardia during surgical removal.

References and Further Reading

1. Aultman AJ 2nd, Genelin M, Gonzalez J. Vagus nerve schwannoma. J Brown Hosp Med. 2024;3(1):89988. https://doi.org/10.56305/001c.89988.
2. Haouimi A. Vagal schwannoma. "Radiopaedia.org". 2023. https://doi.org/10.53347/rID-84674. Accessed 10 June 2023.

Case 37

37

Clinical History

An 18-year-old man with a history of recurrent tonsillitis, presented with recent onset of fever, dysphagia, and trismus.

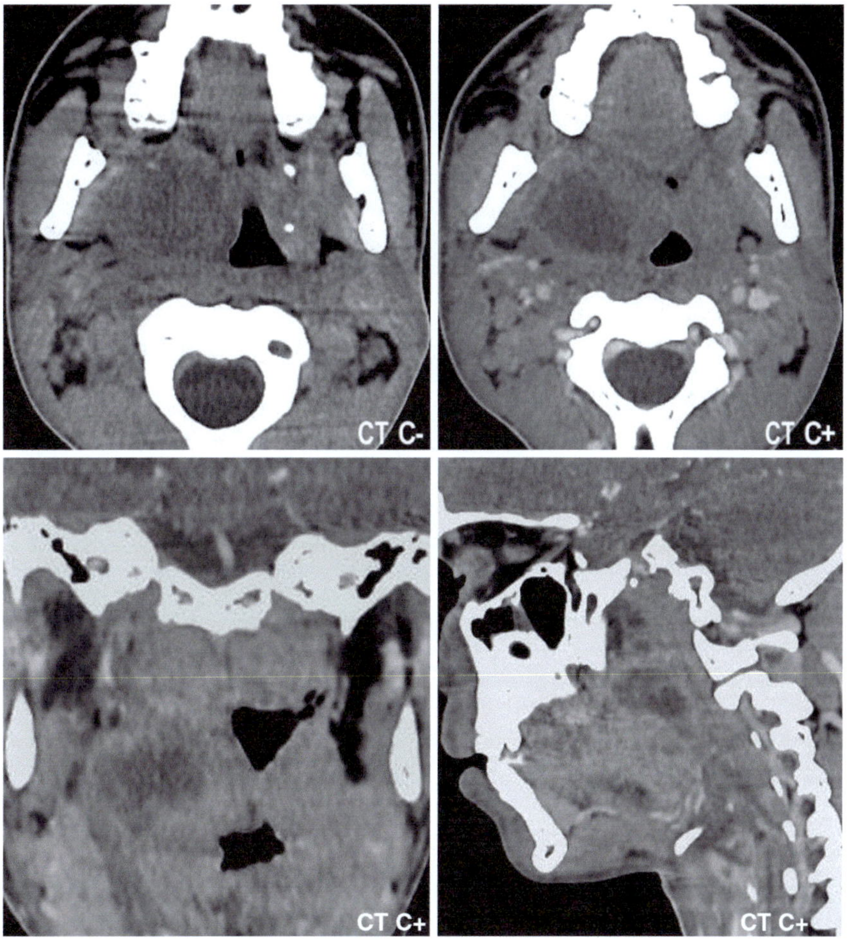

A. Haouimi et al., *Head and Neck Radiology Spot Diagnosis*,
https://doi.org/10.1007/978-3-032-14553-6_37

Findings

Hypodense collection in the right pharyngeal mucosal space neighboring the tonsillar region, extending to the parapharyngeal and submandibular spaces, causing extrinsic compression on oropharyngeal lumen. Faint peripheral enhancement; bilateral reactive lymph nodes.

Diagnosis

Peritonsillar abscess.

Discussion

Peritonsillar abscess, also known as quinsy, is a localized pus collection in pharyngeal mucosal space between the tonsillar capsule and superior constrictor. It is a complication of untreated or poorly treated tonsillitis. It starts as a tonsillar infection progressing to a pus-filled pocket of tonsillar parenchyma.

Clinically, patients present with fever and progressive worsening of symptoms, including difficulty in swallowing. Uvular deviation and trismus suggest possible peritonsillar abscess. The presence of torticollis, severe respiratory distress, stridor, and muffled speech often suggests a possible deep neck space infection.

The diagnosis of peritonsillar abscess is clinical. CT and MRI are indicated when the spread of the infection is suspected beyond the peritonsillar space or concern for complications involving the lateral neck spaces. Both CT and MRI can distinguish between peritonsillar cellulitis and peritonsillar abscess.

Common Differential Diagnosis

- Retropharyngeal abscess: midline lesion with retropharyngeal space epicenter.
- Phlegmonous tonsillitis: no enhancing peripheral rim.
- Non-Hodgkin lymphoma (NHL): bilateral nodal enlargement, systemic involvement.

Management Options

Patients are evaluated on a case-by-case basis. To prevent an abscess formation, initiating immediate appropriate antibiotic therapy is recommended. A delayed initiation of treatment increases the risk of abscess formation. Although most cases are treated conservatively, incision and drainage may be needed in advanced cases. Tonsillectomy might be considered in those with recurrent episodes.

References and Further Reading

1. Gupta G, McDowell RH. Peritonsillar abscess. Stat Pearls Publishing; 2022. Accessed 13 May 2023.
2. Haouimi A. Peritonsillar abscess. Radiopaedia.org. 2019. https://doi.org/10.53347/rID-69226. Accessed 20 Dec 2022.

Case 38

38

Clinical History

A 15-year-old boy presented with a slowly growing, painless left off-midline cervical swelling.

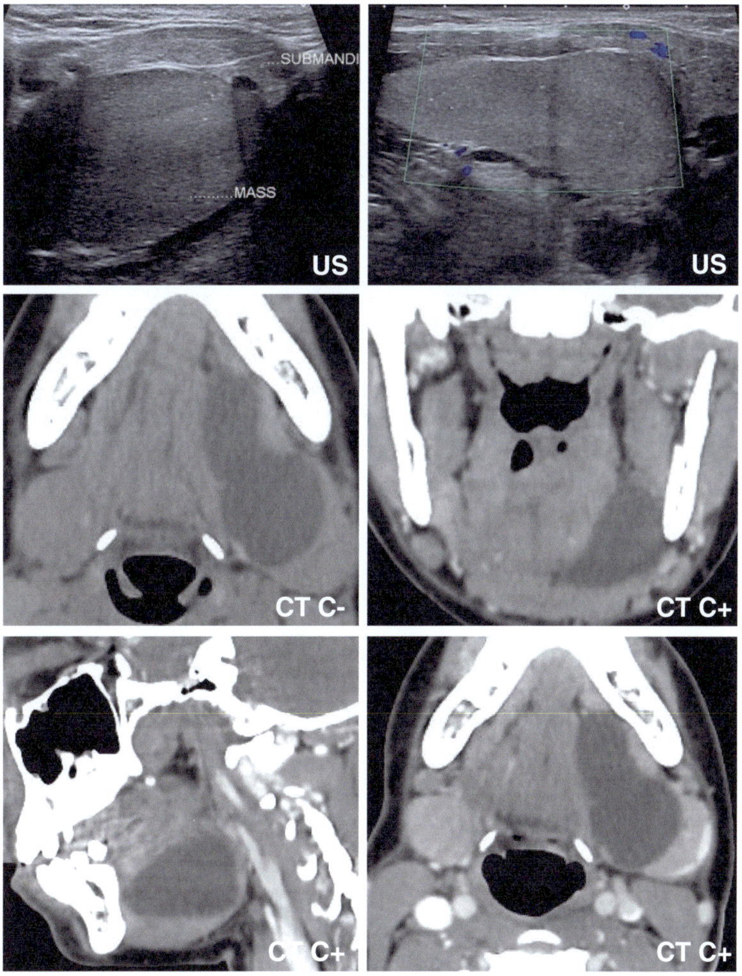

A. Haouimi et al., *Head and Neck Radiology Spot Diagnosis*,
https://doi.org/10.1007/978-3-032-14553-6_38

Findings

A homogeneously echogenic cystic lesion at the floor of the mouth, posteromedial to the normal submandibular gland with no internal vascularity on color Doppler. CT reveals a well-circumscribed low-density off-midline cystic lesion with no enhancement. It is located superior to the floor of the oral cavity with downward displacement of the mylohyoid muscle.

Ultrasound shows the lesion as an avascular cystic lesion occupying both sublingual and submandibular spaces. The lesions are hypodense on CT. On MRI, the diving ranulas can show both the sublingual and submandibular space components as well as extension to the parapharyngeal space. The well-defined lesions are hypointense on T1 and hyperintense on T2 with faint peripheral wall enhancement. Infected lesions may show a thickened, enhanced wall.

Diagnosis

Plunging ranula.

Discussion

Ranulas are a type of retention cyst. The term is derived from the Latin word for frog and the lesion may resemble the underbelly of a frog. Lesions are benign mucoceles at the floor of the mouth resulting from trauma and inflammation. A plunging or diving ranula is a pseudocyst that arises when simple ranula in sublingual space ruptures into the adjacent submandibular space.

Clinically, ranulas appear as a painless bluish lump on the floor of the mouth. They appear as off-midline cervical lesions when they grow bigger in size. The larger-sized diving ranulas can extend to the opposite sublingual space through the anterior isthmus and may have a "horseshoe configuration". The lesions may resolve on their own.

Common Differential Diagnosis

- Thyroglossal duct cyst: often midline and embedded in the strap muscles.
- Second branchial cleft cyst: off-midline cervical lesion mostly in submandibular space.
- Cervical abscess: clinical context, smooth, thick, and regular ring enhancement.

Management Options

Ranulas are "do not touch" lesions. Occasionally, they may require cystectomy or marsupialization.

References and Further Reading

1. Haouimi A. Plunging ranula. Radiopaedia.org. 2019. https://doi.org/10.53347/rID-65538. Accessed 34 Dec 2022.
2. Koch M, et al. Ultrasound in the diagnosis and differential diagnosis of enoral and plunging ranula: a detailed and comparative analysis. J Ultrasound. 2023; https://doi.org/10.1007/s40477-022-00743-7. Accessed 21 Apr 2024.

Case 39

39

Clinical History

A 30-year-old man presented with a right nasal obstruction.

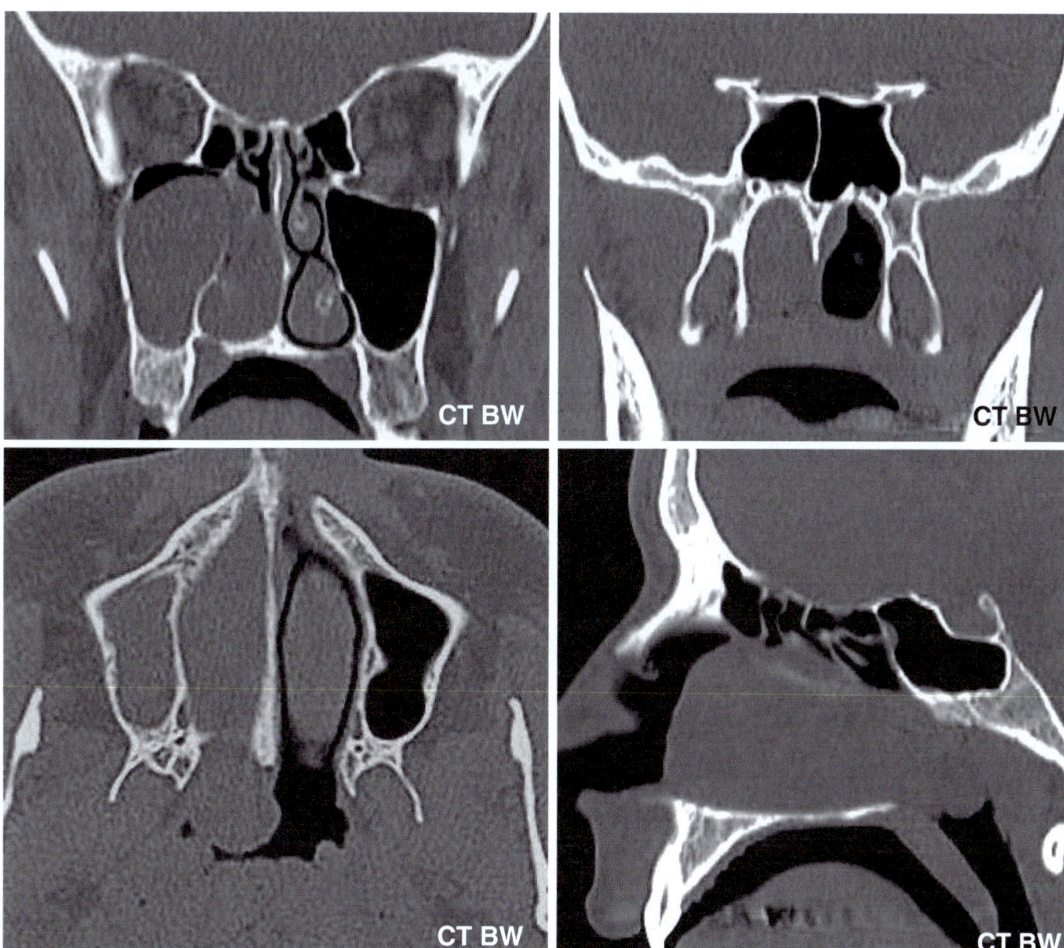

A. Haouimi et al., *Head and Neck Radiology Spot Diagnosis*,
https://doi.org/10.1007/978-3-032-14553-6_39

Findings

Well-defined soft tissue polypoid mass arising from the right maxillary sinus. It extends posteriorly toward the nasopharynx through an enlarged maxillary ostium, obstructing the posterior choana. No associated bony destruction.

Diagnosis

Antrochoanal polyp (Killian polyp).

Discussion

Antrochoanal polyps, also known as Killian polyp, represent up to 6% of all nasal polyps. These non-neoplastic, benign, pear-shaped inflammatory lesions are unilateral and solitary. The stalk arises from the maxillary sinus, but the narrow stalk is difficult to identify. They are seen predominantly in children and young adults. Occasionally, the Killian polyp can be associated with cystic fibrosis.

Most cases emerge through the middle meatus, starting from the zygomatic wall of the maxillary antrum near dental roots. The lesions migrate posteriorly through the nasal cavity to reach the ipsilateral choana. The lesions extrude to a variable distance and occasionally even beyond choana to reach the naso- and/or oropharynx.

Coronal sinus CT is the modality of choice. It shows intramaxillary and intranasal polyp migrating posteriorly toward the choana to a variable distance. There is associated remodeling of sinonasal bones and widening of the ipsilateral infundibulum of the maxillary sinus. Enhanced scan is not necessary, but it may demonstrate peripheral enhancement.

Common Differential Diagnosis

- Inverted papilloma: usually enhances.
- Juvenile nasopharyngeal angiofibroma: sphenopalatine epicenter, younger male patients.
- Maxillary sinus mucocele: rare location, bony erosion.

Management Options

Surgical resection with wide antrostomy. It is important to identify the stalk to prevent recurrence.

References and Further Reading

1. Francisco André E. Antrochoanal Polyp. J Otolaryngol Rhinol. 2018; https://doi.org/10.23937/2572-4193.1510049.
2. Haouimi A. Antrochoanal polyp. Radiopaedia.org. 2022. https://doi.org/10.53347/rID-156775. Accessed 24 Dec 2022.
3. Maldonado M, et al. The antrochoanal polyp. Rhinology. 2004. Accessed 12 June 2025. PMID: 15626248.

Case 40

40

Clinical History

A 50-year-old woman presented with a right-sided hearing loss and dizziness.

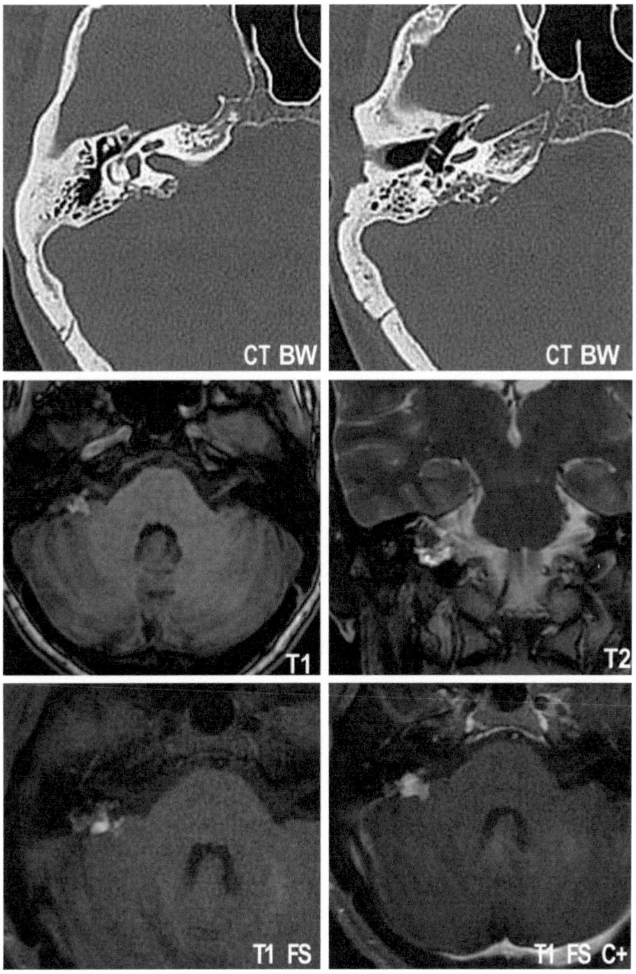

A. Haouimi et al., *Head and Neck Radiology Spot Diagnosis*,
https://doi.org/10.1007/978-3-032-14553-6_40

Findings

A permeative retro-labyrinthine destructive lesion with calcification and spiculated tumoral matrix situated along the cisternal face of the petrous temporal bone. The lesion is epicentered on the vestibular aqueduct along the posterior border of petrous ridge. There is a tiny focal bony wall defect involving the right posterior semicircular canal. The lesion appears ill-defined, expansile, and lobulated with irregular margin on MRI. One component shows intrinsic high signal on T1, T2, and T1 fat sat with no enhancement, and another component having isosignal to the brain tissue on T1, iso-to-low signal on T2 with moderate heterogeneous enhancement.

Diagnosis

Endolymphatic sac tumor.

Discussion

Endolymphatic sac tumors are uncommon, indolent lesions with local aggressivity and very low risk of distant metastasis. They originate from the endolymphatic sac or duct. Most cases are sporadic and bilateral lesions often constitute a component of von Hippel–Lindau disease.

The clinical symptoms are sensory neuronal hearing loss due to the development of endolymphatic hydrops, nonspecific ataxia, vertigo, and tinnitus.

On CT, the lesions appear as a heterogeneously enhancing soft tissue mass with "moth-eaten" type of bony destruction along the posterior petrous ridge and intertumoral bony spiculations. The lesion may extend to the IAC, middle ear, and bony facial canal. These heterogeneously enhancing lesions are hypo-/isointense on T1 and high signal on T2. Scattered foci of T1 high signals in bigger lesions represent methemoglobin, proteinaceous cysts, and cholesterol cleft.

Common Differential Diagnosis

- Jugulo-tympanic paraganglioma: pulsatile tinnitus, intralabyrinthine, not retrolabyrinthine.
- Schwannomas at jugular foramen: enlarged foramen, homogeneous linear enhancement.
- Meningioma: permeative sclerotic bony changes, no flow void.

Management Options

Complete surgical excision with negative margin. Bigger lesions with gross residual volume, positive margin, or unresectable tumor are addressed with radiotherapy or radiosurgery.

References and Further Reading

1. Geng Y, et al. Endolymphatic sac tumour: exploring the role of CT and MRI features in the diagnosis of 22 cases. Clin Radiol. https://doi.org/10.1016/j.crad.2022.04.010. Accessed 11 July 2024. Epub 2022 May 25. PMID: 35643739.
2. Haouimi A. Endolymphatic sac tumour. Radiopaedia.org. 2023. https://doi.org/10.53347/rID-176986. Accessed 31 Oct 2024.

Case 41

41

Clinical History

A 30-year-old woman presented with a slow-growing, painless swelling of the anterior aspect of the roof of the mouth.

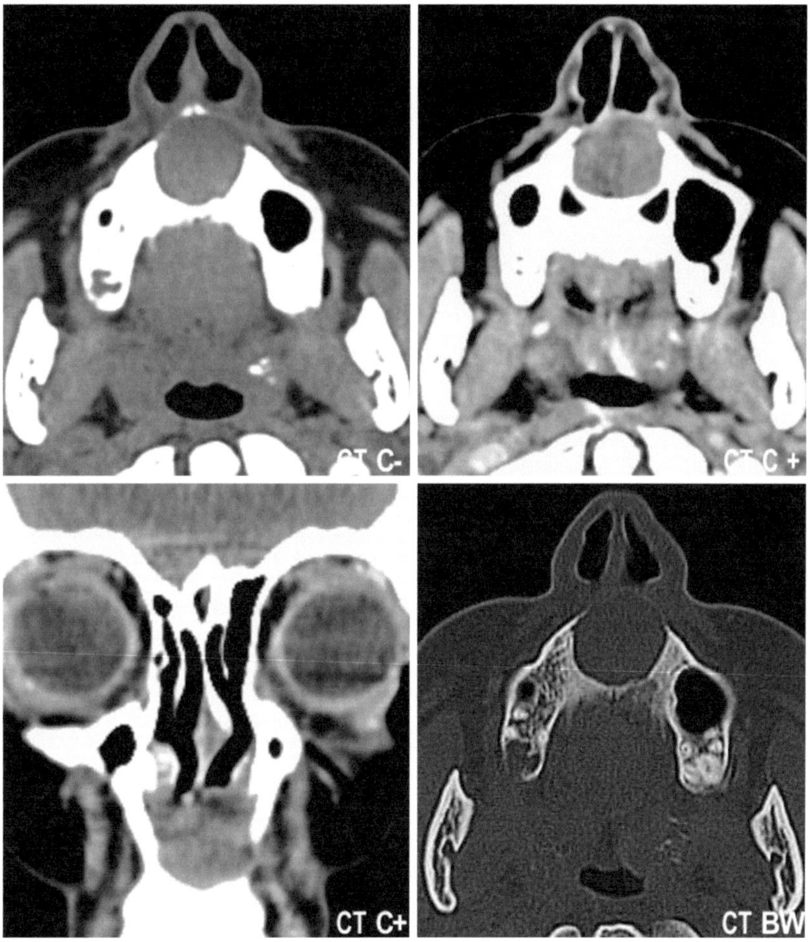

A. Haouimi et al., *Head and Neck Radiology Spot Diagnosis*,
https://doi.org/10.1007/978-3-032-14553-6_41

Findings

A well-defined midline round homogeneous unilocular radiolucent lesion at the anterior aspect of the hard palate centered on the maxillary incisive. No calcification or enhancement. Enlarged oral tonsils with tonsilloliths.

Diagnosis

Nasopalatine duct cyst.

Discussion

Nasopalatine duct cysts, also known as incisive canal cysts, are the most common nonodontogenic fissural cyst of the oral cavity, representing persistent ductal epithelium. The cyst originates from embryogenic remnants of the nasopalatine duct. Pathologically, they contain nonkeratinized stratified squamous epithelium and/or in combination with other epithelia.

The lesions mostly remain asymptomatic. Occasionally, the patients may present with a salty taste in the mouth, pain, and midline swelling at the posterior aspect of superior dental arcade.

Symptoms are not size dependent as patients with smaller cysts may have disproportionately severe symptoms.

CT shows well-defined lucent lesion in the anterior maxilla centered on the incisive canal. A widened incisive canal with diameter of more than 1 cm should be presumed as a nasopalatine duct cyst. Inadvertent root canal therapy can be avoided if the diagnosis of nasopalatine duct cyst can be made with confidence.

Common Differential Diagnosis

- Nasolabial cyst: inferior nasal alar epicenter, scalloping of alveolar process.
- Dentigerous cyst: associated with unerupted or impacted tooth.
- Radicular cyst: associated with infected tooth with alveolar epicenter.

Management Options

Surgical enucleation is recommended only in symptomatic cases.

References and Further Reading

1. Al-Haj Husain A, et al. Appearance of nasopalatine duct cysts on dental magnetic resonance imaging using a mandibular coil: two case reports with a literature review. Imaging Sci Dent. 2023. https://doi.org/10.5624/isd.20220215. Accessed 12 Apr 2024. Epub 2023 Mar 24. PMID: 37405200; PMCID: PMC10315232.
2. Dedhia P, et al. Nasopalatine duct cyst. Case Rep Dent. 2013. https://doi.org/10.1155/2013/869516. Accessed 15 Sept 2024. Epub 2013 Nov 4. PMID: 24307954.
3. Haouimi A. Nasopalatine duct cyst (NPDC). Radiopaedia.org. 2021. https://doi.org/10.53347/rID-94424. Accessed 24 Dec 2022.

Case 42

42

Clinical History

A 25-year-old man presented with a traumatic fracture of the nasal bone and an incidental finding.

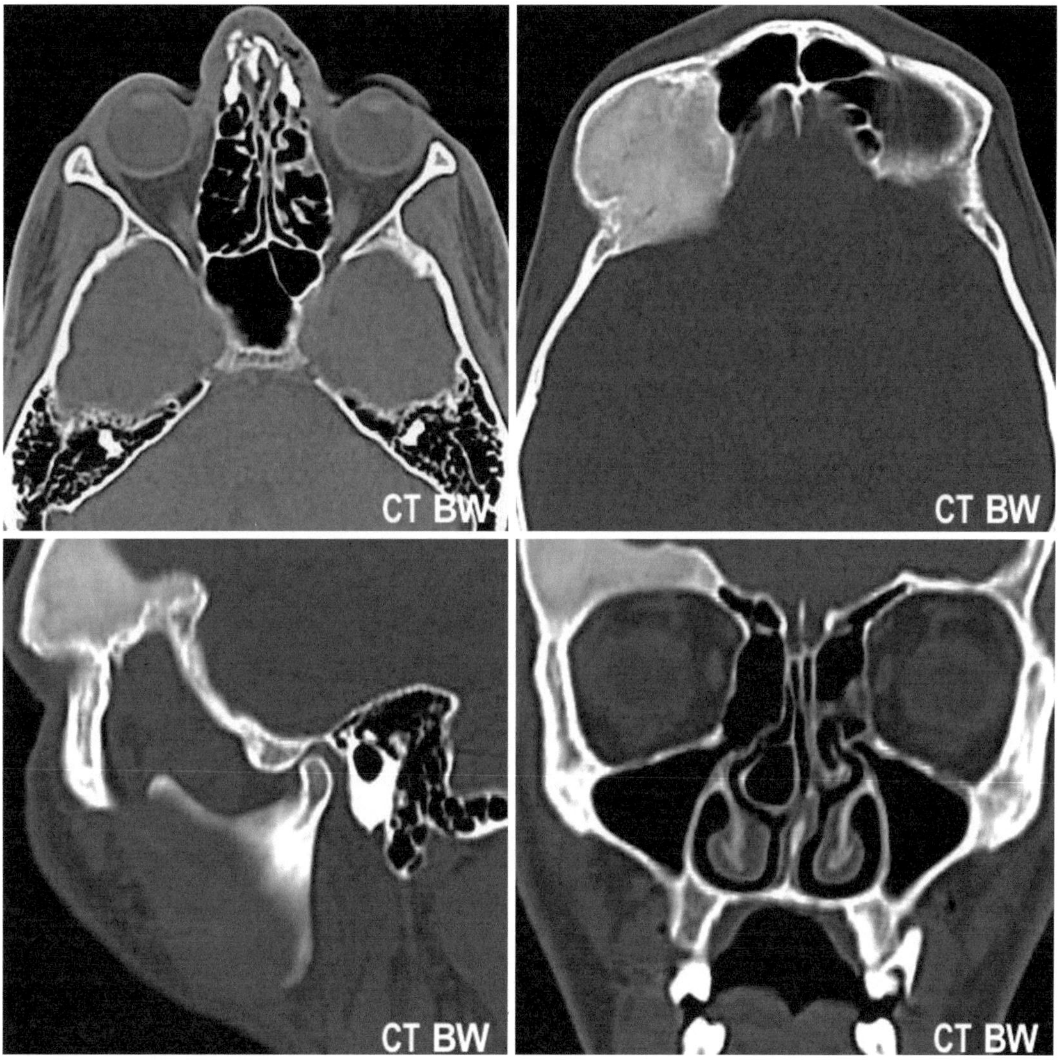

A. Haouimi et al., *Head and Neck Radiology Spot Diagnosis*,
https://doi.org/10.1007/978-3-032-14553-6_42

Findings

Bilateral comminuted displaced nasal bone fractures with soft tissue emphysema. Deviated nasal septum with fracture of its anterior aspect. Concha bullosa.

Homogeneous expansile ground glass appearance of the right orbital roof.

Diagnosis

Craniofacial fibrous dysplasia.

Discussion

Fibrous dysplasia is a benign bony condition arising due to defective osteogenesis with remote malignant potential. The etiology is linked with a missense mutation in the *GNAS1* gene on chromosome 20. Craniofacial fibrous dysplasia mostly involves the facial bones. It is a developmental benign medullary fibro-osseous process where the normal bone is replaced by fibrous tissue. The soft and stringy nature makes the lesion more fragile and vulnerable to fracture.

Patients with monostotic fibrous dysplasia are often asymptomatic. Though lesions initially remain painless, they may present with pain and tenderness, facial deformity, and bony expansion. In monostotic form, however, the lesions can become inactive after puberty. Fracture with minor inciting trauma can also be a first presentation.

On plain film and CT scan, the lesions show an internal "ground glass" matrix. Lesions may show bony expansion, lytic and/or sclerotic components, and possible deformity. Rarely, equivocal cases may require biopsy to rule out malignancy.

Common Differential Diagnosis

- Paget disease: "cotton wool" appearance with deformity mostly involving calvarium.
- Garré sclerosing osteomyelitis: periosteal reaction, nonhomogeneous and sclerotic.
- Cranio-metaphyseal dysplasia: associated with long bone metaphyseal abnormality.

Management Options

Aggressive surgical resection is reserved for symptomatic cases, especially with proptosis, visual loss, and severe deformity. Radiotherapy may precipitate malignant progression. Continued clinical monitoring is essential.

References and Further Reading

1. Haouimi A. Craniofacial fibrous dysplasia. Radiopaedia.org. 2022. https://doi.org/10.53347/rID-96736. Accessed 25 Dec 2022.
2. Szymczuk V, Taylor J, Boyce AM. Craniofacial fibrous dysplasia: clinical and therapeutic implications. Curr Osteoporos Rep. 2023. https://doi.org/10.1007/s11914-023-00779-6. Accessed 24 May 2024. Epub 2023 Feb 28. PMID: 36849642; PMCID: PMC11087144.

Case 43

43

Clinical History

A 1-year-old boy presented with a progressive right facial swelling since birth and a red cutaneous birthmark.

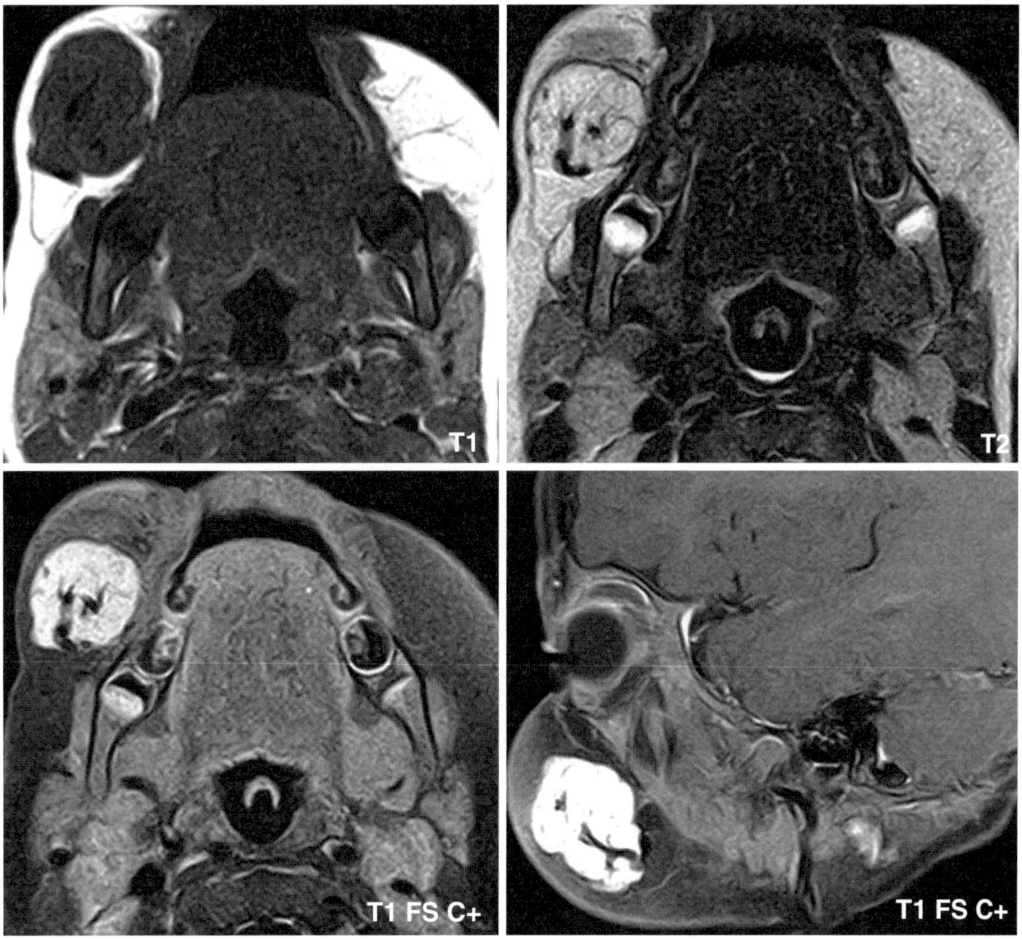

A. Haouimi et al., *Head and Neck Radiology Spot Diagnosis*,
https://doi.org/10.1007/978-3-032-14553-6_43

Findings

A well-defined right facial lobulated soft tissue mass in the right cheek, adjacent to the lateral aspect of the mandible and anterior to the buccal fat pad and masseter. It is isointense to muscle on T1, hyperintense on T2 with intra- and perilesional flow voids (vascular structures). Dilatation of the retromandibular vein and vivid contrast enhancement.

Diagnosis

Facial infantile hemangioma.

Discussion

Facial infantile hemangiomas are the most common infantile tumors and show a Caucasian predilection. They are noncancerous true vascular neoplasms. The proliferative phase continues up to first 6 months as the lesion continues to grow. This is followed by an involutive phase when they will start to shrink and most of those lesions disappear by the age of five years. However, larger lesions may represent a component of PHACE syndrome.

Clinically, facial infantile hemangiomas present as cutaneous bright red or purple bumps, "strawberry marks" or patches, or bluish lumps on the skin surface. Hidden lesions may present with airway obstruction and signs of congestive heart failure.

Most infantile facial hemangiomas do not need imaging for diagnosis. On MRI, the lesions appear as a moderately high-signal lobulated lesion on T2 with intense homogeneous enhancement and intralesional flow voids.

Common Differential Diagnosis

- PHACE syndrome: association of posterior fossa, cardiac, and ophthalmic involvement.
- Cobb syndrome: association of spinal AVM.
- LUMBAR syndrome: involves lower extremities with other tcongenital abnormalities.

Management Options

Infantile hemangiomas are considered "do not touch" lesions. Most lesions regress and/or disappear spontaneously. Occasionally, beta-blockers may be needed to shrink the bigger lesions.

References and Further Reading

1. Chamli A, et al. Hemangioma. Stat Pearls Publishing; 2023. https://www.ncbi.nlm.nih.gov/books/NBK538232/. Accessed 15 Jan 2025.
2. Haouimi A. Facial haemangioma-paediatric. Radiopaedia.org. 2021. https://doi.org/10.53347/rID-96019. Accessed 5 Jan 2023.
3. Inarejos Clemente EJ, et al. Radiologic and clinical features of infantile hemangioma: potential pitfalls and differential diagnosis. Radiographics. 2023. https://doi.org/10.1148/rg.230064. Accessed 12 Apr 2024. PMID: 37883305.

Case 44

44

Clinical History

A 50-year-old man presented with a sudden development of a right-sided indurated soft tissue mass along the carotid axis. Previous history of recurrent migraine.

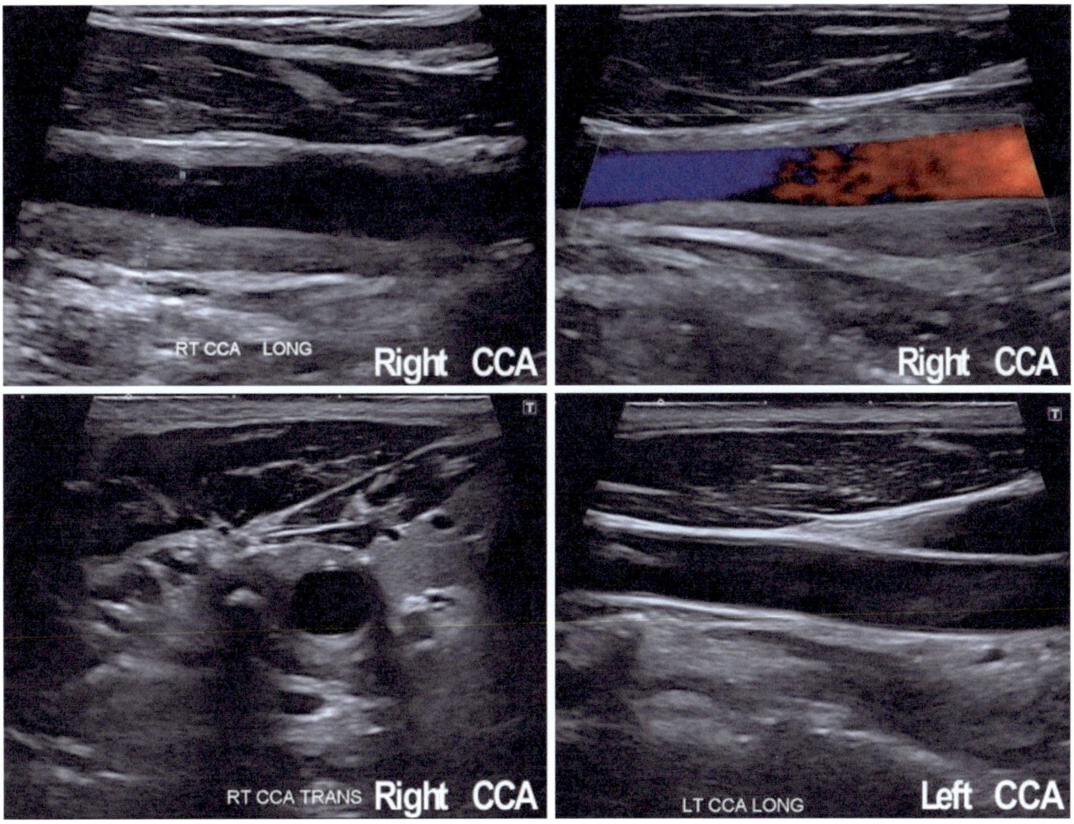

A. Haouimi et al., *Head and Neck Radiology Spot Diagnosis*,
https://doi.org/10.1007/978-3-032-14553-6_44

Findings

Eccentric circumferential thickening of the wall and perivascular soft tissues of the right common carotid artery with no narrowing of the vascular lumen. No significant velocity change on color Doppler. A focal mural calcification on the axial section. Normal left common carotid artery for comparison to the opposite side.

Diagnosis

Carotidynia.

Discussion

Carotidynia, also known as Fay syndrome or transient perivascular inflammation of carotid (TIPIC), is a unilateral self-limiting disorder. The etiology is not clear. Recently, there has been report of an association of COVID-19. Pathologically, this is an inflammation of the vascular and perivascular soft tissues, causing mural and perivascular soft tissue thickening.

Clinically, the patients present with throbbing neck pain along the carotid axis, radiating towards the head. There is an absence of features of active infection, such as chills, lymphadenopathy, erythema, and ear or throat pain. The International Headache Society classified carotidynia as a headache if it is associated with one of the following: (a) Pain, swelling, or increased pulsation on pressure, (b) unilateral neck pain with radiation to the head, (c) exclusion of structural causes, and (d) self-resolution in less than 14 days.

Ultrasound shows mural and perivascular soft tissue thickening without significant luminal narrowing. On MRI, the mural and perivascular soft tissue shows intermediate signal on T1 with marked enhancement.

Common Differential Diagnosis

- Carotid dissection: marked luminal narrowing.
- Extracranial atherosclerosis: narrowing of the proximal ICA.
- Carotid web: fibrous band arising from the posterior carotid bulb, no calcification.

Management Options

The condition is self-limiting and does not require any specific treatment. Symptomatic patients may need analgesics. Some patients may respond well to NSAIDs and corticosteroids.

References and Further Reading

1. Haouimi A. Carotidynia. Radiopaedia.org. 2023. https://doi.org/10.53347/rID-167293. Accessed 15 May 2024.
2. Park JK, et al. CT imaging features of carotidynia: a case report. J Neuroimaging. 2009. https://doi.org/10.1111/j.1552-6569.2007.00232.x. Accessed May 2024. Epub 2008 May 19. PMID: 18494773.

Case 45

45

Clinical History

A 60-year-old woman presented with a left sensory neural hearing loss, otalgia, and vertigo. History of tympanoplasty 1 year prior.

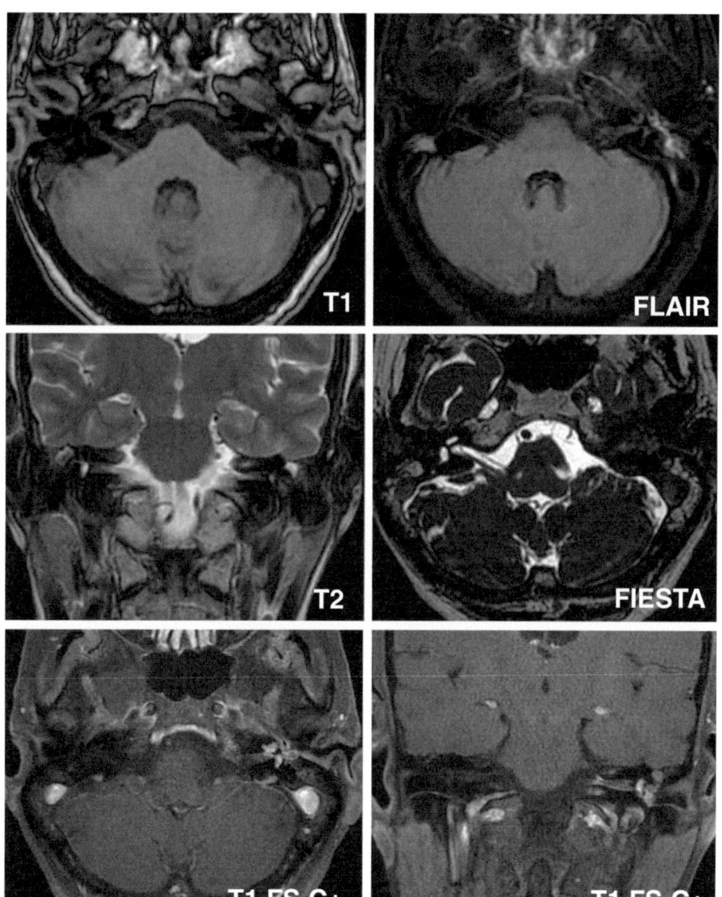

A. Haouimi et al., *Head and Neck Radiology Spot Diagnosis*,
https://doi.org/10.1007/978-3-032-14553-6_45

Findings

Minimal thickening of left acousticofacial bundles and the membranous labyrinth, as well as the superior semicircular canal. The left membranous labyrinth appears isointense on T1, slightly hyperintense on FLAIR, and hypointense on T2 and FIESTA, compared to the contralateral side. Intense enhancement of left vestibulocochlear bundle as well as the membranous labyrinth and semicircular canals. Postsurgical changes of the left middle ear.

Diagnosis

Labyrinthitis with vestibular neuronitis.

Discussion

Labyrinthitis refers to inflammation of the inner ear, the membranous labyrinth in particular. It is a potential complication of acute otomastoiditis following the spread of infection through either the round or oval window. In children, it can be a complication of bacterial meningitis. The inflammation may be triggered by viral infection (Epstein–Barr virus, influenza virus, and herpes simplex virus), autoimmune response, as in Takayasu arteritis, or trauma.

Patients present with sensorineural hearing loss with vertigo, tinnitus, nystagmus, and vomiting.

MRI is the investigation of choice. Initially, there is a preservation of high fluid signal on T2. If there is development of subsequent labyrinthitis ossificans, then the high T2 signal will be replaced with dark signal from fibrosis. The lesions are of isosignal on T1 with intense enhancement of membranous inner ear. Bacterial labyrinthitis may show restricted diffusion due to pus formation.

Common Differential Diagnosis

- Vestibular neuronitis: no labyrinthine involvement.
- Ménière's disease: endolymphatic hydrops.
- Schwannoma: persistent nonregressing lesions following medical treatment.
- Intralabyrinthine hemorrhage: high signal on both T1 and T2.

Management Options

Most cases are managed by medical treatment. Surgical options are reserved for bacterial labyrinthitis. Cochlear implantation is considered for profound deafness.

References and Further Reading

1. Taxak P, Ram C. Labyrinthitis and labyrinthitis ossificans – a case report and review of the literature. J Radiol Case Rep. 2020. https://doi.org/10.3941/jrcr.v14i5.3706. Accessed 21 Apr 2024. PMID: 33082921; PMCID: PMC7536013.
2. Verbist BM. Imaging of sensorineural hearing loss: a pattern-based approach to diseases of the inner ear and cerebellopontine angle. Insights Imaging. 2012. https://doi.org/10.1007/s13244-011-0134-z. Accessed 13 June 2024.

Case 46

46

Clinical History

A 25-year-old woman presented with a right maxillary swelling. The orthopantomogram (OPG) revealed a radiolucent lesion at the right maxillary alveolar process.

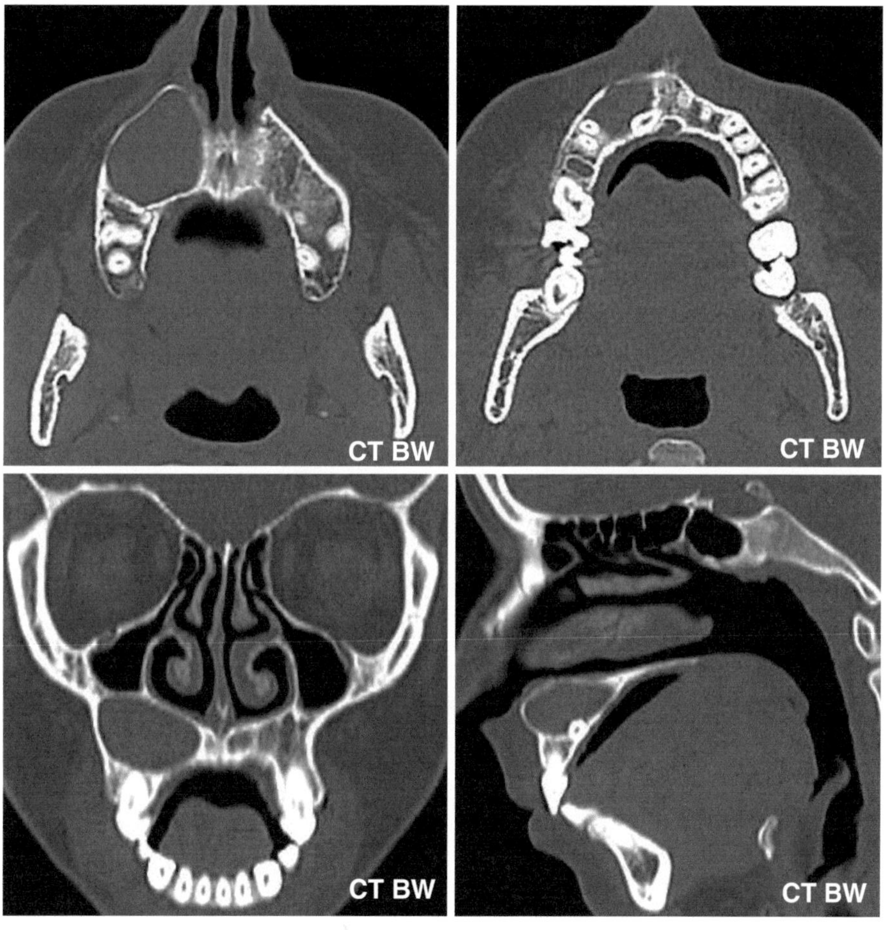

A. Haouimi et al., *Head and Neck Radiology Spot Diagnosis*,
https://doi.org/10.1007/978-3-032-14553-6_46

Findings

An intraosseous homogeneous cystic lesion of the right maxillary alveolar process. No adjacent perilesional soft tissue abnormality. The lesion is unilocular, and there is inclusion of a supernumerary tooth. No bony wall interruption seen on coronal sinus CT sagittal reformation, which shows the unerupted tooth at the floor of the cyst.

Diagnosis

Dentigerous cyst.

Discussion

Dentigerous cyst, also known as follicular cyst, is a benign, slow-growing lesion. They are epithelial-lined developmental anomalies that arise during the process of amelogenesis. The cysts originate from the crown of an unerupted/impacted tooth. It is formed due to hydrostatic pressure exerted by the fluid accumulation between reduced enamel epithelium and the crown of unerupted teeth during amelogenesis.

Dentigerous cysts are the second most common odontogenic cyst after radicular cyst and most remain silent. The patient may present with a concern of delayed tooth eruption. The lesion may become painful when it gets infected.

On plain panoramic view, the cyst appears as a well-defined radiolucent expansile area surrounding the crown of unerupted tooth. Any lucent expansile jaw cyst containing crown of an impacted/unerupted tooth is considered pathognomonic until proven otherwise. CT better explores the lesion. Maxillary lesions can cause bone remodeling.

Common Differential Diagnosis

- Unicystic ameloblastoma: intracystic enhancing nodule on MRI.
- Radicular cyst: dental caries, no impacted or unerupted tooth.
- Aneurysmal bone cyst: multiloculated, fluid–fluid level on MRI.

Management Options

Enucleation of cyst with extraction of unerupted/impacted tooth for symptomatic patients. Marsupialization can be considered for bigger lesions and medically unfit patients.

References and Further Reading

1. Gaillard F, et al. Dentigerouscyst. Radiopaedia.org. 2023. https://doi.org/10.53347/rID-1212. Accessed 6 May 2023.
2. Haouimi A. Dentigerous cyst. Radiopaedia.org. 2023. https://doi.org/10.53347/rID-165081. Accessed 5 May 2023.
3. Wang LL, et al. Odontogenic cysts. Stat Pearls Publishing; 2024. https://www.ncbi.nlm.nih.gov/books/NBK574529/. Accessed 21 June 2025.

Case 47

47

Clinical History

A 70-year-old man presented with a mild decreased visual acuity. Fundoscopy revealed a tiny black lesion at left optic disk.

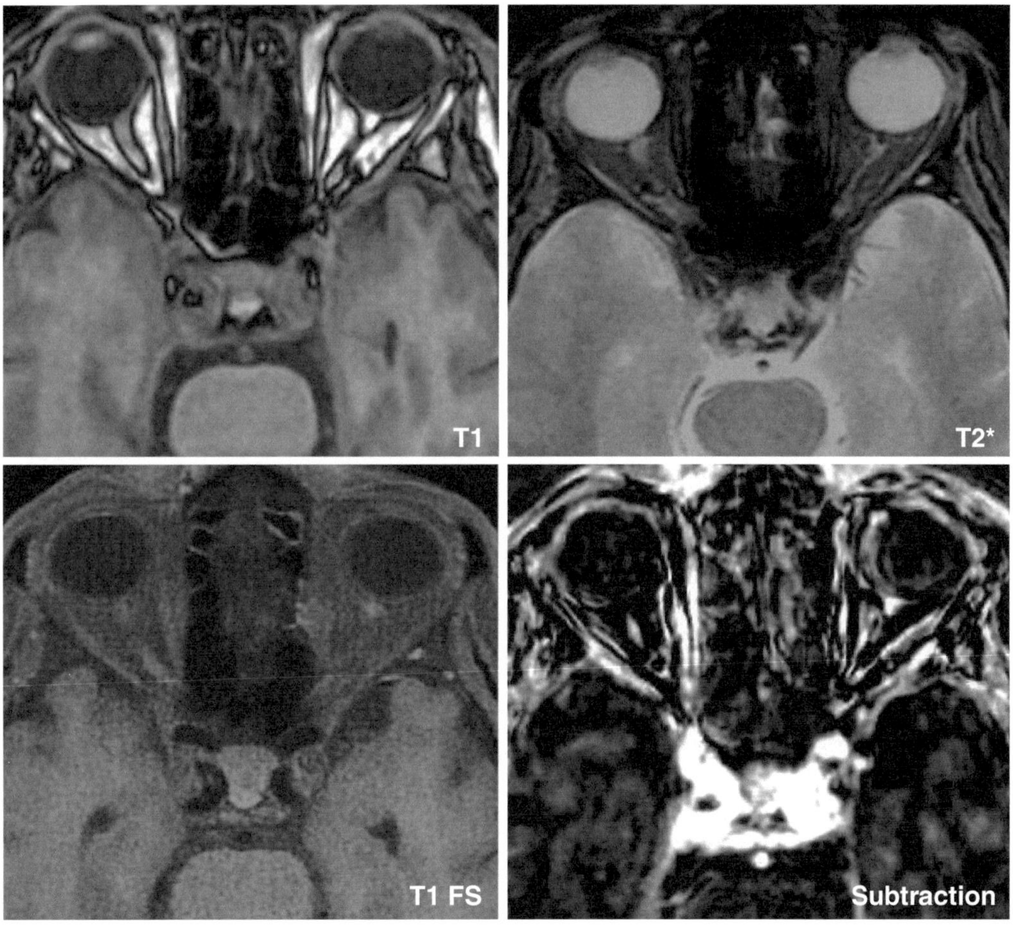

A. Haouimi et al., *Head and Neck Radiology Spot Diagnosis*,
https://doi.org/10.1007/978-3-032-14553-6_47

Findings

A tiny area of the left distal optic nerve and optic disk showing high signal on T1 and T1 fat sat, low signal on T2* with contrast enhancement best seen on subtraction.

Diagnosis

Optic disk melanocytoma.

Discussion

Melanocytoma is a benign hamartomatous lesion arising from optic disk and distal optic nerve with remote malignant potential. Primary optic disk melanoma is extremely rare. The lesions are often unilateral, asymptomatic, and discovered incidentally. However, they can produce secondary symptoms due to central retinal vein obstruction and/or spontaneous tumor necrosis. Melanocytomas are variant of nevus that occur predominantly at optic disk but can also involve the uveal tract. The lesions can also be contiguous with the choroid or sensory retina.

A "dome-shaped" appearance is frequent in melanocytoma on ultrasound. The high internal reflectivity indicates a benign lesion, whereas the low internal reflectivity may be indicative of malignant transformation. However, ultrasound cannot show neovascularization and tumor extension. Other imaging modalities are often needed. On MRI, the lesions are of high signal on T1 and T1 fat sat and low signal on T2* with mild contrast enhancement.

Common Differential Diagnosis

- Retinal pigment epithelium (RPE) hyperplasia: history of trauma, irregular and chorioretinal scarring on fundoscopy.
- Choroidal hemangioma: clinical, dome-shaped isointense lesions on both T1 and T2.
- Retinal hamartoma: juxtapapillary lesion, corkscrew vascular changes on fundoscopy.

Management Options

Annual follow-up fundoscopy and fundal photography. Enucleation is considered in cases with progressive growth and visual symptoms suggesting malignant transformation.

References and Further Reading

1. Haouimi A. Optic nerve melanocytoma. Radiopaedia.org. 2022. https://doi.org/10.53347/rID-158622. Accessed 6 May 2023.
2. Mohmad Z, et al. Melanocytoma of the optic nerve head – a diagnostic dilemma. Clin Pract. 2011. https://doi.org/10.4081/cp.2011.e60. Accessed 16 Feb 2025.
3. Shields JA, et al. Melanocytoma of the optic disk. Indian J Ophthalmol. 2019. https://doi.org/10.4103/ijo.IJO_2039_19. Accessed 21 Mar 2025. PMID: 31755427.

Case 48

48

Clinical History

A 50-year-old man presented with an acute onset of fever and retroauricular swelling. History of repeated right middle ear infection with occasional otorrhea.

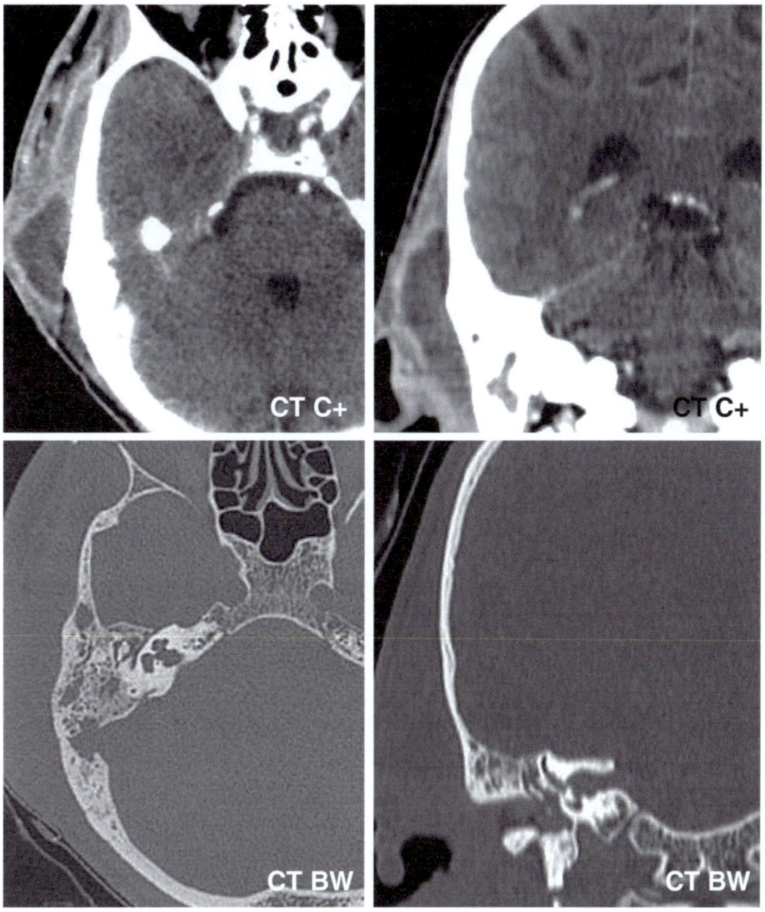

A. Haouimi et al., *Head and Neck Radiology Spot Diagnosis*,
https://doi.org/10.1007/978-3-032-14553-6_48

Findings

Right retroauricular fluid collection with smooth and regular enhancing wall. Complete opacification of the right mastoid air cells, middle ear cavity, and external auditory canal with cortical defect of the mastoid bony wall. Patent right sigmoid sinus (not shown). No adjacent subdural empyema.

Diagnosis

Otomastoiditis with retroauricular subperiosteal abscess.

Discussion

Otomastoiditis is a complication of acute suppurative otitis media. The infection may cause both intra and extracranial complications. Intracranial complications include meningitis, empyema, brain abscesses, and venous sinus thrombosis. Extracranial complications are subperiosteal abscesses and osteomyelitis. The infection causes the mastoid air cells to erode and coalesce into larger, pus-filled cavities. If left untreated, the infection can spread locoregionally. The infection spreads through the tympano-mastoid suture or along the vascular channels in the cribriform area.

Clinically, patients present with fever, ear discharge, pain, and tenderness. Swelling at the MacEwen triangle is highly suggestive of a subperiosteal abscess.

CT is the most common imaging modality used to diagnose otomastoiditis. CT scan demonstrates the opacification of the middle ear, mastoid air cells, as well as the encasement and erosion of the small bones in the middle ear. An MRI can also be used to diagnose otomastoiditis, and itshows the non–CSF-like signal intensity in the mastoid air spaces and the intra- and perimastoid changes.

Common Differential Diagnosis

- Langerhans cell histiocytosis: clinical, often bilateral, +/- additional calvarial lesions.
- Apical petrositis: petrous apex epicenter, walled-off fluid in the petrous apex on MRI.
- Rhabdomyosarcoma: clinical, cranial nerve involvement, and +/- aural polyp.

Management Options

Aggressive intravenous antibiotics. Tympanocentesis and myringotomy tube placement may be needed. Incision and drainage for complicated abscesses.

References and Further Reading

1. Haouimi A. Otomastoiditis with retroauricular abscess. Radiopaedia.org. 2023. https://doi.org/10.53347/rID-164435. Accessed 28 May 2023.
2. Mafee MF, et al. Acute otomastoiditis and its complications. Radiology. 1985. https://doi.org/10.1148/radiology.155.2.3983389. Accessed 18 June 2025.

Case 49

49

Clinical History

A 45-year-old man presented with a gradually increasing painless swelling of left parotid region.

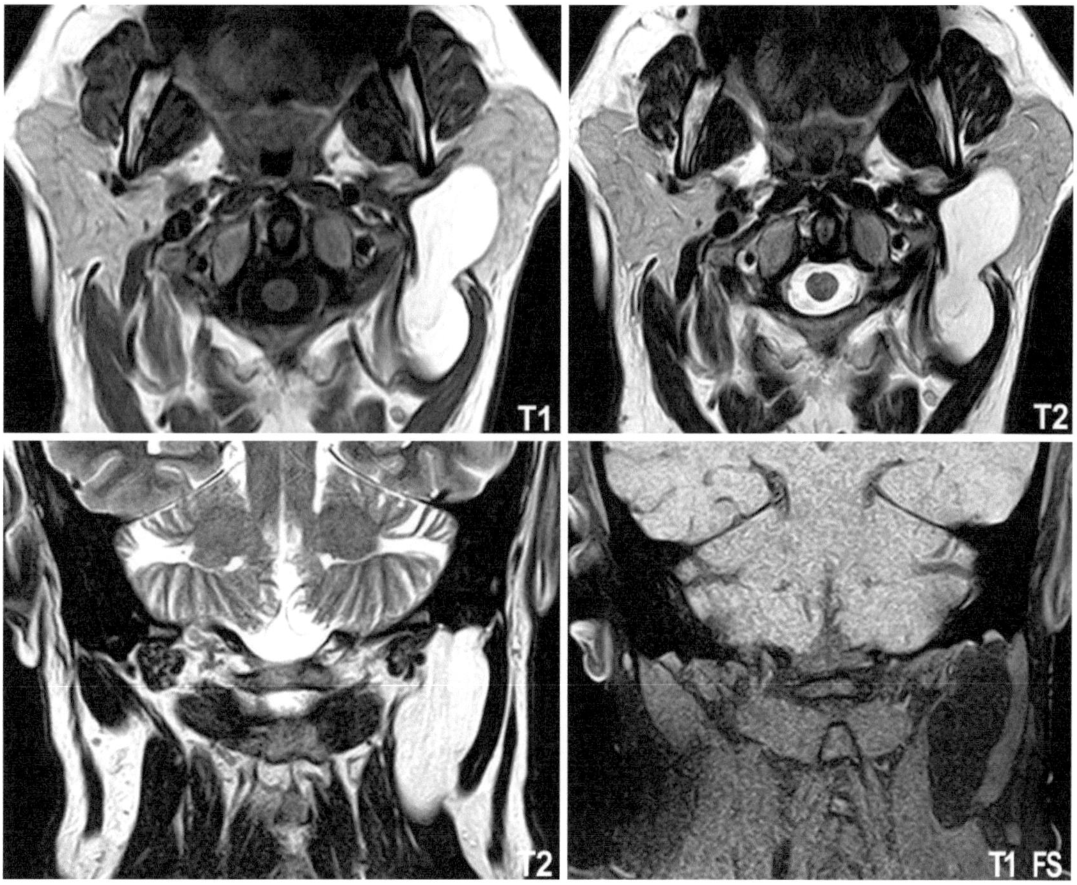

A. Haouimi et al., *Head and Neck Radiology Spot Diagnosis*,
https://doi.org/10.1007/978-3-032-14553-6_49

Findings

Well-encapsulated lobulated soft tissue mass centered on the left posterior cervical space, displacing the adjacent muscles and the parotid gland. It appears high signal on T1 and T2 (isointense to the subcutaneous fat), attenuates on fat-sat sequences with thin internal septations of low signal on T2.

Diagnosis

Soft tissue lipoma of the neck.

Discussion

Lipomas are benign lesions composed of mature adipocytes. Up to 15% of lipomas are seen in the head and neck region. They are commonly found in the posterior cervical and submandibular spaces but can also be trans-spatial. Macroscopically, the lesions are yellow, encapsulated, smooth, or lobulated masses.

Clinically, lipomas appear as asymptomatic, compressible lumps.

On ultrasound, they are well-defined, hyperechoic, homogeneous masses that often reveal echogenic lines parallel to the skin. However, up to 25% of cases may appear as iso or hypoechoic. They show low-density lesions on CT without enhancement. On MRI, lesions are isointense to subcutaneous fat, and the signal can be attenuated by the fat-suppression techniques. On imaging, it is important to differentiate lipomas from atypical well-differentiated liposarcoma (WDL). Thickened intralesional septae and nodules with enhancement and perilesional infiltration are helpful clues to differentiate. Deeply situated lipomas are more likely to be malignant and are considered WDL until proven otherwise.

Common Differential Diagnosis

- Liposarcoma: thick separations: >2 mm, locoregional infiltration, soft tissue nodule.
- Hibernoma: hypointense to subcutaneous fat and hyperintense to muscle on T1, intense enhancement.
- Fat necrosis: irregular with low signal rim, may enhance, calcification +/-.

Management Options

Surgical excision for symptomatic cases with a low chance of recurrence.

References and Further Reading

1. Haouimi A. Soft tissue lipoma-neck. Radiopaedia.org. 2022. https://doi.org/10.53347/rID-151345. Accessed 31 May 2023.
2. Temelkova I, et al. Lipoma of the neck. Open Access Maced J Med Sci. 2018. https://doi.org/10.3889/oamjms.2018.430. Accessed 12 July 2024. PMID: 30455766; PMCID: PMC6236035.

Case 50

50

Clinical History

A 30-year-old asthmatic man presented with a history of chronic sinusitis. Right sinonasal mass found on rhinoscopy.

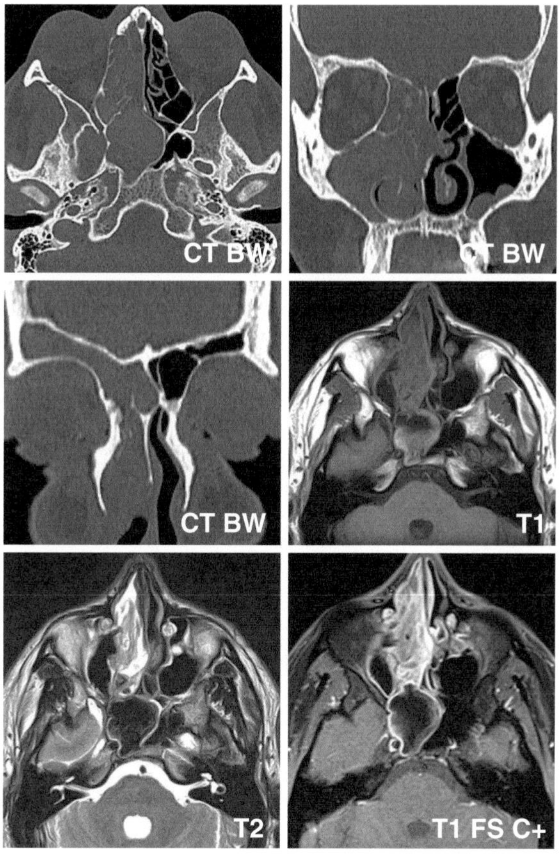

A. Haouimi et al., *Head and Neck Radiology Spot Diagnosis*,
https://doi.org/10.1007/978-3-032-14553-6_50

Findings

Low-density opacification with inspissated material involving the right paranasal sinuses. It extends to the ipsilateral nasal cavity through an enlarged maxillary ostium. Remodeling and thinning of the bony wall of the sinus wall. MRI shows hypointense signal on T1 and markedly hypointense signal on T2, mainly at the sphenoid sinus (due to the high concentration of various metals by the fungal organisms as well as the high protein content). Peripheral inflamed mucosal thickness showing intermediate signal on T1, high signal on T2 with enhancement. The right ethmoid cells and the ipsilateral nasal fossa show areas of low signal on T2.

Diagnosis

Allergic fungal sinusitis.

Discussion

Allergic fungal sinusitis is a severe chronic rhinosinusitis with polyposis. Most cases result from mold and yeast. The disease can arise in nondiabetic and immunocompetent patients. It is commonly found in warm and humid climates and is due to allergic reaction to aerosolized environmental fungi. Patients often have a history of bronchial asthma and hay fever.

The major clinical symptoms are nasal obstruction, headache, and rhinorrhea. Lesions usually involve multiple sinuses, predominantly the maxillary sinus and ethmoid air cells. It can be both uni- and bilateral.

CT shows hyperdense areas within the sinus cavities, outlined by thickened and inflamed hypodense mucosa. Sinus expansion, bony remodeling, and erosive changes of the sinus walls are better seen on CT. MRI signal varies from iso to hypo to signal voids on both T1 and T2, depending on the content. The sinus contents usually do not enhance.

Common Differential Diagnosis

- Sinonasal polyposis: low signal on T1 and high signal on T2.
- Sinus fungal mycetoma: involves only maxillary sinus, calcification +/-.
- Sinonasal mucocele: no bony erosion.

Management Options

Topical steroids are helpful. The results of systemic antifungal drugs are equivocal. Most of the cases are treated by local surgical excision. Relapse is not infrequent.

References and Further Reading

1. Haouimi A. Allergic fungal sinusitis. Radiopaedia.org. 2019. https://doi.org/10.53347/rID-65888. Accessed 1 June 2023.
2. Rowan NR, et al. Radiographic nuances in allergic fungal rhinosinusitis. Am J Rhinol Allergy. 2019. https://doi.org/10.1177/1945892419825695. Accessed 14 July 2024. Epub 2019 Jan 24. PMID: 30674195.

Case 51

51

Clinical History

A 45-year-old woman presented with a left IX, X, and XI cranial neuropathy.

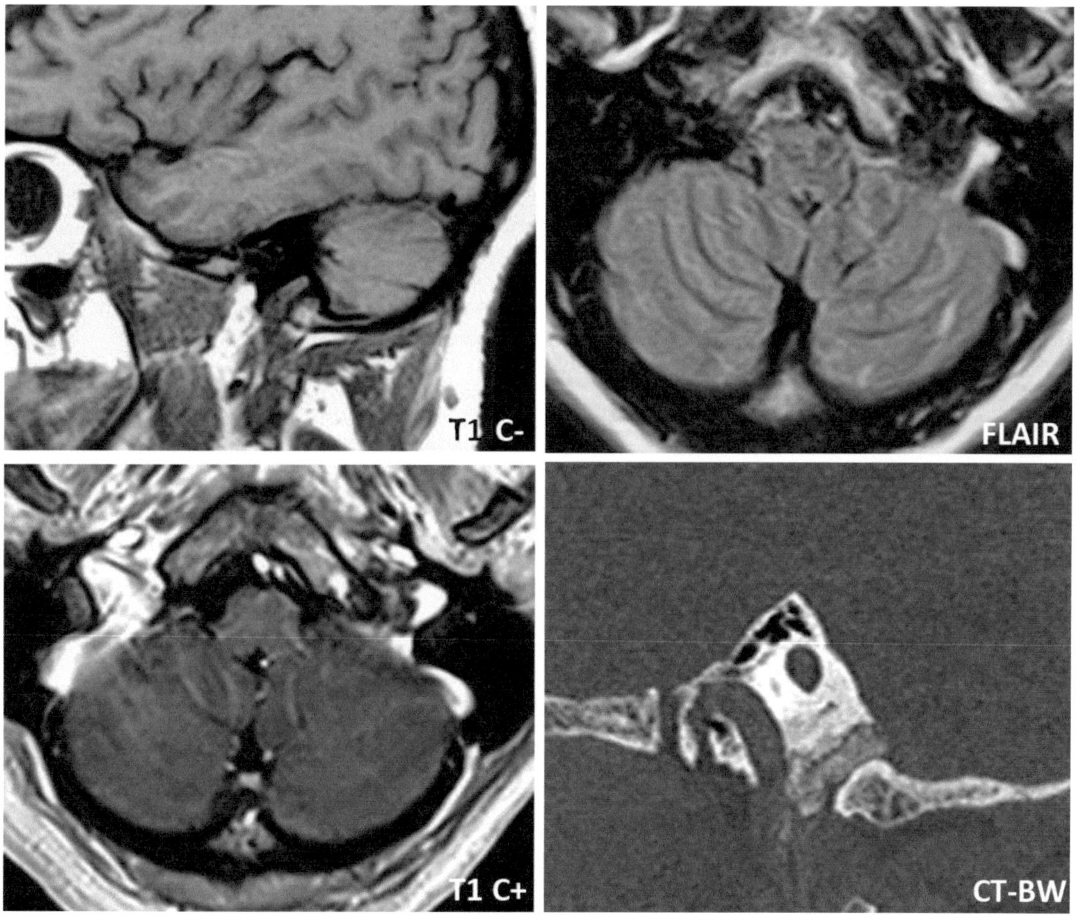

A. Haouimi et al., *Head and Neck Radiology Spot Diagnosis*,
https://doi.org/10.1007/978-3-032-14553-6_51

Findings

A small, ill-defined soft tissue mass centered on the left jugular foramen compressing the jugular bulb. It appears isointense to cortical gray matter on T1 and hypointense on FLAIR with heterogeneous contrast enhancement. Thickening with enhancement of the adjacent dura "dural tail sign." Intracranial extension toward the ipsilateral cerebellopontine angle and an extracranial extension toward the retrostyloid space.

Diagnosis

Left jugular foramen meningioma.

Discussion

Jugular foramen meningiomas are benign, slow-growing extra-axial neoplasms arising from arachnoid cap cells near the jugular foramen. The incidence of jugular foramen meningiomas is rare. It causes symptoms by compressing and invading the lower cranial nerve complex.

Clinically, the patients present with dysphonia, dysphagia, loss of taste, hoarseness of voice, and accessory nerve palsy. Loss of gag reflex, unilateral shoulder weakness, or tongue deviation are occasionally reported. Tinnitus and hearing deficits occur when the vestibulocochlear nerve complex is affected.

The characteristic feature of primary jugular foramen meningiomas is "en plaque" propagation along the dura, but the lesions can also infiltrate surrounding structures in a centrifugal manner. On MRI, the lesions show intermediate signal on T1 and high signal on T2 with intense enhancement. CT can show bony hyperostosis or sclerosis of the jugular foramen. Calcification and "dural tail signs" are important imaging clues.

Common Differential Diagnosis

- Schwannoma: calcification unlikely.
- Glomic tumor: hypervascularized lesion with typical "salt and pepper" appearance.
- Metastatic lesion: known cancer, associated bony erosion.

Management Options

Treatment is mostly surgical. Adjuvant radiosurgery may be needed for incomplete excision.

References and Further Reading

1. Das JM, Al Khalili Y. 2023. Stat Pearls Publishing. https://www.ncbi.nlm.nih.gov/books/NBK549871/. Accessed 30 May 2024.
2. Haouimi A. Radiopaedia.org. 2023. https://doi.org/10.53347/rID-82729. Accessed 19 Mar 2024.
3. Rajesh U, et al. Med J Armed Forces India. 2016. https://doi.org/10.1016/j.mjafi.2016.07.011. Accessed 19 Mar 2022.

Case 52

52

Clinical History

A 3-year-old girl. Incidental finding on ultrasound examination of the neck.

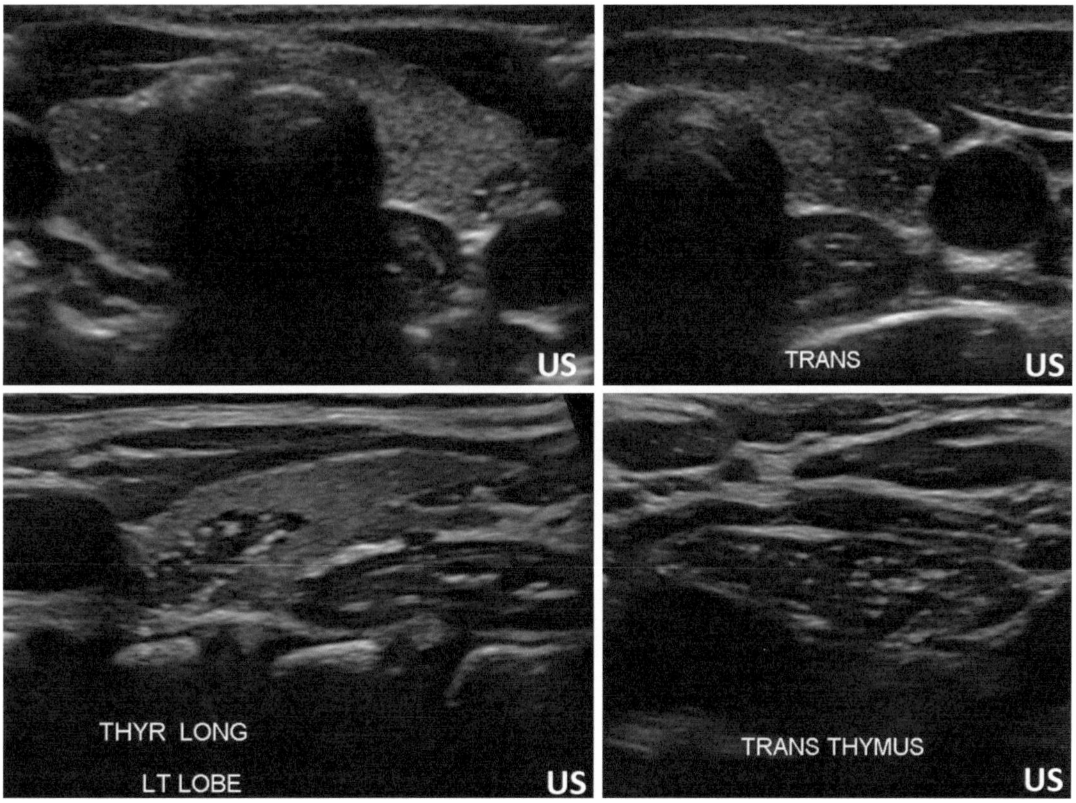

A. Haouimi et al., *Head and Neck Radiology Spot Diagnosis*,
https://doi.org/10.1007/978-3-032-14553-6_52

Findings

A well-defined ovoid hypoechoic area at the lower aspect of the left thyroid lobe containing numerous internal nonshadowing hyperechoic foci. Normal size of the thyroid gland.

Diagnosis

Ectopic thymus within the thyroid gland.

Discussion

The thymus is a primary lymphoid organ. It is physiologically responsible for the maturation and differentiation of T lymphocytes. The organ increases in size and remains active in infants and neonates up to 2–3 years, then gradually begins to involute until it becomes atrophied and is replaced by fatty tissue.

The adult thymus is anatomically situated in the anterior mediastinum. It originates high at the level of pyriform sinus and descends progressively into anterior mediastinum along thymopharyngeal canal. Thymic ectopia can arise due to aberrant thymic caudal migration during embryogenesis. The most common ectopic location is the thyroid gland. Tonsils, submandibular gland, and the skull base are rare locations.

Most cases are asymptomatic and discovered incidentally. On ultrasound, the normal thymus appears as a well-defined ovoid hypoechoic mass containing numerous internal nonshadowing hyperechoic foci. Thyroid nodules are very rare in pediatric population. Appearance of any intrathyroid pseudo-lesion in an asymptomatic patient is highly suggestive of ectopic thymus.

Common Differential Diagnosis

- Benign nodules: cystic or spongiform and size smaller than 2 cm.
- Malignant nodules: microcalcifications, hypoechogenicity, intranodular vascularity.
- Intrathyroid parathyroid: symptoms of primary hyperparathyroidism, separating echogenic line from thyroid, hypervascular, extrathyroid arterial feeder.

Management Options

In asymptomatic cases, a normal ectopic thymus could be confused for a malignant thyroid nodule containing microcalcifications. The familiarity of normal typical echotexture of the thymus often time helps to avoid unnecessary FNAB and surgery in asymptomatic cases.

References and Further Reading

1. Frates MC, et al. Ectopic al thymic tissue mimicking thyroid nodules in children. J Ultrasound Med. 2018. https://doi.org/10.1002/jum.14360. Accessed 20 July 2025. Epub 2017 Aug 29. PMID: 28850707.
2. Haouimi A. Ectopic thymus within the thyroid gland. Radiopaedia.org. 2023. https://doi.org/10.53347/rID-176137. Accessed 31 Oct 2023.

Case 53

53

Clinical History

A 35-year-old man presented with a painless swelling of the left submandibular region.

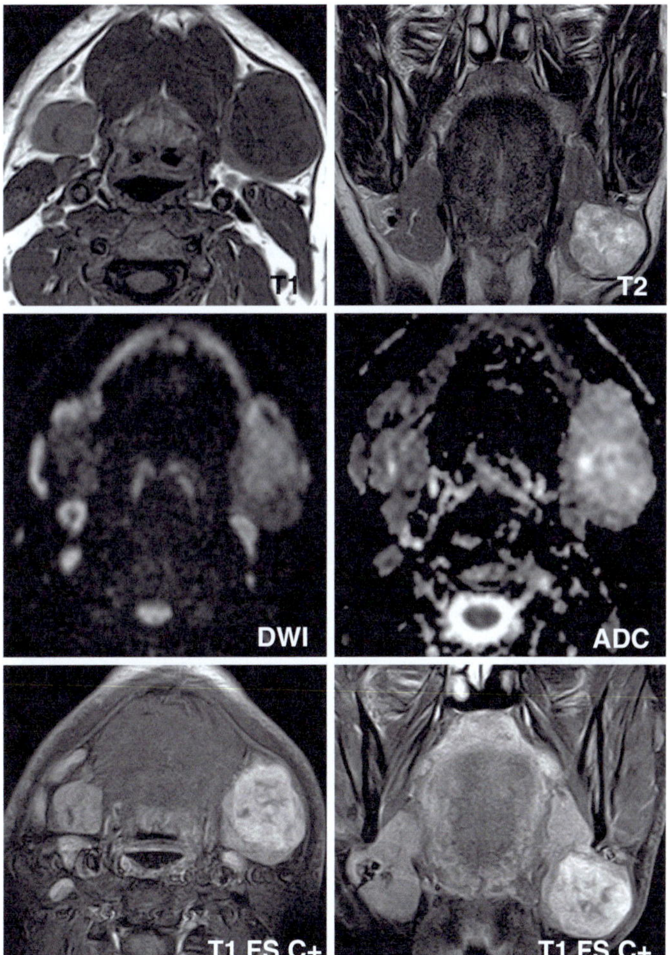

A. Haouimi et al., *Head and Neck Radiology Spot Diagnosis*,
https://doi.org/10.1007/978-3-032-14553-6_53

Findings

A well-encapsulated ovoid lesion at left submandibular gland. It shows a low signal on T1, and an inhomogeneous high signal on T2. The peripheral hypointense rim suggests the presence of a fibrous capsule. Vivid heterogeneous enhancement on postcontrast images. No restricted diffusion. No lymphadenopathy.

Diagnosis

Pleomorphic adenoma of the submandibular gland.

Discussion

Pleomorphic adenoma of the submandibular gland is also known as a benign mixed tumor. They represent less than 10% of all salivary gland tumors. The pathogenesis is poorly explained. It is possibly related to oncogenic simian viral infection or exposure to radiation.

Macroscopically, the lesions are heterogeneous, lobulated, and composed of solid, cystic, and calcified components contained in a fibrous capsule. These benign tumors are made up of epithelial, myoepithelial, and stromal cell components with up to 15% malignant potential if left untreated. Clinically, the patients present with indolent painless nodular swelling in submandibular region. Both CT and MRI are the gold standards to determine the spatial location, their relation, and impact on adjacent structures. Lobulation, homogeneity, and delayed enhancement can be seen in smaller lesions, but larger lesions may develop necrosis, hemorrhage, and calcification, and appear nonhomogeneous. The findings are however not specific. On MRI, smaller lesions show low signal on T1 and a heterogeneously high signal on T2 with heterogeneous enhancement following IV contrast. A rim of decreased signal intensity on T2 represents the fibrous capsule.

Common Differential Diagnosis

- Submandibular gland carcinoma: invasive margins, enlarged lymph nodes.
- Acute submandibular sialadenitis: ductal stone +/-.
- Submandibular mucocele: cystic component, no calcification.

Management Options

Surgical excision accompanied by removal of the submandibular gland in toto is advised to avoid recurrence. For surgically nonresectable cases, radiation therapy is recommended.

References and Further Reading

1. Alves FA, et al. Pleomorphic adenoma of the submandibular gland: clinicopathological and immunohistochemical features of 60 cases in Brazil. Arch Otolaryngol Head Neck Surg. 2002. https://doi.org/10.1001/archotol.128.12.1400. Accessed 13 Nov 2024.
2. Haouimi A. Pleomorphic adenoma-submandibular gland. Radiopaedia.org. 2023. https://doi.org/10.53347/rID-159540. Accessed 31 Oct 2023.

Case 54

54

Clinical History

A 50-year-old obese diabetic woman with hypertriglyceridemia presented with a painless swelling of the parotid glands.

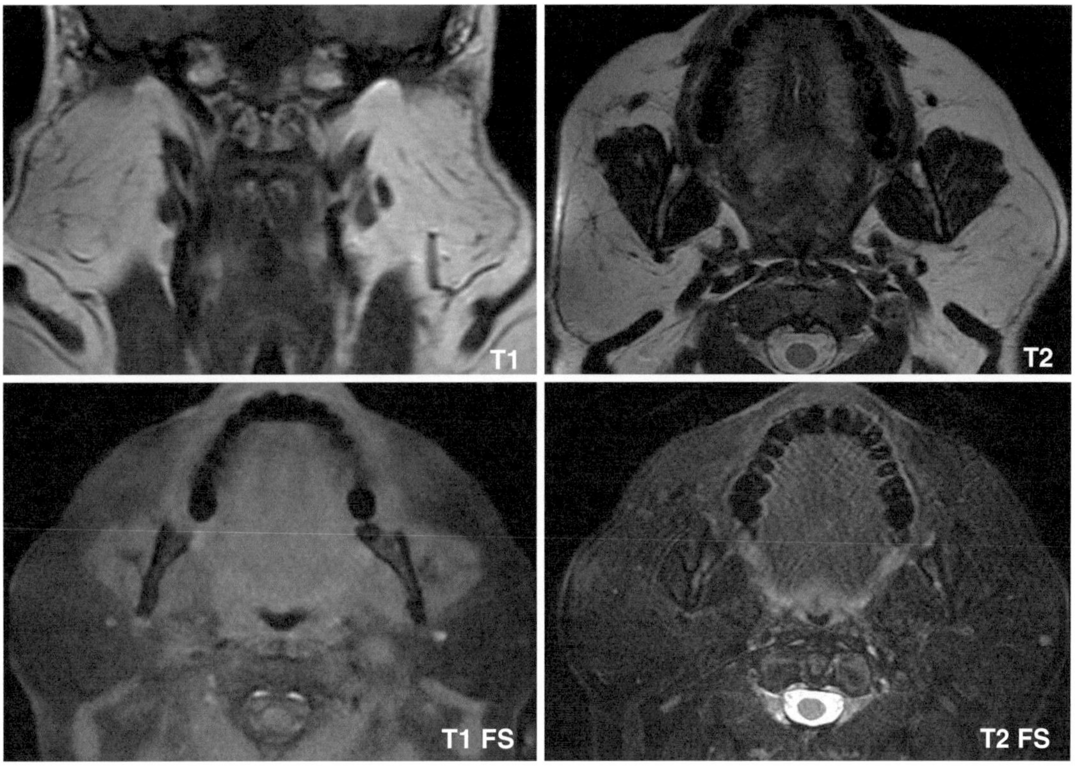

A. Haouimi et al., *Head and Neck Radiology Spot Diagnosis*,
https://doi.org/10.1007/978-3-032-14553-6_54

Findings

Diffusely enlarged parotid glands quasi-completely replaced by fatty tissue, showing high signal on T1 and T2. Signal is attenuated on fat-saturation sequences. No intraglandular focal lesion or cervical lymphadenopathy.

Diagnosis

Parotid liposubstitution.

Discussion

Parotid liposubstitution or fatty degeneration of parotid parenchyma is not an uncommon radiologic finding. Natural physiological degenerative change with normal aging can lead to this condition. The condition can also be secondary to hypertriglyceridemia, Sjögren's syndrome, HIV infection, alcoholism, smoking, and diabetes mellitus may predispose to this condition.

Clinically, most patients are asymptomatic but can present with bilateral enlargement of parotid glands and xerostomia.

On CT, both parotid glands are enlarged in size. Isodense parotid parenchyma is replaced by low-density homogeneous fatty tissue without enhancement. On MRI, the fatty tissue appears as homogeneously high signal on both T1 and T2. The signals are completely suppressed by fat-suppression technique. No contrast enhancement.

Common Differential Diagnosis

- Pleomorphic adenoma: bosselated contour, homo- or heterogeneous enhancement.
- Sjögren's syndrome: leopard skin and honeycomb appearance on ultrasound and MR, respectively.
- Warthin tumor: intraglandular heterogeneous solid-cystic lesion.
- Parotid lipoma: well-circumscribed focal lesion.

Management Options

Parotid fat substitution belongs to "do not touch" lesions.

References and Further Reading

1. Garcia DS, et al. Fat deposition of parotid glands. Braz J Otorhinolaryngol. 2013. https://doi.org/10.5935/1808-8694.20130031. Accessed 30 Apr 2024.
2. Haouimi A. Parotid liposubstitution. Radiopaedia.org. 2023. https://doi.org/10.53347/rID-179004. Accessed 5 Dec 2023.
3. Nicoletti D, et al. Parotid liposubstitution. Radiopaedia.org. 2025. https://doi.org/10.53347/rID-161178. Accessed 27 Oct 2025.

Case 55

55

Clinical History

A 45-year-old woman presented with a right nasal obstruction of 1-year duration.

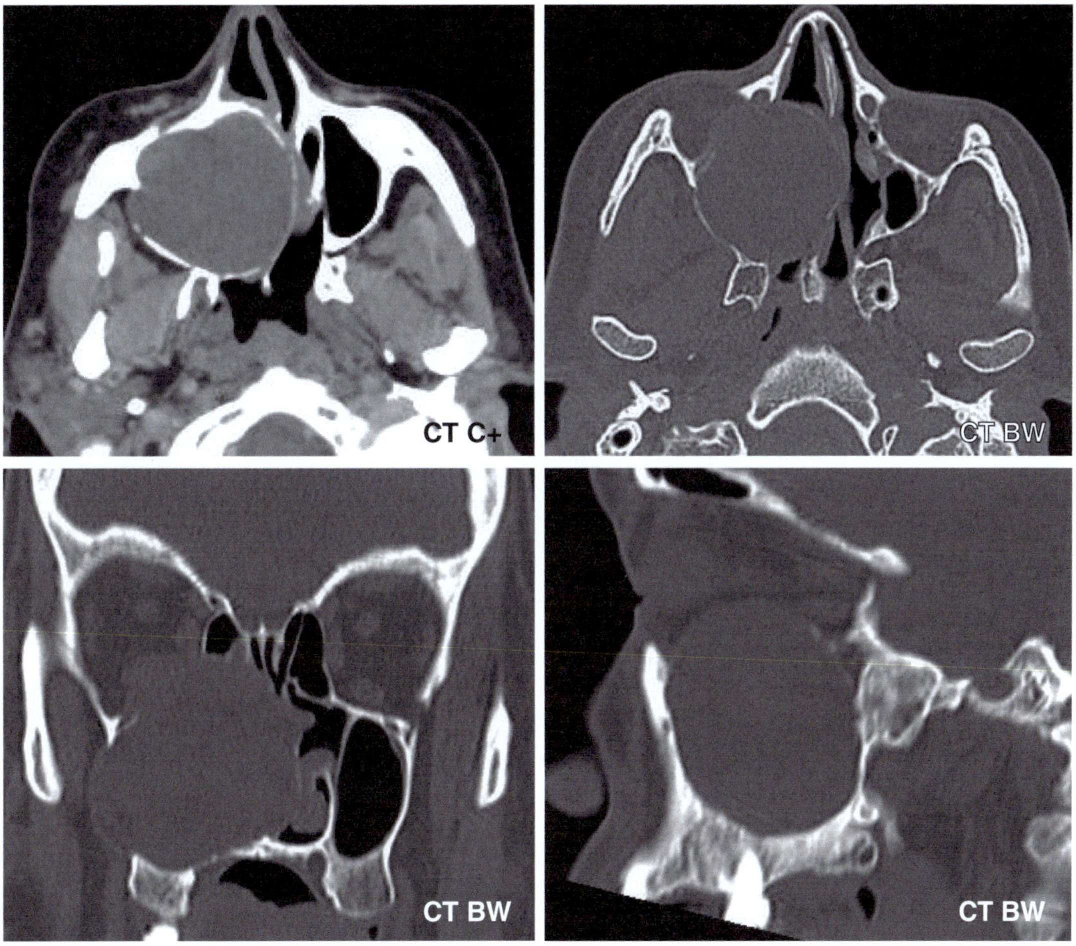

A. Haouimi et al., *Head and Neck Radiology Spot Diagnosis*,
https://doi.org/10.1007/978-3-032-14553-6_55

Findings

An expansile low-density intramaxillary homogeneous lesion in the right maxillary sinus. Obstruction of the ipsilateral nasal fossa with no contrast enhancement. Bony erosion and destruction of anterolateral sinus walls, as well as right orbital floor with intraorbital extension.

Diagnosis

Maxillary mucocele.

Discussion

Maxillary mucoceles are a rare benign slow growing expansile lesion that arises due to ostial blockage. The blockage can occur from multiple sources such as inflammation, malignancy, trauma, postsurgical fibrosis, and bony lesions including osteoma and fibrous dysplasia. Ostial obstruction leads to the accumulation of mucus and the size increases due to intralesional positive pressure. The lesions have the tendency for intraorbital or intracranial extension.

Clinical symptoms are very nonspecific. Most symptoms are due to pressure on surrounding structures. Dental and orbital symptoms including proptosis, diplopia, ophthalmoplegia are late complications.

Plain X-ray can show ballooning of the maxillary sinus with intrasinusal soft tissue density. On CT, mucoceles appear as homogeneous nonenhancing soft tissue density with crescent shaped contour. Bony erosion and remodeling are better seen on CT. Locoregional extension of mucocele can be evaluated both by CT and MRI. Mucoceles show low signal on T1 and high signal on T2. However, MRI signals depend on the nature of the cystic contents. Rich proteinaceous contents may show high signal on T1 and low signal on T2. The lesions can show thin peripheral enhancement.

Common Differential Diagnosis

- Inverted papilloma: usually enhances.
- Antrochoanal polyp: extends posteriorly toward nasopharynx.
- Acute sinusitis: fever, no bony change, fluid level.

Management Options

Though slow growing and benign, the lesions are locally aggressive. Treatment options include marsupialization and Caldwell-Luc procedure, to avoid orbital and dental complications.

References and Further Reading

1. Haouimi A. Maxillary sinus mucocele. Radiopaedia.org. 2023 https://doi.org/10.53347/rID-178959. Accessed 20 June 2024.
2. Ramanadhan S. Maxillary mucocele: a missed out. Caspian J Intern Med. 2023; https://caspjim.com/article-1-3437-en.pdf. Accessed 20 June 2024.

Case 56

56

Clinical History

A 40-year-old man presented with a painless right mandibular hard lump.

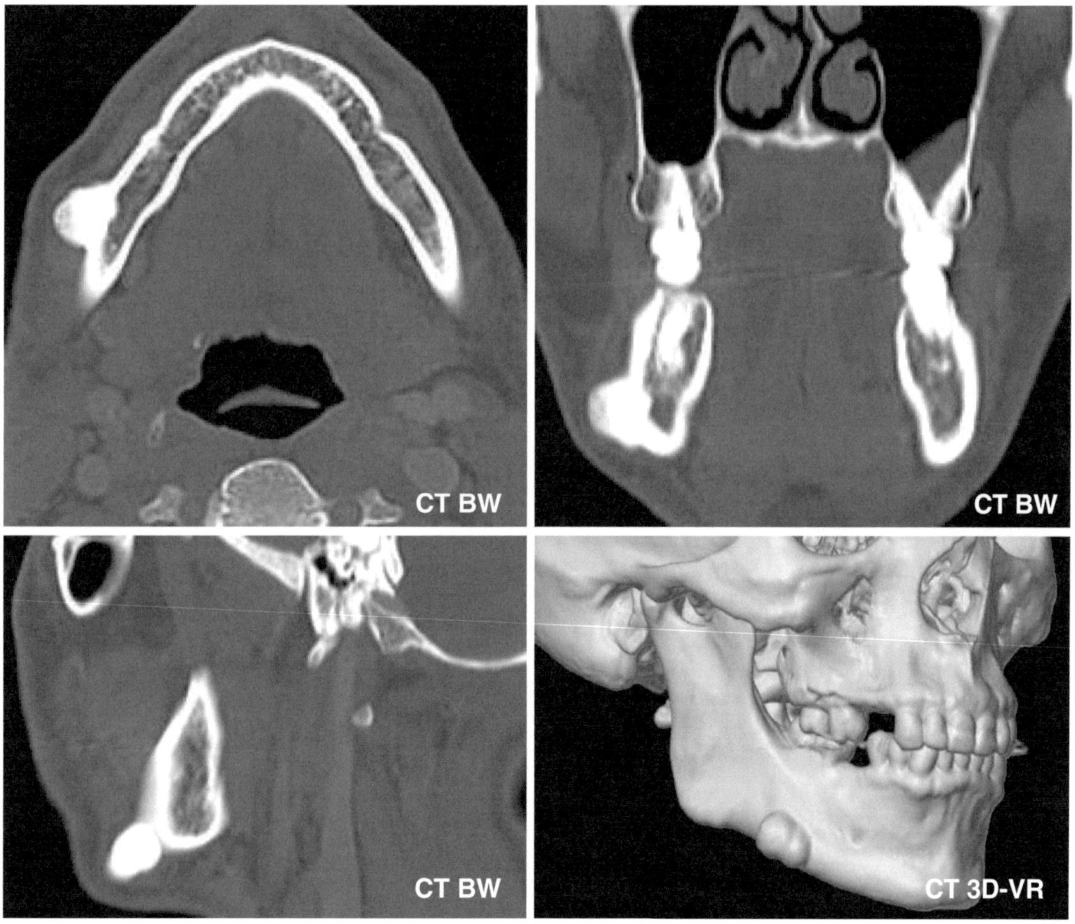

A. Haouimi et al., *Head and Neck Radiology Spot Diagnosis*,
https://doi.org/10.1007/978-3-032-14553-6_56

Findings

A well-defined, broad-based, dense exophytic lesion arising from the buccal aspect of the mandible. No cortical rupture or adjacent soft tissue component.

Diagnosis

Mandibular osteoma.

Discussion

Osteomas are benign indolent osteogenic neoplasms and involvement of mandible is rare. Lesions arise from the proliferation of compact bone and the etiology is poorly understood. However, an association of minor trauma has been hypothesized, which supports a reactive etiology. Subperiosteal hematoma and edema following trauma, as well as muscle traction causing periosteal pulling, which initiates an osteogenic reaction. Most mandibular osteomas are peripheral and involve the lingual aspect of mandible near the mandibular angle. Lesions are often solitary. Multiple osteomas may be a component of Gardner syndrome.

Clinically, small osteomas are asymptomatic but occasionally can cause facial asymmetry. Osteomas involving the mandibular condyle may gradually cause midline deviation. Larger lesions can cause difficulty in mastication.

Osteoma presents as a well-circumscribed dense polypoid or broad-based ivory-like sessile mass. 3D CT scan is the modality of choice in defining the lesion, its relation, and attachment to adjacent bone when surgery is considered.

Common Differential Diagnosis

- Exostosis: clinical features, prepubescent onset, ceasing at adulthood.
- Gardner syndrome: multiple osteomas, numerous colonic polyps, and cutaneous lesions.
- Fibrous dysplasia: ground glass appearance.

Management Options

Osteomas are "do not touch" lesions. Large symptomatic lesions are considered for surgery.

References and Further Reading

1. Haouimi A. Mandibular osteoma. Radiopaedia.org. 2023. https://doi.org/10.53347/rID-173972. Accessed 5 Dec 2023.
2. Ragupathy K, et al. Peripheral osteoma of the body of mandible: a case report. J Maxillofac Oral Surg. 2015; https://doi.org/10.1007/s12663-014-0710-0. Accessed 21 June 2024. Epub 2014 Oct 14.
3. Wolf-Grotto I, et al. Management of giant osteoma of mandible with minor trauma: a case report. J Med Case Rep. 2022; https://doi.org/10.1186/s13256-021-03217-2. Accessed 21 June 2024.

Case 57

57

Clinical History

A 30-year-old pregnant woman at 25 weeks' gestation presented with recurrent epistaxis. ENT examination revealed a small vascular nodule in the left nasal cavity.

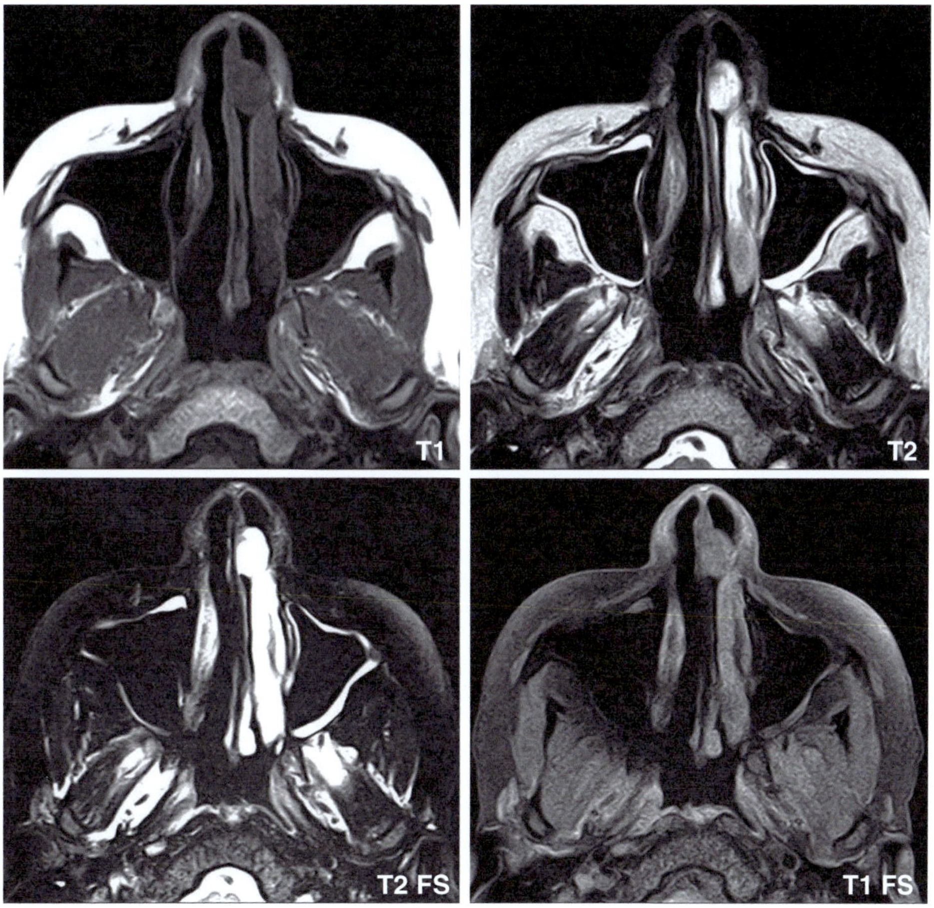

A. Haouimi et al., *Head and Neck Radiology Spot Diagnosis*,
https://doi.org/10.1007/978-3-032-14553-6_57

Findings

A small, well-defined soft tissue nodule at the anterior aspect of the left nasal cavity, having a broad-based attachment to the nasal septum. It shows an intermediate signal on T1 and a very high signal on T2 and T2 fat sat. Normal appearance of the remainder of the nasal cavity. The postcontrast sequences were not performed (pregnant patient), but usually show marked enhancement.

Diagnosis

Nasal pyogenic granuloma gravidarum.

Discussion

Pyogenic granulomas are also known as a "bleeding polyp." They are benign proliferative fibrovascular lesions involving the skin and mucosa of craniofacial region. When the lesion occurs in pregnant woman, it is called pyogenic granuloma gravidarum or "pregnancy tumor." Most pyogenic granuloma gravidarum arise at the anterior nasal septum. The lesions are neither pus-forming nor granulomatous and hence the name is a misnomer. Lobular capillary hemangioma should be the most appropriate terminology.

The pathogenesis remains unclear but has been linked to multiple factors, including minor local trauma, medications such as oral retinoids, altered hormonal activities, and immunosuppression.

Clinically, the lesions present with nasal discharge, repeated epistaxis from a rapidly developing smooth or lobulated vascular nodule from Little's area, making it difficult to differentiate them from malignancy. The diagnosis is clinical. CT scan shows a well-defined unilateral soft tissue density with vivid enhancement without any calcification. On MRI, the lesions are of low signal on T1 and heterogeneously high signal on T2 with a thin peripheral iso- or hypointense rim and intense enhancement following contrast.

Common Differential Diagnosis

- Juvenile angiofibroma: centered at sphenopalatine foramen, male adolescents.
- Antro-choanal polyp: dumbbell-shaped, arising from sinus, intact pterygopalatine fossa.
- Inverted papilloma: centered on middle turbinate, bone remodeling, obstructive sinusitis.

Management Options

Treatment options include surgical excision, embolization, cryotherapy, and silver nitrate cauterization.

References and Further Reading

1. Basiari L, et al. Pyogenic granuloma gravidarum of the nasal cavity causing recurrent epistaxis. Maedica (Bucur). 2024; https://doi.org/10.26574/maedica.2024.19.1.160. Accessed July 2025. PMID: 38736920.
2. Haouimi A. Nasal pyogenic granuloma. Radiopaedia.org. 2022. https://doi.org/10.53347/rID-97988. Accessed 5 Dec 2023.

Case 58

58

Clinical History

A 50-year-old woman presented with a history of dysphonia.

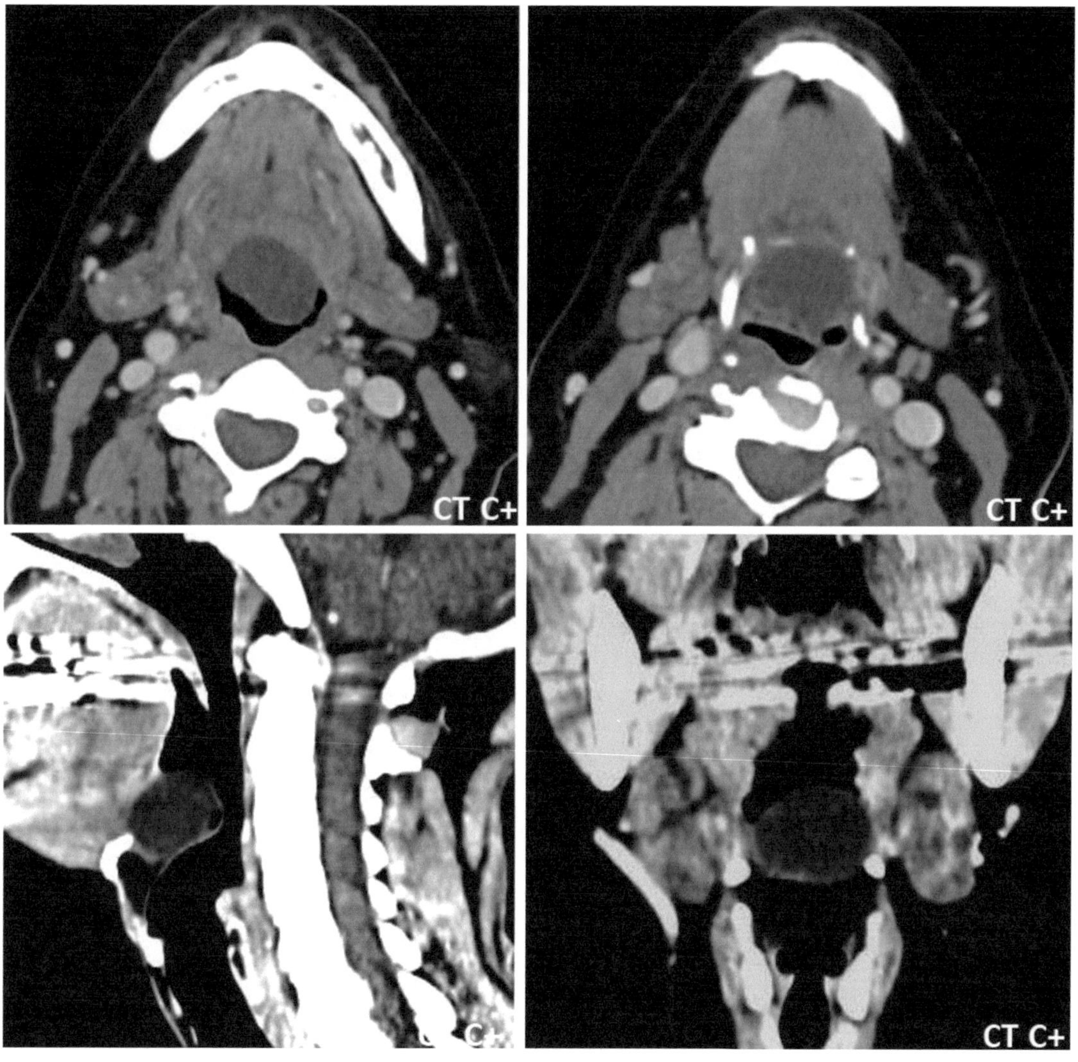

A. Haouimi et al., *Head and Neck Radiology Spot Diagnosis*,
https://doi.org/10.1007/978-3-032-14553-6_58

Findings

A sharply defined, thin-walled, broad-based homogeneous epiglottic cystic lesion arising from its lingual surface. No enhancement, no calcification, and no enlarged cervical lymph node.

Diagnosis

Epiglottic cyst.

Discussion

Epiglottic cysts are rare benign mucus retention cysts which can arise on either the lingual or laryngeal aspect of the epiglottis. They harvest a higher risk of acute airway obstruction with a six-fold increase in the need for acute airway management, particularly when they are infected. The lesions may be complicated, giving rise to an inflammatory epiglottitis or epiglottic abscess which can cause airway obstruction and respiratory arrest.

The cysts are mostly asymptomatic and are discovered incidentally by anesthesiologists, endoscopists, or ENT specialists. The patients may present with nonspecific symptoms. Some patients may complain of laryngeal stridor and dyspnea. Occasionally, significant respiratory obstruction can even lead to death if not properly addressed.

Though epiglottic cysts are mostly discovered by clinical examination without any need for CT or MRI, the radiologist must be vigilant for their presence and be aware of the differential diagnosis. The role of the radiologist is to identify the lesions and to rule out possible airway obstruction.

Common Differential Diagnosis

- Benign squamous papilloma: mostly pedunculated.
- Squamous cell carcinoma: soft tissue density with signs of locoregional invasion.
- Acute epiglottis: clinical history, "thumb sign" on plain lateral view.

Management Options

Once discovered, elective intervention such as endoscopic resection, marsupialization with laser ablation has all been proposed. Recurrence is dependent on remnants of the cyst wall.

References and Further Reading

1. DiMuzio B. Epiglottic cysts. Radiopaedia.org. 2025; https://doi.org/10.53347/rID-24588. Accessed 21 July 2025.
2. Haouimi A. Epiglottic cyst. Radiopaedia.org. 2022; https://doi.org/10.53347/rID-157794. Accessed 10 Dec 2023.
3. Jeng P-H, Huang T-R, Shih C-P. Giant epiglottic cyst: a comprehensive case report and literature review. Ear Nose Throat J. 2024; https://doi.org/10.1177/01455613241259291. Accessed 15 July 2025.

Case 59

59

Clinical History

A 30-year-old woman with a history of chronic headache.

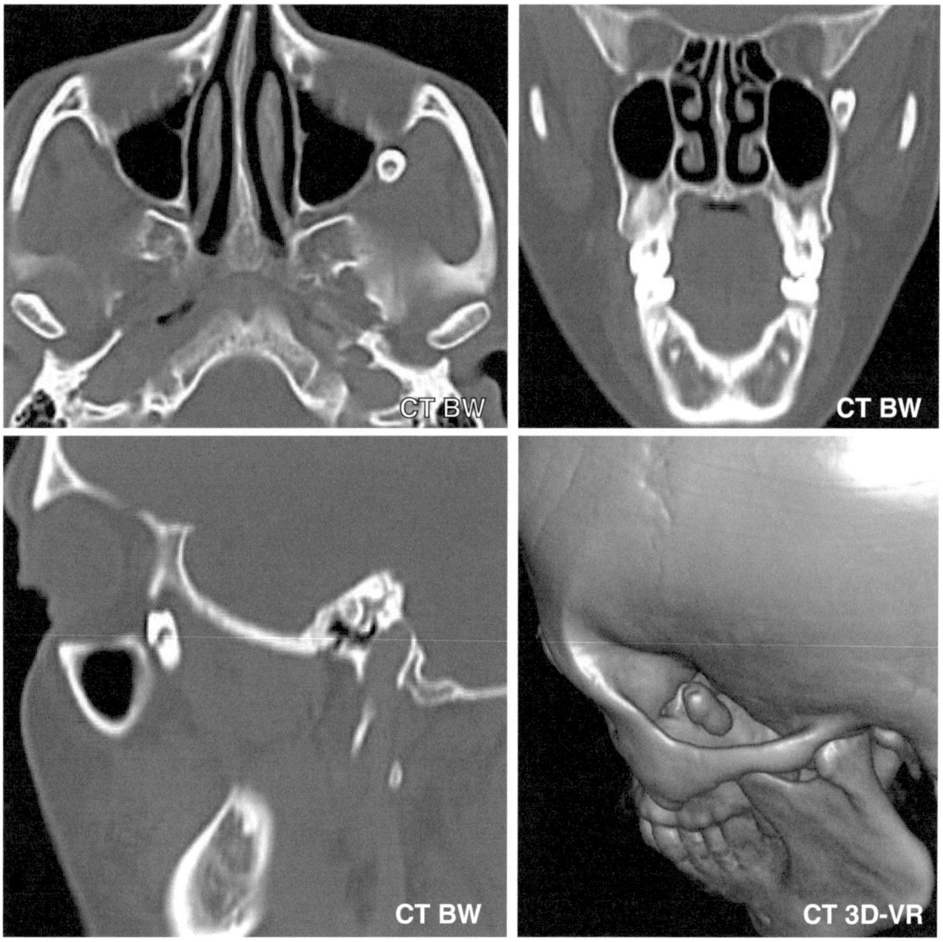

A. Haouimi et al., *Head and Neck Radiology Spot Diagnosis*,
https://doi.org/10.1007/978-3-032-14553-6_59

Findings

A dentiform structure located in the left infratemporal fossa. It is lying posterolateral to the maxillary sinus with no adjacent abscess formation or soft tissue component. The adjacent wall of the maxilla is intact with normal pneumatization of the paranasal sinuses.

Diagnosis

Ectopic tooth in the infratemporal space.

Discussion

The terms ectopic and heterotopic teeth are used interchangeably and often confused. The presence of any tooth outside the dental arcade is considered ectopic. The term heterotopia is reserved for the abnormal tooth position distal to the dental arch. The exact etiology is not clear. Abnormal tissue interaction during odontogenesis may result in ectopic tooth development. Conditions such as cleft palate, trauma, tumors, or cysts may predispose to this condition. Ectopic teeth within the dentate region are common, but the ectopic eruption into the non-dentate region is rare. Ectopia of molar teeth is uncommon.

Ectopic teeth can be completely asymptomatic and discovered incidentally. A tooth in the infratemporal space can lead to symptoms of restricted mouth opening, pain, and swelling.

Panoramic X-rays are of practically no use when ectopic tooth found in temporal space. CT is the modality of choice. 3D CT allows for the precise location of the tooth, which is very important to choose the best surgical approach.

Common Differential Diagnosis

- Tooth-like calcification: prior history of trauma, infection.
- Foreign body: clinical history.

Management Options

Incidentally discovered asymptomatic cases belong to "do not touch" lesions. The treatment is surgical extraction for symptomatic cases.

References and Further Reading

1. Daimi SRH. Bilateral ectopic eruption of a maxillary third molar tooth from the infratemporal surface of the maxilla in a dry human skull. Int J Appl Basic Med Res. 2022; https://pmc.ncbi.nlm.nih.gov/articles/PMC7289208/. Accessed 20 July 2025.
2. Haouimi A. Ectopic tooth-infratemporal fossa. Radiopaedia.org. 2022. https://doi.org/10.53347/rID-157906. Accessed 10 Dec 2023.
3. Mishri SR, et al. Ectopic third molar tooth on the infratemporal surface of maxilla. Italian J Anat Embryol. 2016; https://pubmed.ncbi.nlm.nih.gov/28872802/. Accessed 20 July 2025

Case 60

60

Clinical History

A 65-year-old man presented with a progressively increasing painless nuchal mass over a span of 25 years.

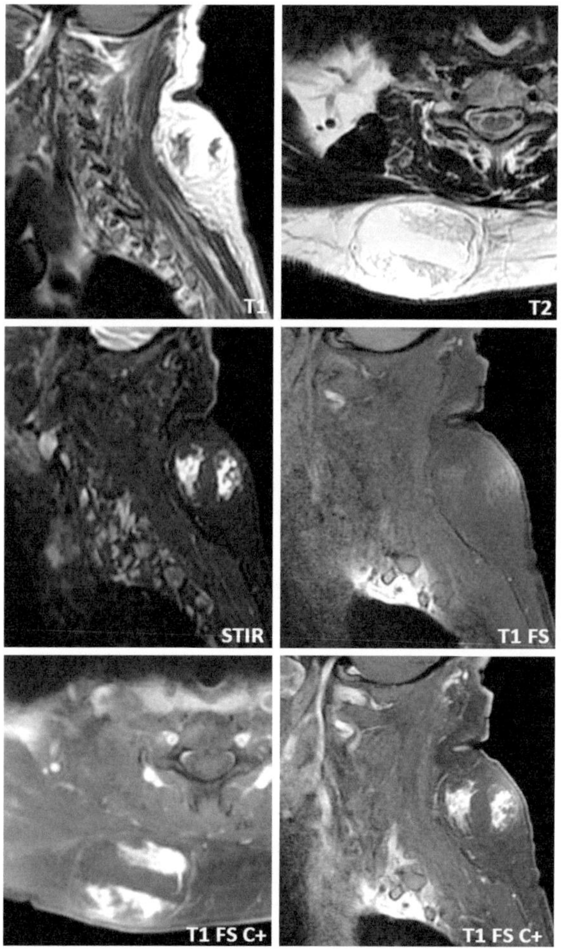

A. Haouimi et al., *Head and Neck Radiology Spot Diagnosis*,
https://doi.org/10.1007/978-3-032-14553-6_60

Findings

A subcutaneous well-defined encapsulated nuchal lesion of complex signal intensity. There are fatty components showing high signal on both T1 and T2 with suppression of signal on fat-suppression sequences. The soft tissue component is of low signal on T1, intermediate signal on T2, and high signal on STIR with vivid enhancement on postcontrast images. No invasion of the adjacent structures.

Diagnosis

Hemangiolipoma.

Discussion

Hemangiolipomas are benign tumors composed of mature adipocytes and thin-walled branching blood vessels. The exact etiology of hemangiolipoma is not known. They usually occur in adolescents and young adults with slight male predominance.

There are infiltrating and noninfiltrating subtypes. Noninfiltrating types are more common, and they do not extend deep into the skin. However, they may be painful. Infiltrating hemangiolipomas extend into deeper soft tissue but are usually painless.

The blood vessels are often fibrin-packed thrombi responsible for MRI high signal on both T1 and T2. The patients usually complain of slow-growing, painless subcutaneous nodule. Occasionally, they can also cause severe pain. Histologically, they can mimic Kaposi's sarcoma, especially in the presence of scanty fatty component.

Common Differential Diagnosis

- Lipoma: homogeneous T1, and T2 high signal, suppression on fat sat sequences.
- Liposarcoma: thick septa, nodularity, invasive lesion.
- Kaposi's sarcoma: HIV positive or in AIDS patient, clinically showing purplish masses.

Management Options

Complete excision is considered curative in symptomatic cases with excellent prognosis. Incomplete resection may lead to recurrence.

References and Further Reading

1. Haouimi A. Haemangiolipoma. Radiopaedia.org. 2022; https://doi.org/10.53347/rID-158215. Accessed 21 Feb 2022.
2. Haouimi A. Soft tissue haemangiolipoma. Radiopaedia.org. 2022; https://doi.org/10.53347/rID-152007. Accessed 21 Feb 2023.
3. Pourbagher A, et al. MRI manifestations of soft-tissue haemangiomas and accompanying reactive bone changes. Br J Radiol. 2011; https://doi.org/10.1259/bjr/58308513. Accessed 14 Jan 2024. Epub 2010 Dec 1. PMID: 21123304; PMCID: PMC3473825.

Case 61

61

Clinical History

A 65-year-old woman presented with a painless swelling of the right nasal region.

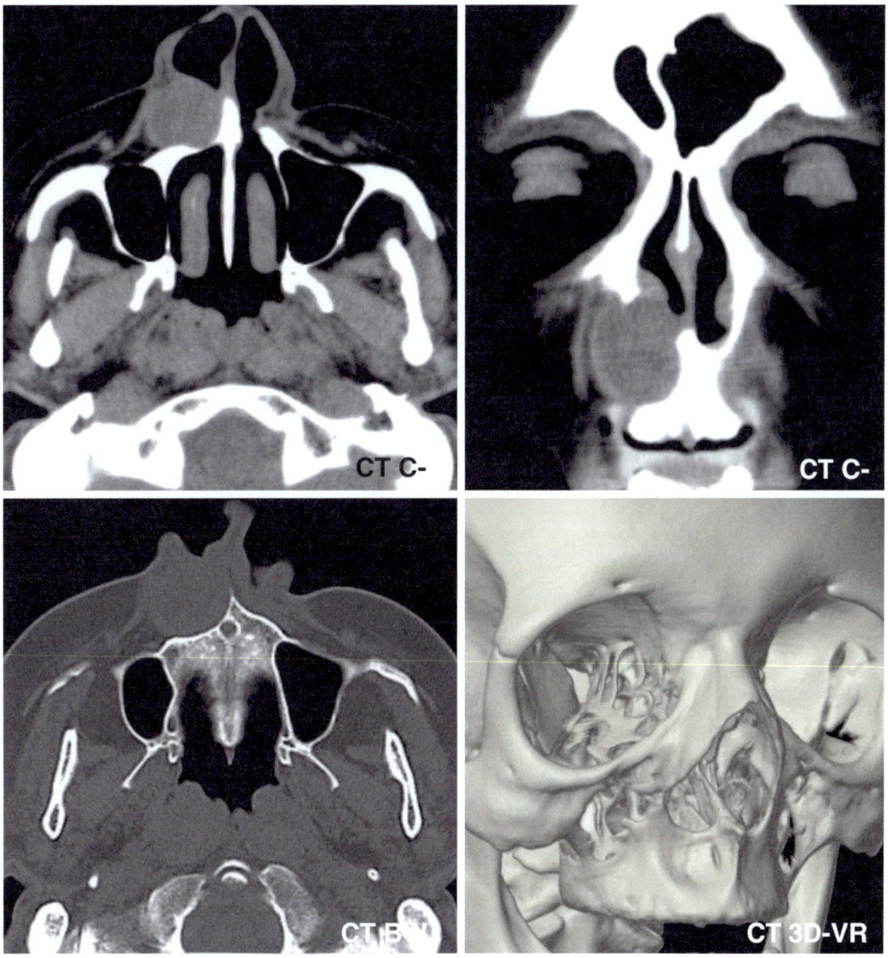

A. Haouimi et al., *Head and Neck Radiology Spot Diagnosis*,
https://doi.org/10.1007/978-3-032-14553-6_61

Findings

A well-defined, rounded cystic mass at the right nasal alar region. Cortical scalloping of the adjacent maxilla well visualized on bone window and 3D-VR images.

Diagnosis

Nasolabial cyst or Klestadt cyst.

Discussion

Nasolabial cysts are also known as Klestadt cysts. These slow-growing non-odontogenic developmental cysts are epicentered at the ala nasi. Lesions are anatomically interposed between the inferior nasal meatus posteriorly and labiogingival fold anteriorly. Lesions are mostly seen in female adults. They may represent the sequelae of sequestration of embryological epithelial tissue in facial fissure or remnant of nasolacrimal duct.

Clinically, nasolabial or Klestadt cysts present as painless unilateral swelling near alar base or nasogenian fold. Occasional pain and nasal obstruction have been reported.

On CT, these well-defined off-midline round lesions are seen posterior to the labiogingival sulcus, anterior to the piriform aperture. The lesions appear low-density, homogeneous, and nonenhancing. Bone windows may reveal remodeling and scalloping of the adjacent maxillary sinus wall. On MRI, the nasolabial cysts appear as homogeneously intermediate signal on T1 and high signal on T2. The cysts themselves do not enhance, although a fine, thin wall enhancement can be observed.

Common Differential Diagnosis

- Nasopalatine cyst: intraosseous, hard palate epicenter, high signal on both T1 and T2.
- Minor salivary gland tumors: usually solid, not completely cystic.

Management Options

Klestadt cysts are "do not touch" lesions. Surgical enucleation is reserved for cases that cause cosmetic concerns and for symptomatic patients.

References and Further Reading

1. Haouimi A. Nasolabial cyst. Radiopaedia.org. 2020; https://doi.org/10.53347/rID-73717. Accessed 10 Dec 2023.
2. Kumar AV, et al. Lestadt's cyst with radiographic contrast medium: a case report. J Clin Diagn Res. 2014; https://doi.org/10.7860/JCDR/2014/9743.5070. Accessed 10 Dec 2023. Epub 2014 Oct 20. PMID: 25478470.
3. Tiago RS, et al. Nasolabial cyst: diagnostic and therapeutical aspects. Braz J Otorhinolaryngol. 2008; https://doi.org/10.1016/s1808-8694(15)30749-7. Accessed 10 Dec 2023. PMID: 18392500; PMCID: PMC9452201.

Case 62

62

Clinical History

An 85-year-old woman presented with a painless left orbital swelling.

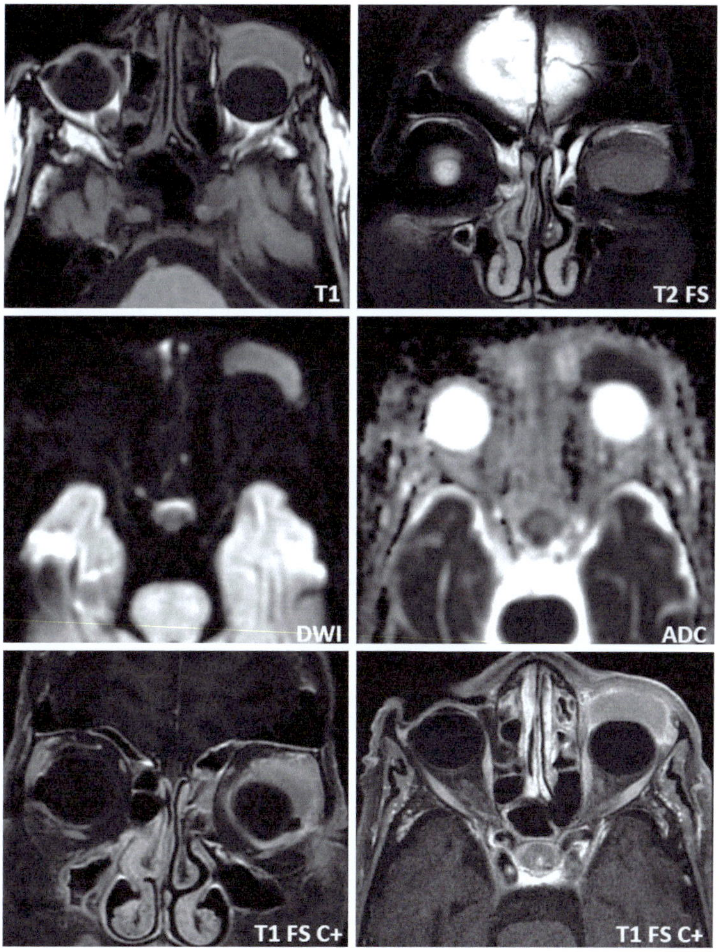

A. Haouimi et al., *Head and Neck Radiology Spot Diagnosis*,
https://doi.org/10.1007/978-3-032-14553-6_62

Findings

A left orbital well-circumscribed lesion anterior to the globe and posterior to the superior palpebra. It is isointense to muscles on both T1 and T2 with restricted diffusion. Moderate homogeneous enhancement with posterior and lateral displacement of globe and lacrimal gland, respectively.

Diagnosis

Orbital MALT lymphoma.

Discussion

Orbital lymphomas represent approximately 50% of all primary orbital malignancies in adults between 50 and 70 years of age. Histologically, orbital MALT lymphomas are B-cell non-Hodgkin lymphomas. The exact etiology is not known. A combination of genetic and inflammatory factors has been proposed. The relationship between *Chlamydia psittaci* infection and orbital lymphoma has also been postulated.

Many lesions are asymptomatic. Depending on the location, patients may complain of fullness in the eyelid, orbital mass, proptosis, and diplopia.

The lesions are markedly hypoechoic on ultrasound and may contain fine linear echogenic strands. Color Doppler images reveal internal vascularity. On CT, they appear as a well-defined iso- or minimally hyperdense homogeneous masses that may mold around the adjacent ocular structures without bony involvement. On the MRI, they are iso- or hypointense on T1 and iso- or hyperintense on T2 with restricted diffusion. Both CT and MRI show mild to moderate enhancement.

Common Differential Diagnosis

- Rhabdomyosarcoma: mostly in children.
- Orbital pseudotumor: retrobulbar, associated thickened extraocular muscles (myositis).
- Diffuse lymphangioma: no or heterogeneous enhancement.

Management Options

The treatment options are surgery, radiotherapy, chemotherapy, and immunotherapy.

References and Further Reading

1. Bayraktar S, et al. Primary ocular adnexal mucosa-associated lymphoid tissue lymphoma (MALT): single institution experience in a large cohort of patients. Br J Haematol. 2011; https://doi.org/10.1111/j.1365--2141.2010.08429.x. Accessed 10 Dec 2023.
2. Haouimi A. Orbital lymphoma (MALToma). Radiopaedia.org. 2023; https://doi.org/10.53347/rID-160601. Accessed 10 Dec 2023.
3. Jakobiec FA, et al. Clinicopathologic and magnetic resonance imaging analysis of a multifocal orbital lymphoid tumor. Ocul Oncol Pathol. 2018; https://doi.org/10.1159/000478731. Accessed 15 June 2025. Epub 2017 Aug 23. PMID: 30320086.

Case 63

63

Clinical History

A 40-year-old woman presented with a history of acute onset of left orbital pain, mild proptosis, and diplopia.

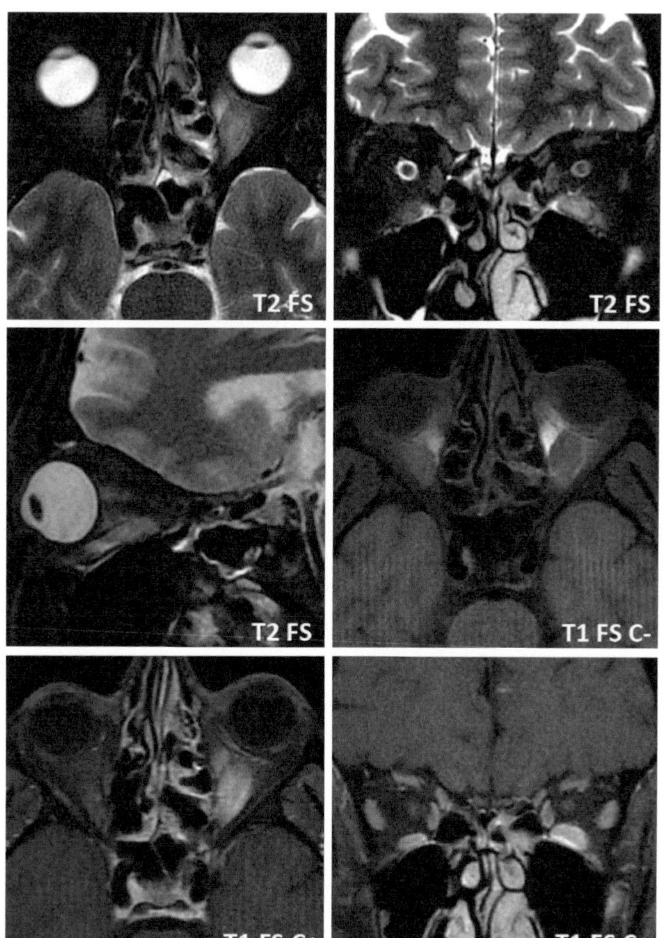

A. Haouimi et al., *Head and Neck Radiology Spot Diagnosis*,
https://doi.org/10.1007/978-3-032-14553-6_63

Findings

Grade I proptosis with a fusiform swelling of the left inferior rectus muscle involving its tendinous insertion. It shows a high signal on T2 fat sat with relatively homogeneous enhancement. Mild inflammatory changes of the adjacent orbital fat. Normal appearance of the other extraocular muscles and lacrimal gland.

Diagnosis

Myositic orbital pseudotumor.

Discussion

Orbital pseudotumor or "idiopathic orbital inflammatory syndrome" is a benign, nonspecific nonneoplastic inflammatory condition. They can be diffuse or localized, causing orbital myositis, dacryoadenitis, scleritis, uveitis, and Tolosa–Hunt syndrome (affecting the superior orbital fissure and cavernous sinus). Orbital myositis may involve a single or multiple extraocular muscles and their tendons. Immune-mediated process and viral infection are two likely mechanisms.

Clinically, patients present with acute onset of unilateral painful proptosis, diplopia, conjunctival chemosis, and periorbital edema. Bilateral involvement is rarely seen.

CT and MRI show evidence of a single or multiple extraocular muscle thickening involving both the muscle belly and its tendons with blurring of muscle contour and spillover inflammatory edema in the adjacent orbital fat. MR enhancement of the optic nerve sheath in contrast to the central hypodense nerve may create a positive "tram track sign."

Common Differential Diagnosis

- Grave's disease: bilateral, thyroid dysfunction, no tendon involvement, "coke bottle sign."
- Dacryoadenitis: involvement of lacrimal gland, may show signs of sinusitis.
- Tolosa–Hunt syndrome: involves orbital apex and cavernous sinus.
- Orbital lymphoma: monoclonal proliferation.

Management Options

Mostly treated with systemic corticosteroids in the form of oral or intravenous administration.

References and Further Reading

1. Bakan S, et al. Myositic type of idiopathic orbital pseudotumor in a 4-year-old child: a case report. Case Rep Med. 2012; https://doi.org/10.1155/2012/473856. Accessed 12 Apr 2024. Epub 2012 Jun 10. PMID: 22719772; PMCID.
2. Chaudhry IA, et al. Orbital pseudotumor: distinct diagnostic features and management. Middle East Afr J Ophthalmol. 2008; https://doi.org/10.4103/0974-9233.53370. Accessed 10 Dec 2023. PMID: 20379424; PMCID: PMC2848795.
3. Haouimi A. Myositic orbital pseudotumour-inferior rectus muscle. Radiopaediaorg. 2022. https://doi.org/10.53347/rid-79130. Accessed 10 Dec 2023.

Case 64

64

Clinical History

A 30-year-old woman complains of headache following history of tooth extraction. The patient has previous history of middle turbinectomy.

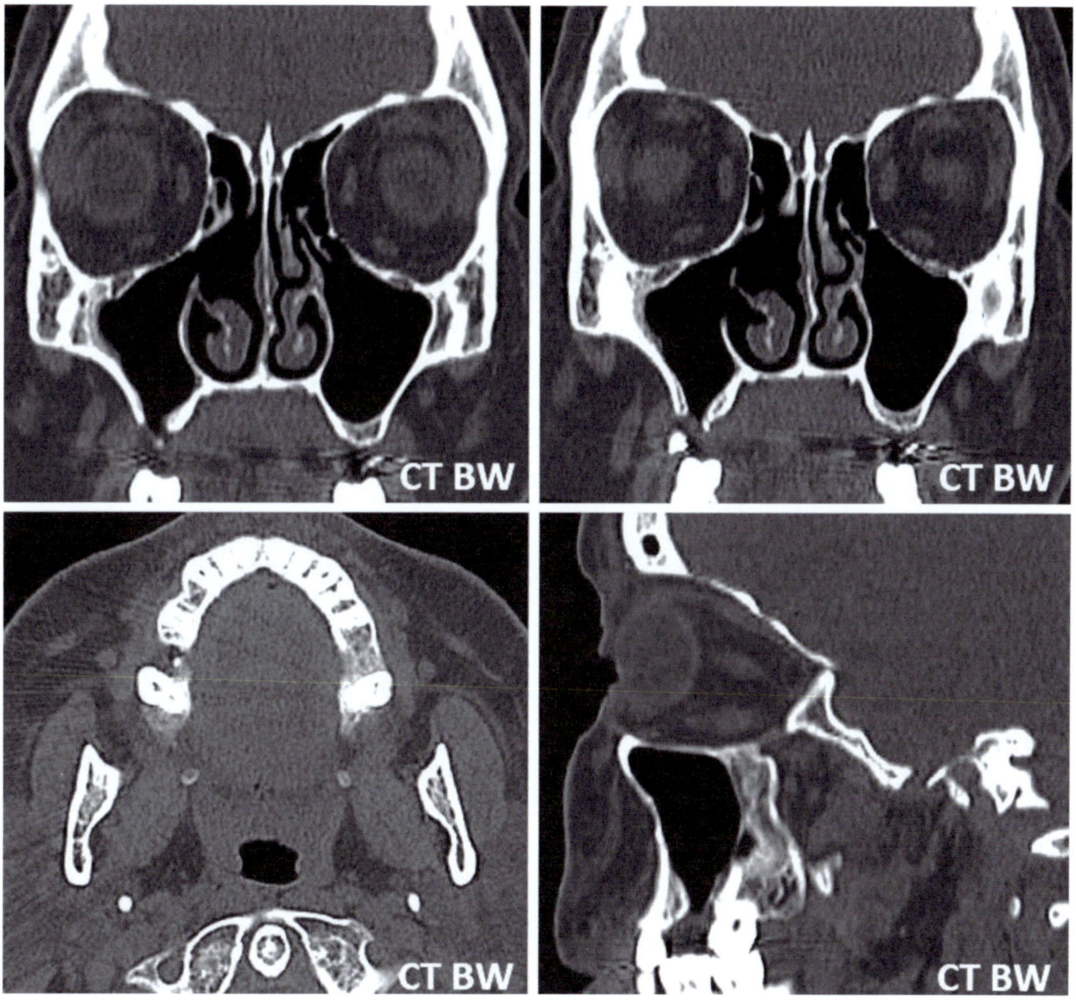

A. Haouimi et al., *Head and Neck Radiology Spot Diagnosis*,
https://doi.org/10.1007/978-3-032-14553-6_64

Findings

A bony defect of the floor of the right maxillary sinus, creating a fistulous communication between the right maxillary antrum and the oral cavity. The defect in the alveolar process of the right maxillary sinus is created secondary to extraction of tooth (#16). No other bony abnormality. Postsurgical aspect of right nasal fossa better seen on axial and coronal slices.

Diagnosis

Oroantral fistula.

Discussion

Oroantral communications and fistulae are frequently encountered by oral and maxillofacial surgeons. These occur due to abnormal communication between the oral cavity and the maxillary antrum, typically as complications of maxillary tooth extraction, the first molar in particular. Smaller lesions (<2 mm) generally heal spontaneously. But larger defects often fail to heal on their own, leading to epithelialization and formation of an oroantral fistula.

Clinical symptoms include unilateral nasal discharge, pain, purulent discharge, altered nasal resonance, difficulty in sucking through a straw, and a whistling sound while speaking. During clinical examination, a hissing noise through the maxillary sinus can be heard when performing a Valsalva maneuver.

The bony hiatus at the alveolar process and the fistulous communication can be easily demonstrated on CT scans. CT is superior to panoramic radiographs in detecting the presence of dental roots, implants, or any dislodged antral foreign body, as well as associated sinusitis.

Common Differential Diagnosis

- Osteomyelitis: modification of bony architecture.
- Trauma: positive clinical history.
- Osteoradionecrosis: positive clinical history, known cancer.

Management Options

Numerous surgical procedures have been proposed, including rotating or advancing buccal, lingual, and palatal flaps.

References and Further Reading

1. Bodner L, Gatot A, Bar-Ziv J. Oroantral fistula: improved imaging with a dental computed tomography software program. Br J Radiol. 1995;68(815):1249–50. https://doi.org/10.1259/0007-1285-68-815-1249.
2. Haouimi A. Oroantral fistula. Radiopaedia.org. 2023; https://doi.org/10.53347/rID-172162. Accessed 10 Dec 2023.
3. Khandelwal P, Hajira N. Management of oro-antral communication and fistula: various surgical options. World J Plast Surg. 2017; Accessed 10 Dec 2023. PMID: 28289607; PMCID: PMC5339603.

Case 65

65

Clinical History

A 60-year-old woman presented with a history of orbital pain and episodic right visual loss.

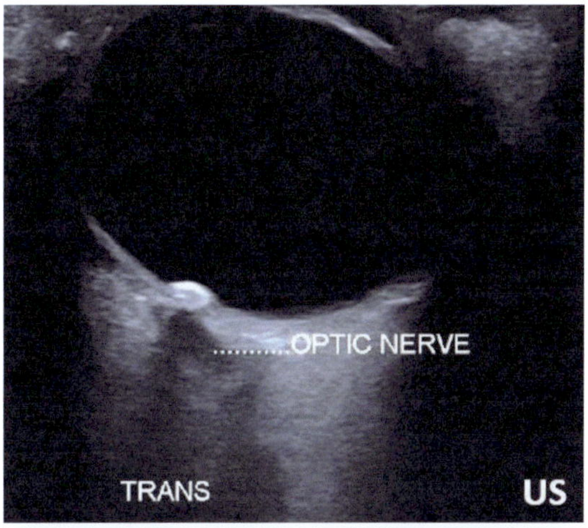

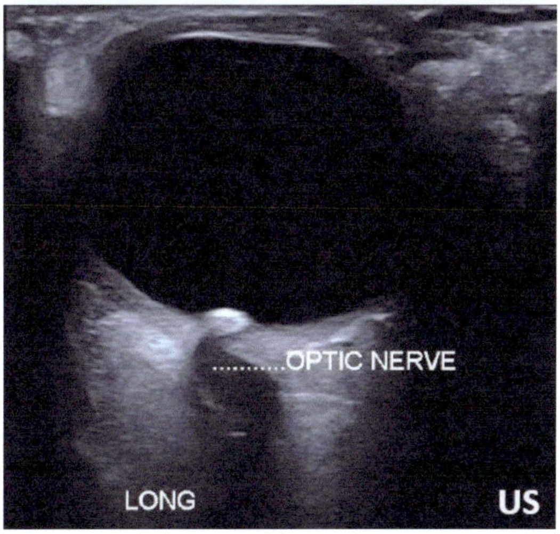

A. Haouimi et al., *Head and Neck Radiology Spot Diagnosis*,
https://doi.org/10.1007/978-3-032-14553-6_65

Findings

Small echogenic focus with posterior acoustic shadowing (calcification) at the optic nerve head of the right eye.

Diagnosis

Optic disc drusen.

Discussion

Optic nerve drusen are usually bilateral and composed of proteinaceous material, calcium salts, and cellular debris. The word "drusen" comes from the German word meaning geode. According to some estimates, optic nerve drusen arise in about 1% to 2% of the US population, more common in Caucasians than Afro-Americans. Anatomically, optic disc drusens are subretinal yellow deposits of varying sizes. They may be inherited, appear in children, and are not related to aging. Inherited dysplasia of the optic disc with compromised blood supply, leads to reduced axoplasmic flow and formation of calcific deposits. Conditions such as retinitis pigmentosa, glaucoma, β-thalassemia, and idiopathic intracranial hypertension can be associated with optic nerve drusen.

On fundoscopy, optic disc drusen have a "lumpy-bumpy" appearance. The lesions mostly do not affect vision, but some patients complain of transient visual obscuration and visual field defects.

On ultrasound, tiny echogenic focus with posterior acoustic shadow can be seen on the surface of optic nerve head. On CT, drusen is seen as a small calcific focus with smooth border. The diagnosis is mostly straightforward on imaging and fundoscopy.

Common Differential Diagnosis

- Retinoblastoma: mass with calcification, often not located on optic disc.
- Astrocytic hamartoma: retinal detachment, unilateral, neurocutaneous syndrome.

Management Options

Optic disc drusen are considered a "do not touch" lesion.

References and Further Reading

1. Costello F. Optic disc drusen studies consortium. Diagnosing optic disc drusenin the modern imaging era: a practical approach. Neuroophthalmology. 2020; https://doi.org/10.1080/01658107.2020.1810286. Accessed 10 Dec 2023. PMID: 33762782; PMCID: PMC7946029.
2. Haouimi A. Optic disc drusen. Radiopaedia.org. 2023; https://doi.org/10.53347/rID-171290. Accessed 10 Dec 2023.
3. Tuğcu B, Özdemir H. Imaging methods in the diagnosis of optic disc drusen. Turk J Ophthalmol. 2016; https://doi.org/10.4274/tjo.66564. Accessed 12 Sept 2024.

Case 66

66

Clinical History

A 14-year-old girl presented with a history of purulent discharge from a left submandibular cutaneous nodule.

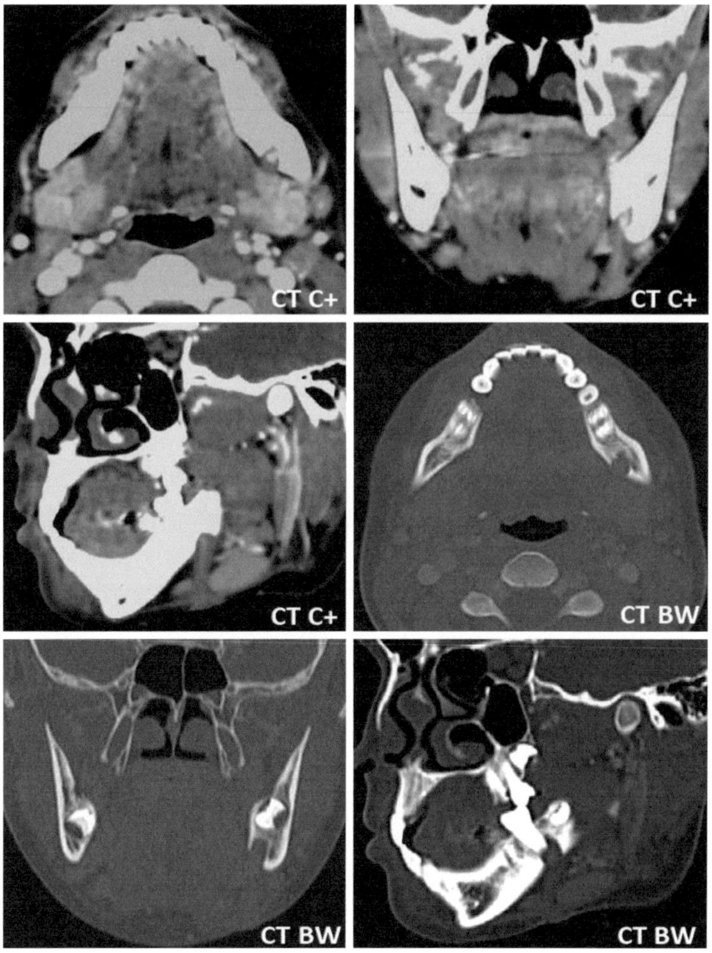

A. Haouimi et al., *Head and Neck Radiology Spot Diagnosis*,
https://doi.org/10.1007/978-3-032-14553-6_66

Findings

Left submandibular enhancing fistulous tract extending up to a periapical lucency of the root of tooth 37, through a bony defect of the adjacent mandibular cortex (better seen on sagittal oblique reformation). No associated soft tissue abscess.

Diagnosis

Odontogenic cutaneous fistula.

Discussion

Odontogenic cutaneous fistulas result from chronic dental and periodontal infection, pulpal degeneration following tooth fracture and residual tooth. Pulpal infection causes a breach in enamel and dentin. Fistulas are characterized by the presence of a draining sinus originating from a localized pus-filled focus related to the affected tooth. About two-thirds of fistulas originate from the teeth of lower jaw, and the remaining one-third originate from upper jaw teeth. The most frequent teeth involved are the molar teeth. The internal opening is seen at the gingival area, whereas the external opening often appears as a suppurative dimple/nodule in the cheek.

Most patients complain of purulent discharging facial nodule and/or abscess with no obvious dental problems. Absence of dental problems can lead to misdiagnosis.

Odontogenic infections appear as periapical lucency of the affected tooth on dental X-rays. Contrast CT may show the fistulous tract. Apart from delineating the fistulous tract on T2 and postcontrast T1 as high signal, MRI can show both the external cutaneous nodule/abscess and affected internal area in the alveolar margin of the infected tooth.

Common Differential Diagnosis

- Neoplastic processes: no dental abnormality, no fistulous tract, no history of trauma.
- Subcutaneous mycoses: deeper involvement, no dental abnormality, history of trauma.

Management Options

The treatment is typically centered on removal of the source of the infection by root canal treatment or extraction of the affected tooth.

References and Further Reading

1. Abdelrahman A, et al. Odontogenic cutaneous fistula. Radiopaedia.org. 2022. Accessed 31 Dec 2022. https://doi.org/10.53347/rID-82533.
2. Haouimi A. Odontogenic cutaneous fistula. Radiopaedia.org. 2022. https://doi.org/10.53347/rID-156966. Accessed 31 Dec 2022.
3. Lee EY, et al. Clinical characteristics of odontogenic cutaneous fistulas. Ann Dermatol. 2016; https://doi.org/10.5021/ad.2016.28.4.417. Accessed 31 Dec 2022. Epub 2016 Jul 26. PMID: 27489421; PMCID: PMC4969468.

Case 67

67

Clinical History

A 70-year-old woman complaining of oropharyngeal pulsatile sensation.

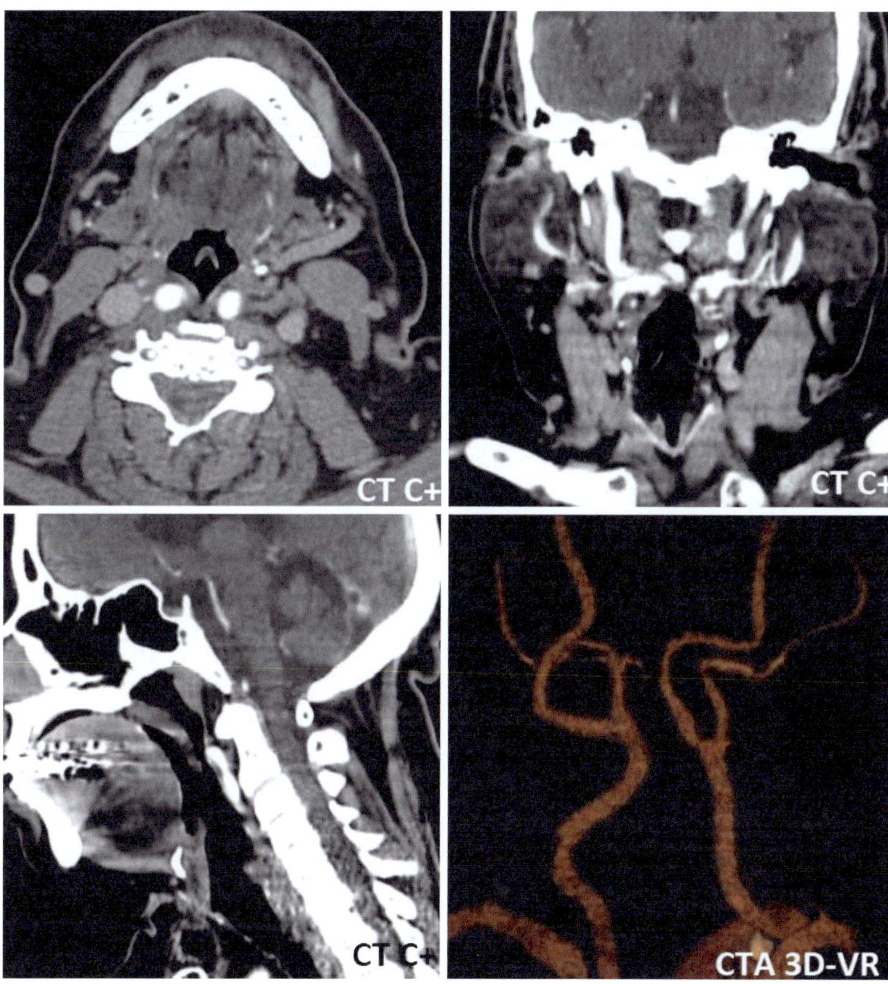

A. Haouimi et al., *Head and Neck Radiology Spot Diagnosis*,
https://doi.org/10.1007/978-3-032-14553-6_67

Findings

Aberrant course of the common carotid arteries, as well as the right and left internal carotid arteries, at the retropharyngeal space in an extreme close quasi-midline apposition. The arteries appear to be tortuous.

Diagnosis

Kissing carotids.

Discussion

Midline course or deviation of tortuous, elongated, or kinked carotids has been termed "kissing carotids." It is indeed a romantic term with extreme surgical importance. Anatomical variation of both internal and external carotid arteries is seen in up to 10% of the normal population. Aberrant internal carotid arteries arise from the persistence of angulation during embryonic descent (from third aortic arch and the dorsal aortic root toward the chest). The preferred anatomical kissing spot is retropharyngeal space. However, they can even kiss the parapharyngeal wall, inside the sella turcica and sphenoid sinus. The internal carotid arteries can change their position to kiss each other on short-interval imaging studies, particularly in elderly and even during certain respiratory movements in younger patients, as well as in hypertensives.

Clinical presentation ranges from an asymptomatic incidental finding to a throbbing throat sensation, dysphagia, and sleep apnea. Kissing carotids in the sphenoid region may produce signs of endocrinopathy.

CT scan shows narrowing of oropharyngeal lumen due to presence of retropharyngeal and/or peritonsillar soft tissue density. Buckled or tortuous internal carotid arteries in close apposition on enhanced postcontrast images. MRI reveals kissing signal voids.

Common Differential Diagnosis

- An anatomical variant: no differential to propose.
- Retropharyngeal abscess: clinical history, normal carotid positions, no flow void.

Management Options

Tracheal injury during intubation, nasogastric tube placement, or introduction of transesophageal ultrasound probes poses a high risk of vascular injury when the kissing site is submucosal (occasionally it may even be <1 mm). Once identified, the radiologists must inform all members of the team, including all concerned surgeons and anesthetists ASAP.

References and Further Reading

1. Haouimi A. Retropharyngeal carotid arteries-kissing carotids. "Radiopaedia.org". 2024. Accessed on 6 Jan 2024. https://doi.org/10.53347/rID-160939.
2. Rafailidis V et al. Kissing carotids: a lovely term for an anatomic variant "Eurorad case". 2023. Accessed on 21 Jan 2025. https://doi.org/10.1594/EURORAD/CASE.13010.

Case 68

68

Clinical History

A 16-year-old boy complaining of rapidly progressing nasal obstruction with snoring.

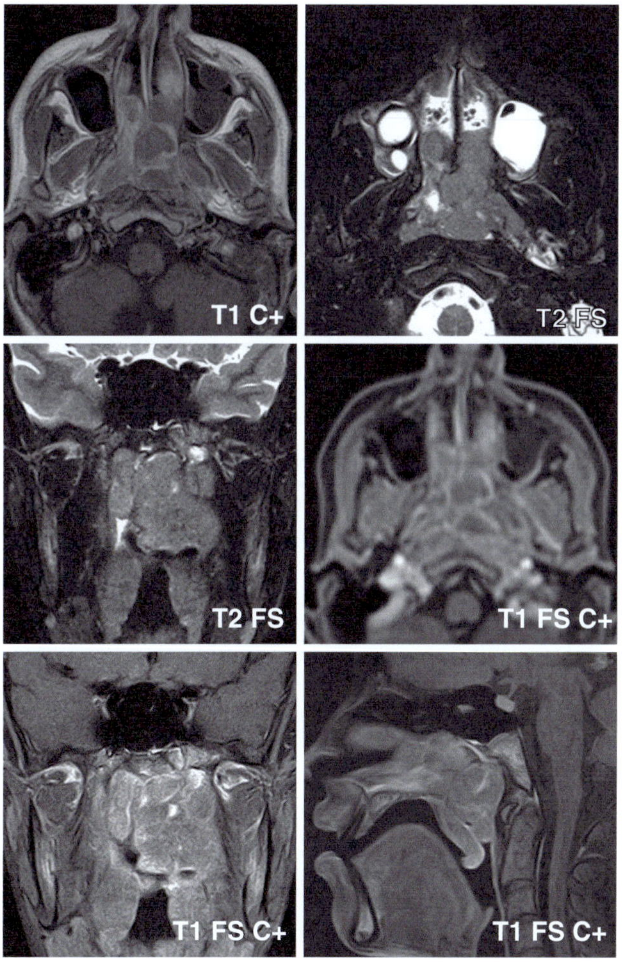

A. Haouimi et al., *Head and Neck Radiology Spot Diagnosis*,
https://doi.org/10.1007/978-3-032-14553-6_68

Findings

A large lobulated nasopharyngeal soft tissue mass causing bilateral obliteration of the fossae of Rosenmüller and Eustachian tube openings. It is iso- or slightly low signal to muscles on T1, intermediate signal on T2 fat-sat with moderate heterogeneous enhancement. The anterior extension of the lesion causing obstruction of the choanae and downward displacement of soft palate. Signs of left-sided secondary otomastoiditis. Mild maxillary sinusitis with bilateral mucus retention cysts.

Diagnosis

Nasopharyngeal Burkitt lymphoma (BL).

Discussion

Burkitt lymphoma is an aggressive type of mature B-cell non-Hodgkin lymphoma. The rapid doubling time of 24–48 h, makes it one of the fastest-growing tumors in humans. The incidence of nasopharyngeal involvement is very rare. WHO classifies BL into three clinical groups: (a) endemic, (b) sporadic, and (c) immunodeficiency related. The endemic cases seen in Africa and Papua New Guinea, where malaria and EBV are prevalent. Sporadic cases are mostly seen in North America and countries in the European Union. A few BL are seen in HIV infection, especially when CD4 count greater than 200 and no opportunistic infection.

Many BL symptoms resemble common illnesses. The symptoms appear suddenly and can rapidly worsen. Waldeyer's ring involvement can cause dysphagia, dyspnea, wheezing, and even airway obstruction, which may be potentially life-threatening.

Both CT and MRI are useful for evaluating locoregional extension: CT is mainly for evaluating bony erosion at the nasopharynx and skull base. Soft tissue is better evaluated on MR.

Common Differential Diagnosis

- Nasopharyngeal carcinoma: fossa of Rosenmüller epicenter, unilateral, perineural spread.
- Chordoma: spheno-occipital epicenter, "thumb sign" +/−, calcification +/−.
- Enlarged adenoids: no bony erosion.

Management Options

The management options are surgery, radiotherapy, chemotherapy, and radio-immunotherapy. Burkitt lymphomas are highly chemosensitive, which is the modality of choice in children.

References and Further Reading

1. Goel Alexander, N et al. Burkitt lymphoma of the nasopharynx causing life-threatening airway obstruction: a case report. Am J Otolaryngol. 2021. Accessed on 6 Jan 2024. https://doi.org/10.1016/j.amjoto.2021.102977.
2. Haouimi A. Burkitt lymphoma. "Radiopaedia.org". 2024. Accessed on 6 Jan 2024. https://doi.org/10.53347/rID-159530.

Case 69

69

Clinical History

A 65-year-old man presented with a painful right orbital swelling.

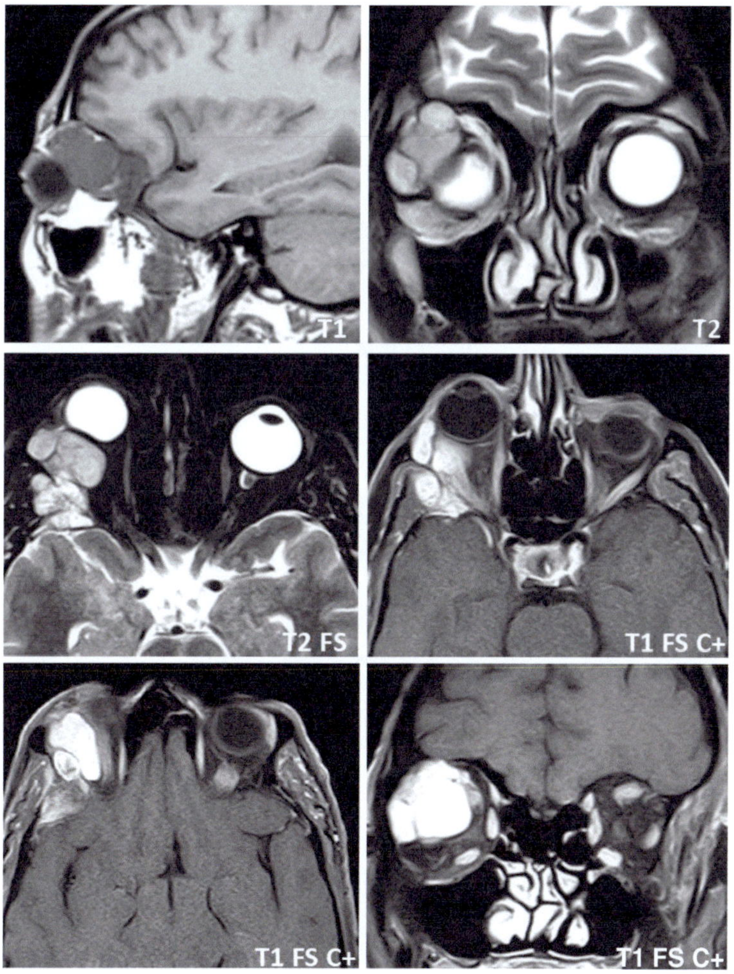

A. Haouimi et al., *Head and Neck Radiology Spot Diagnosis*,
https://doi.org/10.1007/978-3-032-14553-6_69

Findings

A large extraconal soft tissue mass of the right orbit, epicentered at the lacrimal gland. It shows an isosignal to the cortical gray matter on both T1 and T2 with intense enhancement. The extrinsic compression displaces the lateral and superior rectus muscles, ocular globe, and optic nerve, creating grade 2 proptosis. Also, there is invasion of greater wing of sphenoid, extra-axial anterior temporal soft tissue, and temporalis muscle.

Diagnosis

Adenoid cystic carcinoma (ACC) of the lacrimal gland.

Discussion

Adenoid cystic carcinomas are a rare invasive lacrimal gland malignancy with poor overall prognosis. ACC represent only 1% of all head and neck malignancies but is the commonest primary malignant epithelial tumor of the lacrimal gland. Tumors are locally very aggressive with the tendency for locoregional invasion and perineural spread.

Clinically, patients present with insidious onset of painful ophthalmoplegia with periorbital paresthesia. Later ptosis, ophthalmoplegia, and proptosis can appear.

Lacrimal ACC often show an "almond-shaped" extension toward the orbital apex. CT reveals lobular, homogeneous isodense lesion with bony erosion of the neighboring skull base. These lesions are of low signal on T1 with moderate to marked enhancement. On T2, lesions are iso- to low signal.

Common Differential Diagnosis

- Sjögren's syndrome: fatty component +, associated salivary gland involvement.
- Sarcoidosis: painless, bilateral, no bony erosion, ocular lesions.
- Dermoid, epidermoid: bony remodeling, no erosion.

Management Options

Surgical exenteration may or may not be followed by radiotherapy.

References and Further Reading

1. Benali, K et al. Lacrimal gland adenoid cystic carcinoma: report of an unusual case with literature review. Radiat Oncol J. 2021. Accessed on 23 Jan 2024. https://doi.org/10.3857/roj.2021.00122. Epub 2021 Jun 28. PMID: 34619831; PMCID.
2. Gu, A et al. A rare case of orbital adenoid cystic carcinoma mimicking as optic nerve glioma. Cureus. 2022. Accessed on 23 Jan 2024. https://doi.org/10.7759/cureus.25863. PMID: 35836445; PMCID: PMC9274972.
3. Haouimi A. Adenoid cystic carcinoma of lacrimal gland. "Radiopaedia.org". 2024. Accessed on 23 Jan 2024. https://doi.org/10.53347/rID-174477

Case 70

70

Clinical History

A 25-year-old man presented with a painless swelling of the right supraclavicular region.

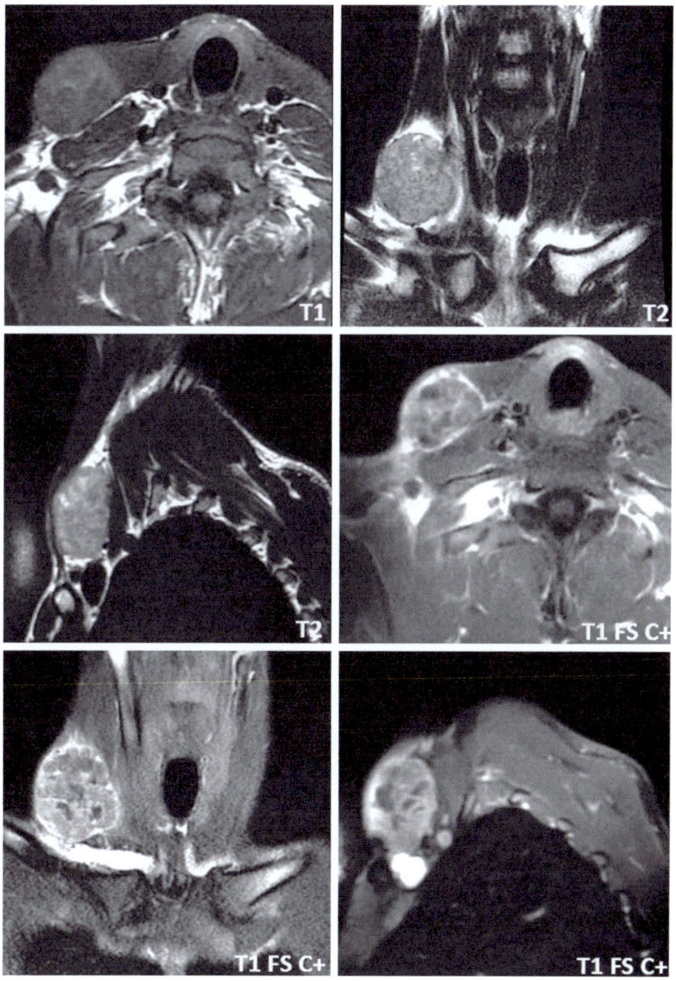

A. Haouimi et al., *Head and Neck Radiology Spot Diagnosis*,
https://doi.org/10.1007/978-3-032-14553-6_70

Findings

A well-defined ovoid soft tissue mass at the right supraclavicular region, interposed between the sternocleidomastoid and anterior scalenus. It is iso- to hyperintense on T1 and an inhomogeneously hyperintense on T2. Heterogeneous enhancement with central areas of necrosis and enhanced peripheral capsule. No cervical lymphadenopathy.

Diagnosis

Clear cell sarcoma (CCS) of soft tissue of the neck.

Discussion

Clear cell sarcomas are rare, highly invasive mesenchymal tumor with melanocytic differentiation. They are seen mostly involving the distal tendons and aponeurosis of the lower extremity. There is morphological overlap with malignant melanoma. Uniformly arranged nests of dense transparent cells and scattered "wreath-like" multinucleated giant cells are seen histologically, which remain separated by fibrous tissue septae.

Clinically, larger lesions present as a subcutaneous lump (with or without pain).

CT shows homogeneously isodense soft tissue lump but can be heterogeneous in presence of necrosis. Up to 40% of cases show enlarged lymph nodes. Unlike other types of sarcomas, the lesions show high signal on T1 and low signal on T2 (due to the presence of melanin). However, low melanin content may not result in high T1 signal.

Common Differential Diagnosis

- Neurofibromas: target sign, perilesional edema-like zone, fascicular sign +/−.
- Hemangioma: presence of phlebolith +, no locoregional invasion.
- Malignant schwannoma: ill-defined, heterogeneous, linear septa, low signal on T2.

Management Options

The treatment options of CCS are lumpectomy and removal of involved lymph nodes along with adjuvant chemo- and radiotherapy.

References and Further Reading

1. Feasel, P C. et al. Primary clear cell sarcoma of the head and neck: a case series withreview of literature. J CutanPathol. 2016. Accessed on 23 Jan 2024. https://doi.org/10.1111/cup.12755. Epub 2016 Jul 15. PMID: 27264732.
2. Haouimi A. Clear cell sarcoma of soft tissue – neck. "Radiopaedia.org". 2024. Accessed on 23 Jan 2024. https://doi.org/10.53347/rID-174362
3. Liu, CC et al. Primary clear cell sarcoma of soft tissue in the posterior cervical spine invading the medulla oblongata: a case report. World J Clin Cases. 2022. Accessed on 23 Jan 2024. https://doi.org/10.12998/wjcc.v10.i21.7571. PMID: 36158008.

Case 71

71

Clinical History

An 85-year-old woman with a history of chronic headache. Incidental CT finding.

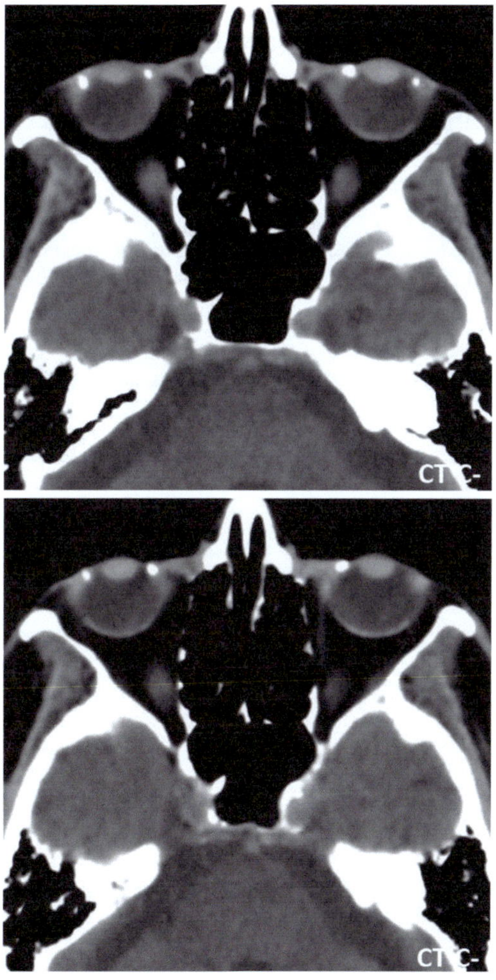

A. Haouimi et al., *Head and Neck Radiology Spot Diagnosis*,
https://doi.org/10.1007/978-3-032-14553-6_71

Findings

Small ovoid bilateral calcifications of the anterior globe, at the insertion of both recti (medial and lateral).

Diagnosis

Senile calcific scleral plaques.

Discussion

Senile scleral plaques are frequently seen in elderly persons above 70 years of age. They are either incidentally seen on CT or during transscleral intravitral injection of antivascular endothelial growth factor (VEGF) therapies for maculopathy. They are oblong well-demarcated slate-gray areas, posterior to the limbus and anterior to the insertions of the medial and lateral rectus muscles, caused by hyaline degeneration. Up to 50% of the cases may calcify. The pathogenesis remains unclear. Atherosclerotic ischemia, repetitive mechanical stress due to ocular movement, and exposure to solar ultraviolet radiation have been hypothesized. On clinical examination, these are vertical, sharply demarcated greyish elliptical foci, averaging 2 mm in width and 5–6 mm in height in a specific location (posterior to limbus and anterior to the horizontal recti).

Common Differential Diagnosis

- Optic disc drusen: location at the optic nerve head.
- Choroidal osteoma: arciform posterior globe calcification sparing optic disc, younger age.
- Trochlear calcification: location, medially.
- Foreign body: positive history, unilateral.

Management Options

Incidental asymptomatic cases are considered "do not touch" lesions. Considering the high risk of spontaneous perforation in scleromalacia, graft placement over the defect can be considered.

References and Further Reading

1. Beck M et al. Senile scleral plaques imaged with enhanced depth optical coherence tomography. Acta Ophthalmologica. 2014. Accessed on 25 Jan 2024. https://doi.org/10.1111/aos.12547
2. Gordon RN et al. Calcified scleral plaquesimaged onorbital computed tomography. AmJ Ophthalmol. 1999. Accessed on 25 Jan 2024. https://doi.org/10.1016/s0002-9394(98)00379-1. PMID: 10218703.
3. Haouimi A. Senile calcific scleral plaques. "Radiopaedia.org". 2024. Accessed on 25 Jan 2024. https://doi.org/10.53347/rID-172543

Case 72

72

Clinical History

A 60-year-old man with a history of acute pain and blurring of vision in the right eye immediately after pounding a metal object with a metal chisel.

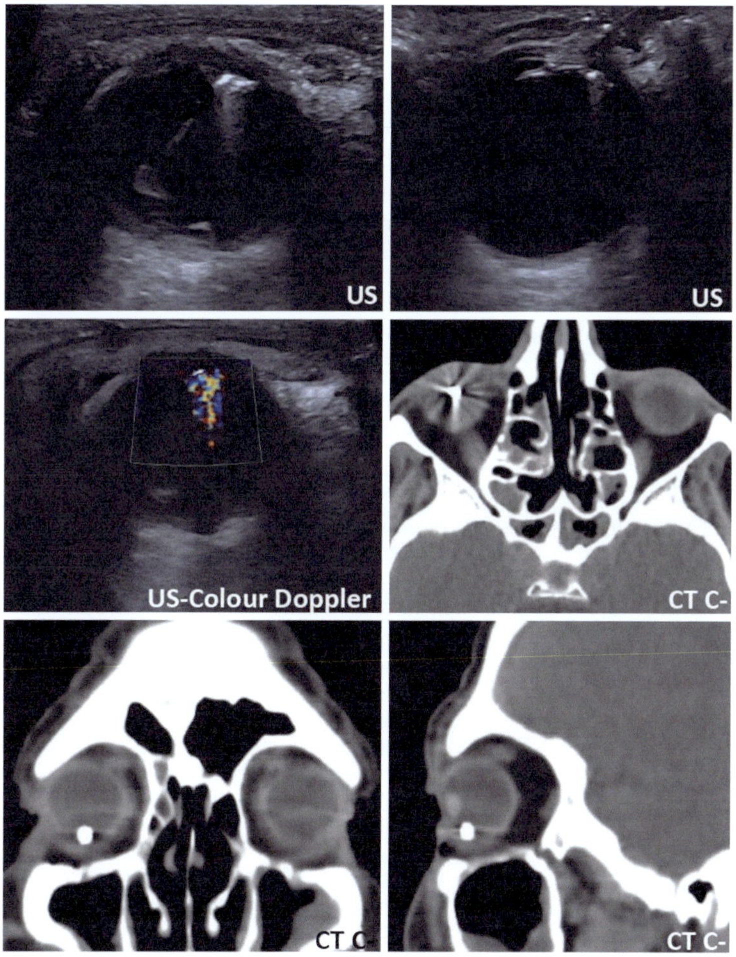

A. Haouimi et al., *Head and Neck Radiology Spot Diagnosis*,
https://doi.org/10.1007/978-3-032-14553-6_72

Findings

A small echogenic foreign body within the inferior wall of the right globe with a twinkling artifact on color flow Doppler. Echogenic material within the vitreous chamber, which was mobile with the extraocular movements of the globe in keeping with vitreous hemorrhage. The nonenhanced CT confirmed the presence of a metallic foreign body within the inferior wall of the globe producing streak.

Diagnosis

Intraocular foreign body (IOFB).

Discussion

IOFBs are a common ocular injury and can be seen in up to 40% of eyes with penetrating injuries. A vast majority of cases occur in workplaces and are more prevalent in the young age group. Up to 90% of intraocular foreign bodies are metallic and most of those are ferromagnetic. Ocular damage from foreign bodies depends on multiple factors, including the composition of the foreign body, size, and shape, as well as the projectile force during impact.

Plain X-rays can demonstrate radiodense IOFB. CT is the investigation of choice and can reveal ferro-positive metallic bodies above 1 mm. However, infra-millimetric and radionegative foreign bodies, as well as those adjacent to the sclera, can be missed on CT. Ultrasound can detect both radiolucent and radiodense foreign bodies. MRI can theoretically show wooden or plastic foreign bodies. Because of the strong magnetic field, there is a high risk of movement of IOFB, which can cause further irreversible damage to intraocular contents. MRI is absolutely contraindicated for patients with an intraocular ferromagnetic metallic foreign body.

Common Differential Diagnosis

- Optic disc drusen: location at optic nerve head, calcific, not metallic.
- Trochlear calcification: location, medially, extraocular, no history of eye injury.
- Senile calcific scleral plaques: specific location, calcific, not metallic, extraocular.

Management Options

All traumatized eyes with open globe penetrating injury must be considered to contain intraocular foreign bodies until proven otherwise, no matter the external appearance of the injury. Immediate appropriate measures must be in accordance with ophthalmologist's advice.

References and Further Reading

1. Gupta A Tripathy K. Intraocular Foreign Body. Stat Pearls Publishing. 2024. Accessed on 25 Jan 2024. https://www.ncbi.nlm.nih.gov/books/NBK576415/.
2. Haouimi A. Orbital foreign body. "Radiopaedia. org". 2024 Accessed on 25 Jan 2024. https://doi.org/10.53347/rID-169064.

Case 73

73

Clinical History

A 25-year-old man with a history of subtotal thyroidectomy 3 months prior, presented with fever and a painful swelling of the right cervical region.

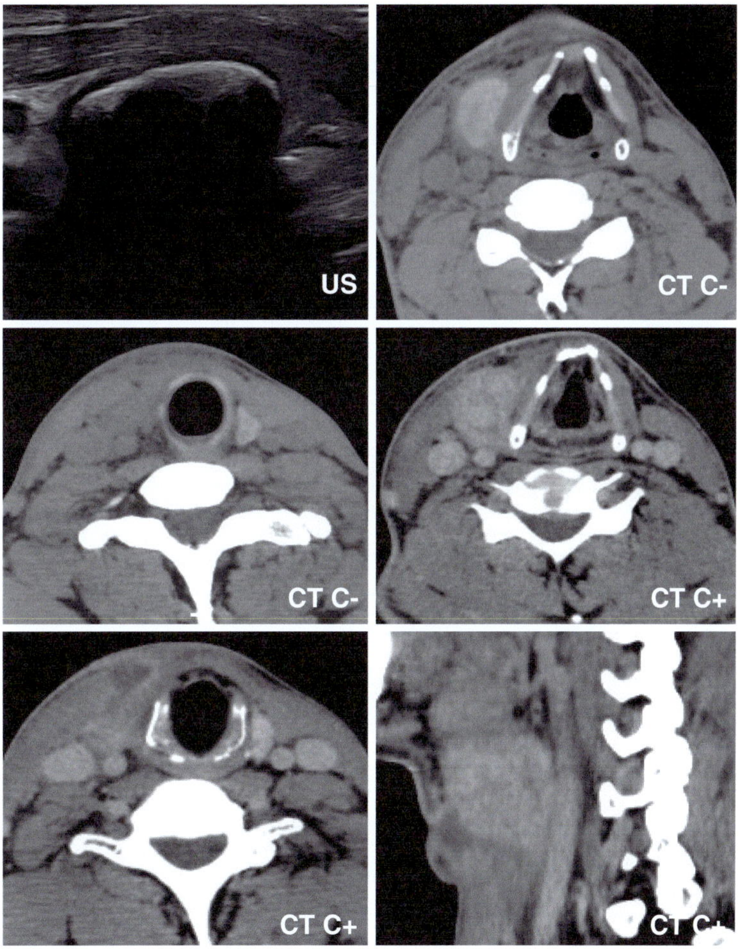

A. Haouimi et al., *Head and Neck Radiology Spot Diagnosis*,
https://doi.org/10.1007/978-3-032-14553-6_73

Findings

An arciform echogenic mass with posterior acoustic shadow seen on ultrasound. CT shows a spontaneously hyperdense, well-defined ovoid structure without any contrast enhancement in the right thyroid bed. Inflammatory changes of the neighboring subcutaneous fat along with small pocket of collection inferolateral to it. A fistulous communication is seen extending from the ovoid structure reaching the skin, better seen in parasagittal reformatted image. Associated ipsilateral reactive cervical lymphadenopathy.

Diagnosis

Infected gossypiboma of the neck.

Discussion

Gossypiboma, also known as textiloma, is a mass of cotton matrix that is inadvertently forgotten and buried during surgery. They cause foreign body–like reactions. An acute presentation can lead to a septic course, resulting in the formation of an abscess or granuloma. Delayed presentations may occur months or years after the original surgery, with adhesion and encapsulation. Prolonged infection can even lead to fistulization. Occasionally, gossypibomas can mimic tumors. Delayed diagnosis is problematic and can lead to increased mortality and morbidity rates. The cases are underreported due to the medicolegal implications. Clinical history is a crucial factor in diagnosis.

Gossypibomas appear as spongiform, low-density masses with gas bubbles on CT with or without a thin enhancing capsule. Chronic cases may show calcifications along the surgical sponge architecture. Gossypibomas generally show low signal on both T1 and T2 with a central whorled appearance.

Common Differential Diagnosis

- Tumor recurrence: nonhomogeneous enhancement.
- Abscess: peripheral enhancement.
- Postradiation status: prior history of radiation.

Management Options

Surgical removal.

References and Further Reading

1. Adonis M, et al. Imaging of gossypibomas: pictorial review. Am J Roentgenol. 2012;193(6_supplement) https://doi.org/10.2214/AJR.07.7132.
2. Haouimi A. Gossypiboma - neck. "Radiopaedia.org". 2024 Accessed on 25 Jan 2024. https://doi.org/10.53347/rID-169762.
3. Kim, KJ et al. Gossypiboma of the neck mimicking an isolated neck recurrence. Clin Exp Otorhinolaryngol. 2013. Accessed on 25 Jan 2024. https://doi.org/10.3342/ceo.2013.6.4.269. Epub 2013 Nov 29. PMID: 24353871; PMCID:

Case 74

74

Clinical History

A 16-year-old adolescent presented with a history of vertigo and loss of equilibrium.

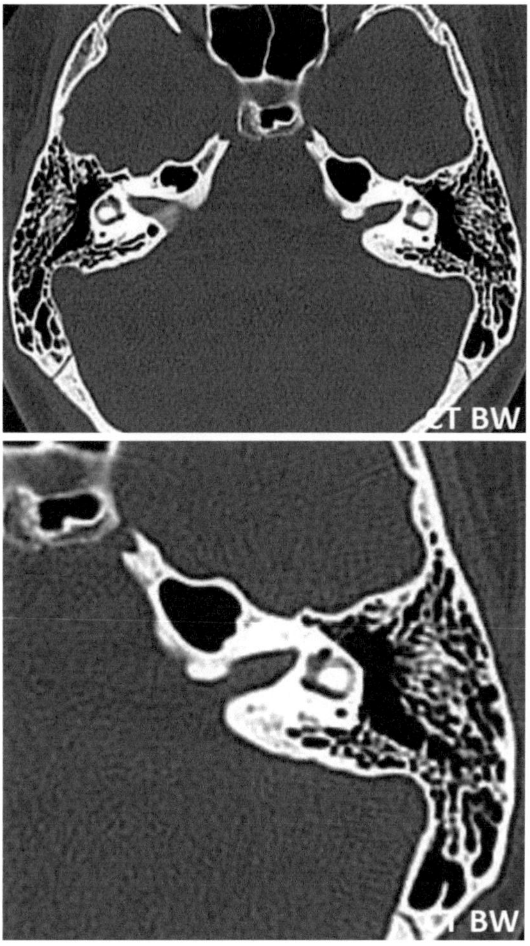

A. Haouimi et al., *Head and Neck Radiology Spot Diagnosis*,
https://doi.org/10.1007/978-3-032-14553-6_74

Findings

Broad-based bony growth arising from the anterosuperior aspect of the left internal auditory canal. It is protruding into its lumen, causing narrowing of the porus acousticus.

Diagnosis

Internal auditory canal (IAC) exostosis.

Discussion

Internal auditory canal (IAC) exostosis is a very rare focal bony overgrowth in the internal auditory meatus. Most cases are asymptomatic, but occasionally they may present with disabling symptoms such as vertigo, dizziness, hearing loss, and vestibular dysfunction due to extrinsic compression on vestibular and facial nerves. This can severely compromise quality of life.

High-resolution infra-millimetric CT remains the most effective modality to identify bony lesions such as osteomas and exostoses. Internal auditory canal exostoses are usually seen as broad-based bony growths without any pedunculated attachment, causing focal narrowing of the canal. On MRI, internal auditory canal exostoses are broad-based bony growths that are intensely seen on both T1 and T2 without any contrast enhancement. MRI is superior in demonstrating extrinsic nerve compression and ruling out other potential pathologies.

Common Differential Diagnosis

- Schwannoma: enlargement of the canal, involvement of nerve sheath, enhancement +/−.
- Paget's disease: bone deformity, generalized involvement, "cotton wool" appearance.
- Fibrous dysplasia: "ground glass" matrix.

Management Options

The slow-growing nature of these lesions allows watchful waiting. Surgery is mainly reserved for severe cases with neurologic deficits.

References and Further Reading

1. García-Moncó Fernández C et al. Internal auditory canal exostosis. "Radiopaedia.org". 2023. Accessed on 03 Nov 2024. https://doi.org/10.53347/rID-100076.
2. Haouimi A. Internal auditory canal exostosis. "Radiopaedia.org". 2024. Accessed on 25 Jan 2024. https://doi.org/10.53347/rID-181437
3. Mubita L et al. Internal auditory canal exostosis: a technical case report. Surg Neurol Int. 2018. Accessed on 25 Jan 2024. https://doi.org/10.4103/sni.sni_412_17. PMID: 29629231; PMCID: PMC5875108.

Case 75

75

Clinical History

A 13-year-old girl presented with a painless right cheek swelling.

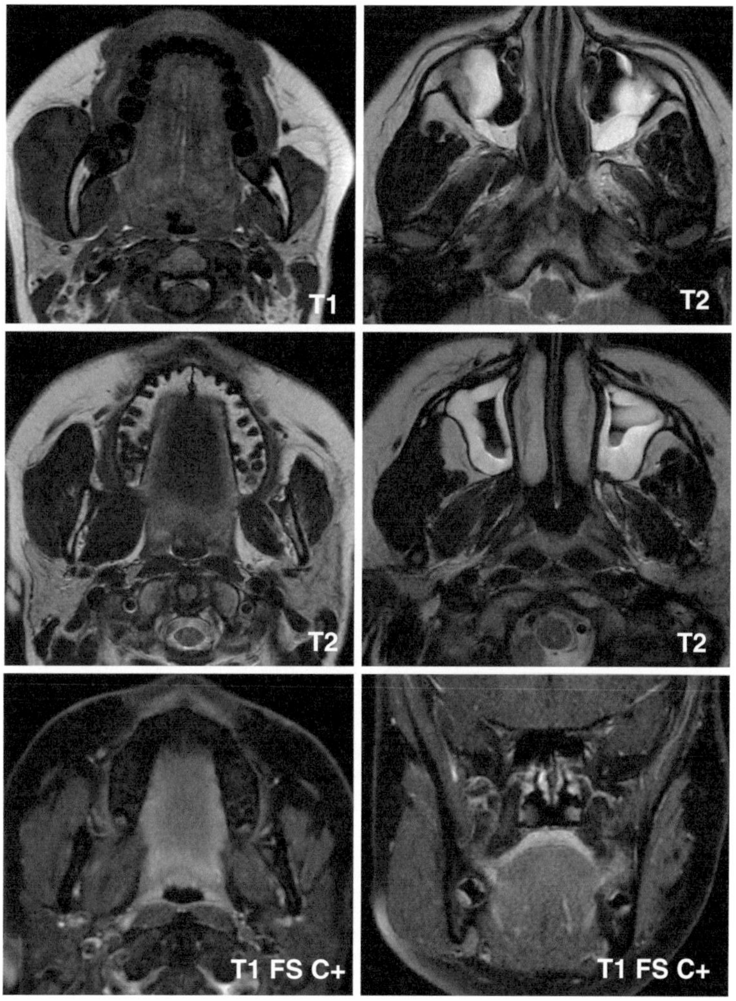

A. Haouimi et al., *Head and Neck Radiology Spot Diagnosis*,
https://doi.org/10.1007/978-3-032-14553-6_75

Findings

Unilateral hypertrophy of right temporalis, masseter, medial, and lateral pterygoid muscles with preserved signal intensity. No abnormal enhancement.

Diagnosis

Unilateral masticator muscles hypertrophy (MMH).

Discussion

Masticator muscles hypertrophy is an uncommon condition due to benign enlargement of the volume of masticator muscles. It can be both uni- or bilateral associated with or without mandibular hyperostosis. The condition was first described in 1880 by an English physician, J.W. Legg.

In general, MMH is a rare condition of unknown etiology. The possible causes include inhabitual chewing, nocturnal involuntary teeth grinding (bruxism), use of anabolic steroids, and trauma. It is typically encountered in adults between 20 and 40 years of age with no gender predominance.

Patients with masticator muscle hypertrophy may present with facial asymmetry and concerns regarding cosmesis. However, occasionally patients may present with pain, dysfunctional mastication, and signs of Minotaur syndrome. Pathology involving the parotid space needs to be ruled out as a cause for those with facial asymmetry.

CT shows volumetric enlargement of the muscles of mastication "ensemble" or in isolation (uni or bilateral). 3D images can show the "threatening" appearance of the face. MRI shows no signal abnormality. It allows comprehensive soft tissue evaluation of masticator and parotid space.

Common Differential Diagnosis

- Hypotrophy/atrophy of counterpart: opposite-sided atrophy of the muscles of mastication.

Management Options

The treatment for MMH depends on the severity of the case. It can involve conservative treatment with antispasmodic, anxiolytic drugs, and analgesics, surgery, or a combination.

References and Further Reading

1. Haouimi A. Unilateral masticator muscles hypertrophy. "Radiopaedia.org". 2024. Accessed on 25 Jan 2024. https://doi.org/10.53347/rID-182328
2. Kebede B, Megersa S. Idiopathic masseter muscle hypertrophy. Ethiop J Health Sci. 2011. Accessed on 12 June 2025:https://pubmed.ncbi.nlm.nih.gov/22435002/ PMID: 22435002; PMCID: PMC3275871.
3. Opeyemi O et al. Unilateral masticator muscle hypertrophy with mandibular ramus hyperostosis. Int J Pediatr Otorhinolaryngol. 2011. Accessed on 25 Jan 2024. https://doi.org/10.1016/j.pedex.2011.06.001

Case 76

76

Clinical History

A 13-year-old boy presented with a history of chronic nasal discharge with fetid odor.

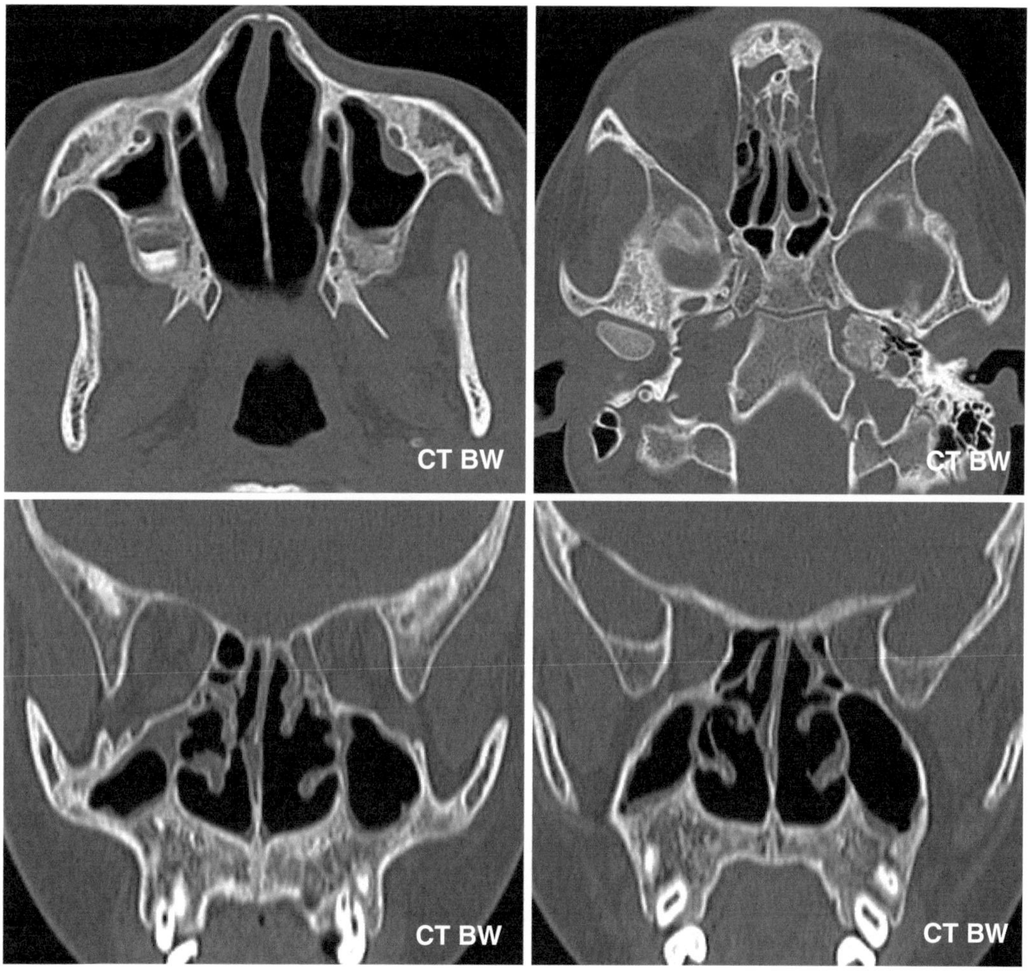

A. Haouimi et al., *Head and Neck Radiology Spot Diagnosis*,
https://doi.org/10.1007/978-3-032-14553-6_76

Findings

Enlarged nasal cavities with mild bowing of lateral nasal walls. Bilateral atrophy of all turbinates with bony resorption. Loss of definition of the ostiomeatal complex. Hypoplasia of the paranasal sinuses with mucoperiosteal thickening.

Diagnosis

Atrophic rhinitis.

Discussion

Atrophic rhinitis is a chronic nasal condition leading to shrinkage of nasal contents, particularly the nasal mucosa. Primary atrophic rhinitis or ozena is rare (less than 1%) and typically afflects middle-aged adults, more common in women. The possible causes of primary atrophic rhinitis are allergy, estrogen imbalance, and avitaminosis A and D. Secondary atrophic rhinitis is mostly due to postsurgical intervention. Other causes include post-radiation, sarcoidosis, syphilis, granulomatosis with polyangiitis (GPA), and autoimmune conditions. Rhinitis medicamentosa is another category of atrophic rhinitis resulting from chronic nasal decongestant use.

Clinically, patients with atrophic rhinitis often complain of the triad of fetor, crusting, and spacious nasal cavities with perceived congestion. Nasal dryness, halitosis, and anosmia can also be present.

Coronal sinus CT is the investigation of choice. The CT findings include loss of definition of the ostiomeatal complex, resorption of the ethmoid bulla, and uncinate process. CT also shows enlargement of the nasal cavities with erosion and bowing of the lateral nasal wall, bony resorption, and mucosal atrophy of the inferior and middle turbinates. Mucosal thickening of the paranasal sinuses and hypoplasia of the maxillary sinuses can sometimes be seen.

Common Differential Diagnosis

- Turbinectomy: clinical history, surgical amputation, not atrophy.

Management Options

Nasal moisturizing agents and regular nasal rinsing with saline water are recommended. Antibiotics are prescribed when there are signs of infection.

References and Further Reading

1. Bist SS et al. Primary atrophic rhinitis: a clinical profile, microbiological and radiological study. ISRNOtolaryngol. 2023. Accessed on 26 Jan 2024. https://doi.org/10.5402/2012/404075.
2. Haouimi A. Atrophic rhinitis. "Radiopaedia. org". 2024. Accessed on 26 Jan 2024. https://doi.org/10.53347/rID-182643.
3. Pace-Balzan, A et al. Computed tomographic findings in atrophicrhinitis. J Otolaryngol. 1991. Accessed on 26 Jan 2024. https://pubmed.ncbi.nlm.nih.gov/1774803/.

Case 77

77

Clinical History

A 90-year-old man presented with a left hemifacial painless swelling.

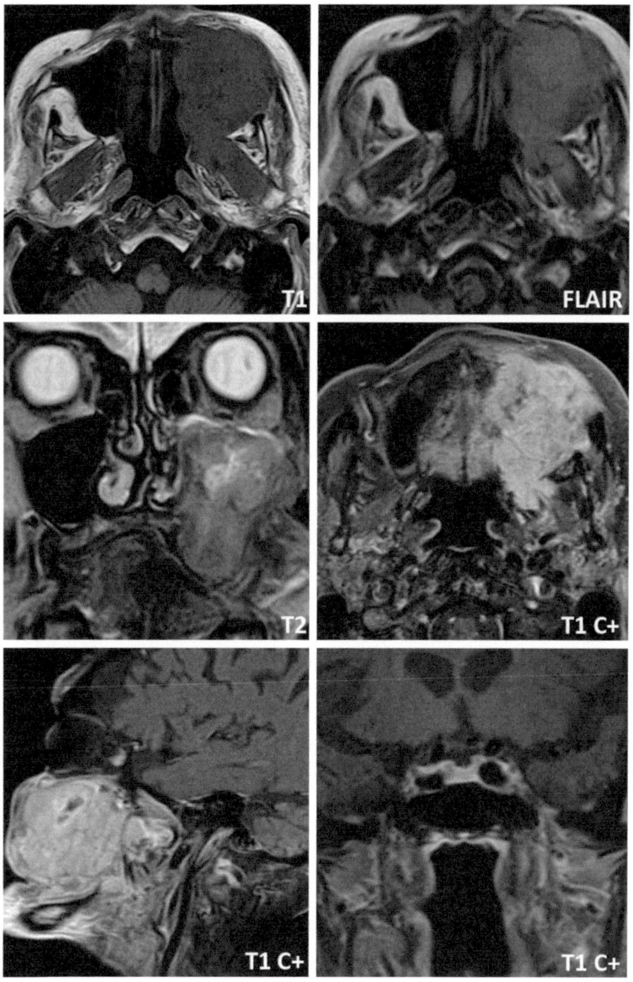

A. Haouimi et al., *Head and Neck Radiology Spot Diagnosis*,
https://doi.org/10.1007/978-3-032-14553-6_77

Findings

A poorly defined left maxillary soft tissue lesion showing a low signal intensity on T1 and intermediate to high signal on T2 and FLAIR with slightly heterogeneous enhancement. Extensive circumferential locoregional extension to the cheek, nasal cavity, inferior aspect of the left orbit, and hard palate. Posterior extension to adjacent pterygopalatine fossa, buccal fat pad, both pterygoids and masseter muscles. Perineural extension through left mandibular nerve.

Diagnosis

Adenoid cystic carcinoma of the maxillary sinus.

Discussion

Maxillary sinus adenoid cystic carcinomas are uncommon, malignant, aggressive lesions originating from minor salivary glands. They have poor long-term prognosis and a predisposition for perineural invasion. The lesions are characterized by indolent growth, a tendency to recur, locoregional invasion, and distant metastasis. It contributes to less than 1% of all head and neck malignancies and around 5% of paranasal sinus malignancies. The lesions are usually diagnosed in the elderly at advanced stage with a 10-year survival rate of 37–65%. Locoregional extension involves adjacent soft tissues, orbit, masticator space, and nasal cavity.

Clinically, the patients present with nasal obstruction, facial pain, swelling, and epistaxis. CT reveals bony destruction, and MRI shows the extent of locoregional invasion.

Common Differential Diagnosis

- Squamous cell carcinoma: rapid growth, typically lacks perineural extension.
- Juvenile nasopharyngeal angiofibroma: highly vascular, seen in adolescent males.
- Esthesioneuroblastoma: epicenter at cribriform plate of ethmoid "figure of 8" lesions.

Management Options

The treatment is surgical with or without radiation.

References and Further Reading

1. Gurung S et al. Adenoidcystic carcinoma of maxillary antrum: a casereport. Int J Surg Case Rep. 2022. Accessed on 08 Dec 2024. https://doi.org/10.1016/j.ijscr.2022.107055.
2. Haouimi A. Adenoid cystic carcinoma of the maxillary sinus. "Radiopaedia.org". 2024. Accessed on 08 Dec 2024. https://radiopaedia.org/cases/193227
3. Koeller KK. Radiologic features of sinonasal Tumors. Head Neck Pathol. 2016. Accessed on 14 Apr 2024: https://doi.org/10.1007/s12105-016-0686-9. Epub 2016 Feb 1. PMID: 26830408; PMCID: PMC4746141.

Case 78

78

Clinical History

A 45-year-old man presented with a painless swelling of the left side of the buccal cavity.

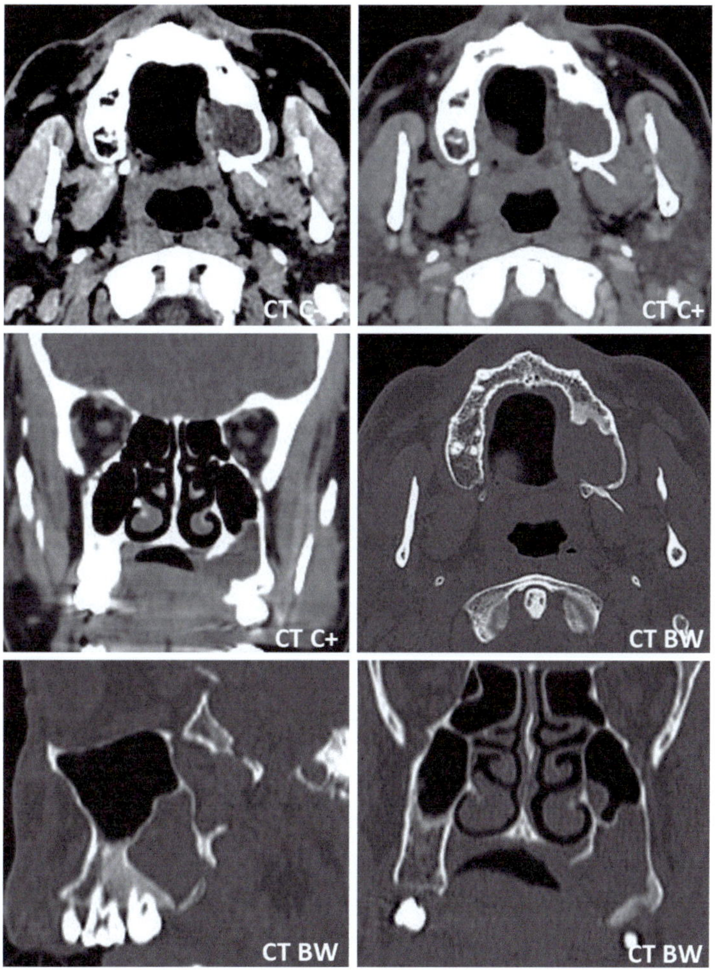

A. Haouimi et al., *Head and Neck Radiology Spot Diagnosis*,
https://doi.org/10.1007/978-3-032-14553-6_78

Findings

An expansile lytic lesion with hypodense internal content involving the left maxilla, adjacent to the root of the tooth #26 and tooth #27 on CT scan. Quasi-complete destruction of the medial wall of the maxilla, upward elevation of the floor of the maxillary sinus with an anterior sclerotic rim. No adjacent soft tissue component.

Diagnosis

Odontogenic fibromyxoma of the maxilla.

Discussion

Odontogenic fibromyxomas are slow-growing benign aggressive lesions of the jaw, mostly affecting the mandible. They arise mostly in females in their 20s and 30s. They are rarely seen in children or adults after 50 years. The lesions never metastasize to the lymphatics. Lesions are composed of mucus or gelatinous grayish white material containing collagen fibers in myxoid stroma. They are believed to originate from the mesenchymatous dental follicle, gingiva, and periodontal ligament. They replace the spongy bone and displace the cortical bone.

Clinically, small lesions are asymptomatic. Larger lesions can present as painless jaw expansion and facial deformity.

CT scan can show radiolucency of the alveolar processes with or without trabeculations. The appearance resembles "honey combing," "soap bubble," or "tennis racket." The cortical plate may be perforated. On MRI, the lesions are of low signal on T1 and high signal on T2. However, depending on cellularity, viscosity, protein, and hemoglobin breakdown products, the lesions can show high signal on T1.

Common Differential Diagnosis

- Ameloblastoma: curviform septa, multilocular, strong enhancement, low signal on T1.
- Fibrous dysplasia: ground glass appearance.
- Aneurysmal bone cyst: fluid–fluid levels, variable signal on T1, and high signal on T2.

Management Options

Smaller lesions are managed conservatively and need monitoring. For larger lesions, the options are enucleation, curettage, and radical surgery.

References and Further Reading

1. Dietrich EM et al. Odontogenic fibromyxoma of the maxilla: a case report and review of the literature. Case Rep Med. 2011. Accessed on 26 Jan 2024. https:/doi.org/10.1155/2011/238712. Epub 2011 May 2. PMID: 21629853; PMCID:
2. Haouimi A. Odontogenic fibromyxoma - maxilla. "Radiopaedia.org". 2024. Accessed on 26 Jan 2024. https://doi.org/10.53347/rID-180345.

Case 79

79

Clinical History

A 16-month-old boy presented with absent eyes since birth. No similar family history.

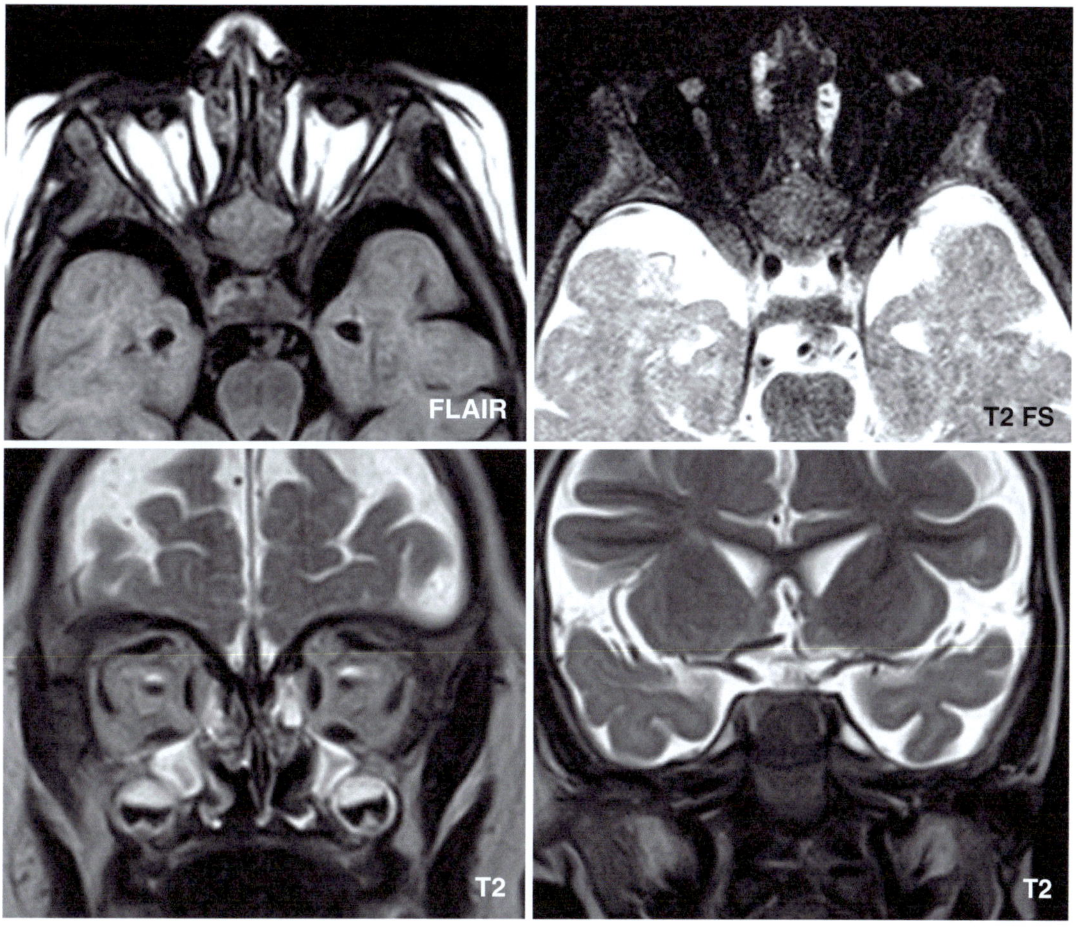

A. Haouimi et al., *Head and Neck Radiology Spot Diagnosis*,
https://doi.org/10.1007/978-3-032-14553-6_79

Findings

Bilateral absence of ocular globes, replaced by a residual soft tissue with thin hypoplastic optic nerves, optic chiasma, as well as the orbital muscles.

Diagnosis

Bilateral anophthalmia.

Discussion

Congenital anophthalmia or missing eyes refers to complete uni- or bilateral absence of the eye structures derived from the neural ectoderm. It is a rare genetic disorder. In many instances, they seem sporadic. This condition may be associated with other systemic malformations. In most of the cases, the eyelids, lacrimal apparatus, as well as conjunctiva are present. Anophthalmia is the severe form of microphthalmia and is the result of arrest of globe development during organogenesis.

This etiology is believed to be due to a combination of genetic and chromosomal changes coupled with environmental factors. Other predisposing factors may include the effects of thalidomide during pregnancy, maternal infection with rubella and toxoplasmosis, and radiation exposure. Anophthalmia can be either isolated or syndromic, and is associated with Aicardi, CHARGE, De Morsier, Hallermann–Streiff, and Norrie syndromes.

The diagnosis is clinical after birth but can also be detected during intrauterine life by fetal MRI. A 3D "reverse face" view on ultrasound can also be used for evaluation of the fetal orbits.

Common Differential Diagnosis

- The diagnosis is straightforward and no differential consideration.

Management Options

There cannot be a replacement for eye with a child born with micro or anophthalmia. Conforming devices including prosthetic eyes can help address cosmetic concerns as well as the development of orbits and facial bones.

References and Further Reading

1. Bridge H et al. Imaging studies in congenital anophthalmia reveal preservation of brain architecture in 'visual' cortex. Brain. 2009. Accessed on 17 July 2024: https://doi.org/10.1093/brain/awp279. PMID: 19892766.
2. Halilbasic M et al. Congenital bilateral anophthalmia: a case reportand review of literature. Med Arch. 2018. Accessed on 27 Jan 2024. https://doi.org/10.5455/medarh.2018.72.300-302. PMID 30515001 PMCID.
3. Haouimi A. Bilateral anophthalmia. "Radiopaedia.org". 2024. Accessed on 27 Jan 2024. https://doi.org/10.53347/rID-164313.

Case 80

80

Clinical History

A 5-year-old girl presented with a history of recurrent episodes of difficulty in breathing.

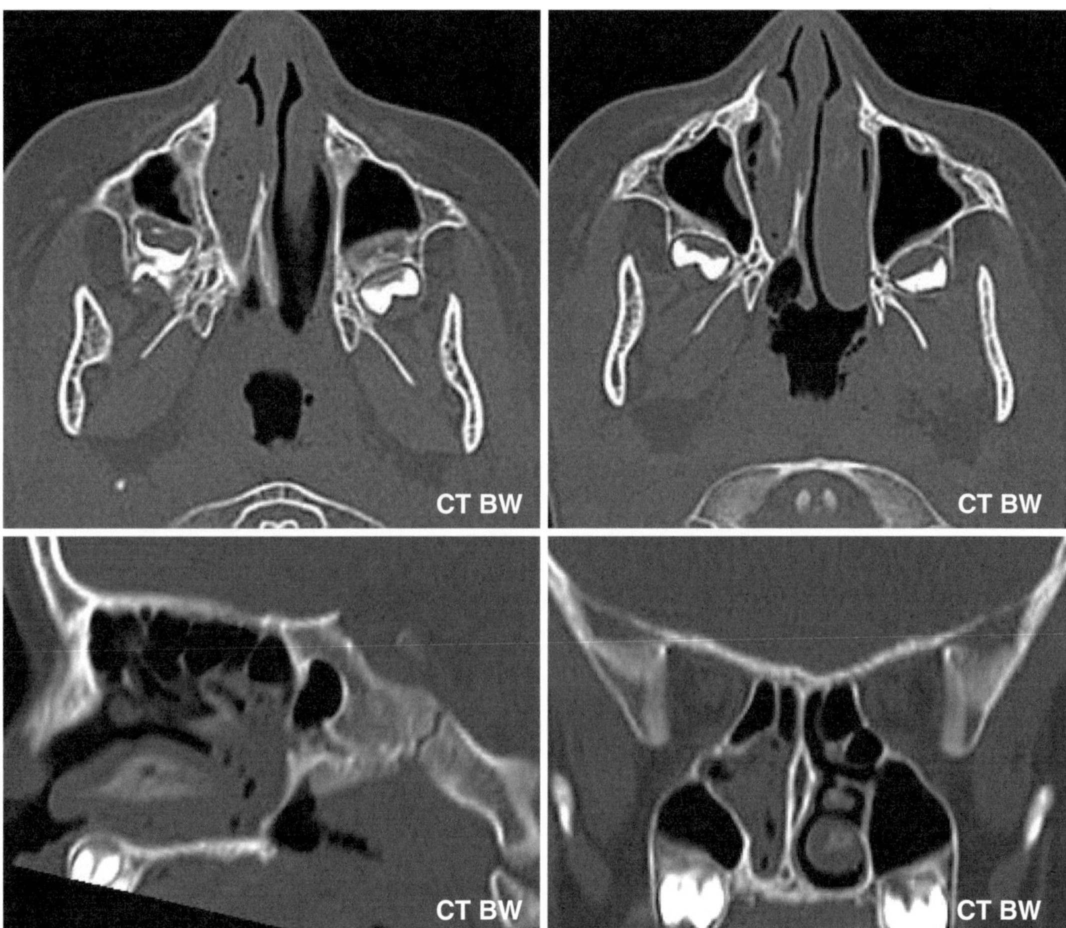

A. Haouimi et al., *Head and Neck Radiology Spot Diagnosis*,
https://doi.org/10.1007/978-3-032-14553-6_80

Findings

Complete obstruction of the posterior aspect of the right nasal cavity with bony wall and retained secretions in the right nasal cavity.

Diagnosis

Unilateral choanal atresia.

Discussion

The choana is considered the entrance to the nasopharynx. Failed recanalization of the nasal fossa during fetal development leads to choanal atresia, which occurs when bone, mucous membrane, or both are involved. This condition can be either unilateral or bilateral. It is typically syndromic and associated with Tessier, CHARGE, and Treacher Collins syndromes.

Bilateral choanal atresia causes infants to breathe only through their mouths when they cry. Acute breathing problems in bilateral choanal atresia result in cyanosis, and such infants may require resuscitation during the postnatal period. The chest retracts unless the child is crying. The severity of the symptoms is less and non-life-threatening for unilateral cases.

A 2-mm thin reformed coronal sinus CT scan can easily demonstrate thickening of the anterior portion of the pterygoid plates, thickening of the vomer, and medial bowing of the posterior maxilla, with or without membranous involvement.

Common Differential Diagnosis

- Choanal stenosis: narrowed choana, not occluded.
- Bilateral dacryocystocele: cystic lesions at both inferior meatus.
- Pyriform aperture stenosis: stenosis of anterior nasal opening.

Management Options

Bilateral choanal atresia in an infant with airway obstruction is a perinatal emergency. The goal of treatment is to maintain an adequate airway via the oral route. Surgical correction of bilateral cases should be considered as soon as possible.

References and Further Reading

1. Andaloro C La, Mantia I ChoanalAtresia. Stat Pearls Publishing. 2023. Accessed on 27 Jan 2024. https://www.ncbi.nlm.nih.gov/books/NBK507724/.
2. Haouimi A. Choanal atresia. “Radiopaedia.org”. 2024. Accessed on 27 Jan 2024. https://doi.org/10.53347/rID-181594.
3. Kwong KM. Current updates on choanal atresia. Front Pediatr. 2015. Accessed on 27 Jan 2024. https://doi.org/10.3389/fped.2015.00052. PMID: 26106591; PMCID: PMC4460812.

Case 81

81

Clinical History

A 1-year-old girl presented with a progressively increasing swelling of the left frontal region since birth.

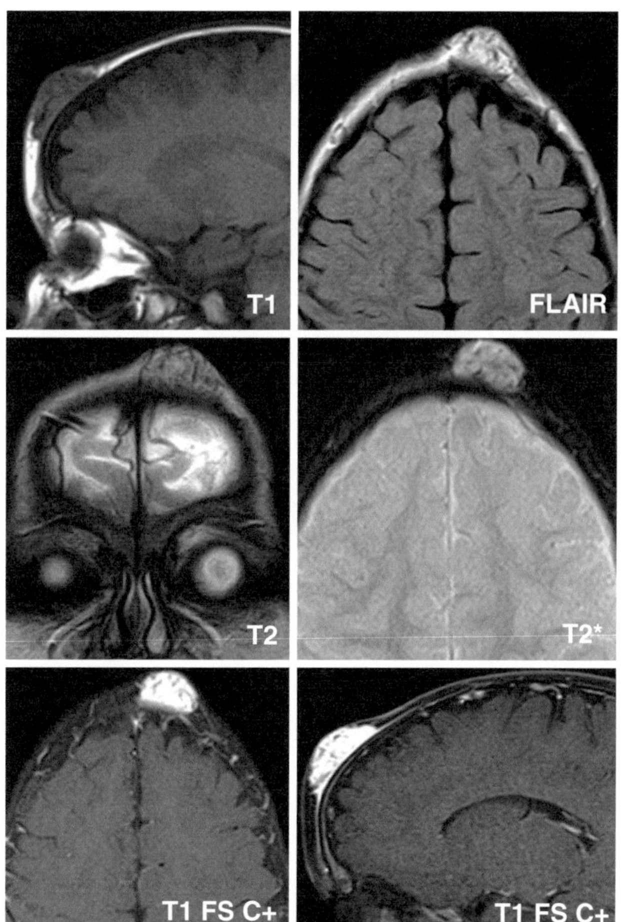

A. Haouimi et al., *Head and Neck Radiology Spot Diagnosis*,
https://doi.org/10.1007/978-3-032-14553-6_81

Findings

Left frontal off-midline well-defined subcutaneous soft tissue mass. It demonstrates intermediate signal on T1, high signal on T2, and FLAIR with internal flow void indicating vascular structures. Vivid homogeneous enhancement. Intact adjacent external table of the skull, no intracranial extension.

Diagnosis

Infantile scalp hemangioma.

Discussion

Infantile hemangiomas, also known as "strawberry" birthmarks, are benign self-limiting vascular neoplasms that usually resolve on their own by 10 years without treatment. They may occur in up to 5% of infants. Most lesions are not present at birth but appear within weeks following birth. They grow rapidly during first 3 months and usually complete growing by the fifth month. Lesions are more common in Caucasian twins, and in low birthweight premature infants.

Lesions appear as a red cutaneous patch or as focal cutaneous bump. More deeply seated hemangiomas may appear bluish. Larger lesion size, raised periorbital, perioral, and diaper area lesions, bleeding open sore hemangiomas, and those with more than five hemangiomas are considered higher risk. Those infants need special medical attention. The lesions can present as a component of PHACES, LUMBAR, and Kasabach–Merritt syndrome.

The diagnosis is straightforward. No radiological investigation except in high-risk hemangiomas. Ultrasound and color Doppler show a well-defined echogenic mass with prominent internal vascularity. On CT, the lesions are isodense with intense enhancement without any phleboliths. On MRI, these show an isosignal on T1 and high signal on T2 with homogeneous enhancement.

Common Differential Diagnosis

- AVM: bigger size, multiple flow voids.
- Veno-lymphatic malformation: mostly cystic, no or very minimal enhancement.
- Angiosarcoma: aggressive growth, intense contrast pulling, heterogeneous enhancement.

Management Options

Infantile hemangiomas are "do not touch" lesions. Some physicians prefer to treat with beta blockers such as propranolol. High-risk cases need multidisciplinary care and referral to specialists.

References and Further Reading

1. Haouimi A. Infantile haemangioma of th escalp. "Radiopaedia.org". 2024. Accessed on 27 Jan 2024. https://doi.org/10.53347/rID-94478.
2. Larson, AS et al. Imaging of benign cervicofacial vascular anomalies and associated syndromes. Interv Neuroradiol. 2022. Accessed on 12 May 2024: https://doi.org/10.1177/15910199211034989.

Case 82

82

Clinical History

A 60-year-old man presented with a history of right-sided reduced visual acuity.

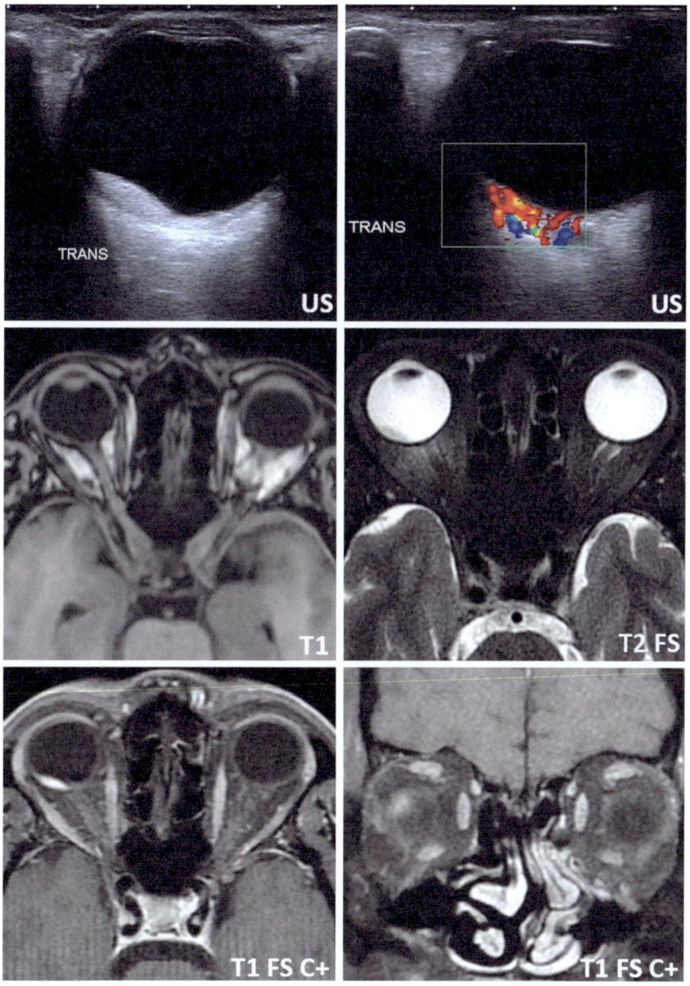

A. Haouimi et al., *Head and Neck Radiology Spot Diagnosis*,
https://doi.org/10.1007/978-3-032-14553-6_82

Findings

Ultrasound shows an echogenic dome-shaped lesion with a broad choroidal base in the posterior temporal quadrant of the right eye. The lesion shows prominent internal vascularity on color Doppler. On MRI, this choroidal mass demonstrates intermediate signal on T1, slightly low signal on T2 with vivid and homogeneous enhancement. No extraocular extension.

Diagnosis

Choroidal hemangioma.

Discussion

Choroidal hemangiomas are rare benign vascular hamartomas, usually seen in middle-aged Caucasians with no appreciable gender predilection. Circumscribed lesions are usually elevated, "orange red" or "salmon colored," situated posterior to the equator, and remain contained in one region. Diffuse choroidal hemangiomas appear as ill-defined "splashed ketchup" spots. The diffuse choroidal hemangiomas involve more than one zone or adjacent quadrants. Most of the diffuse choroidal hemangiomas are associated with Sturge–Weber syndrome. Clinically, the patient complains of painless, progressive, blurred vision with visual field defect, floaters, and metamorphopsia. Symptoms are caused by the accumulation of subretinal serous fluid or degenerative changes in the macula or both.

Ultrasound shows the lesion as a dome-shaped mass with broad choroidal base, isoechoic to normal choroid. On MRI, lesions appear as high signal on T1 and iso or hyperintense on T2.

Common Differential Diagnosis

- Choroidal melanoma: high signal on T1 and low signal on T2.
- Choroidal metastasis: history, low signal on T1 and high signal on T2.
- Sturge–Weber syndrome: brain changes like tram-track calcification, cerebral hemiatrophy.

Management Options

Asymptomatic cases are usually monitored periodically. Treatment options include photodynamic and radiation therapy or anti-VEGF injections. The endpoint is resolution of fluid and not complete tumor regression.

References and Further Reading

1. Haouimi A. Choroidal haemangioma. "Radiopaedia.org". 2019. Accessed on 27 Jan 2024. https://doi.org/10.53347/rID-72469.
2. Lupidi M et al. New insights on circumscribed choroidal hemangioma: "bench to bedside". Graefes Arch Clin Exp Ophthalmol. 2024. Accessed on 18 June 2025: https://doi.org/10.1007/s00417-023-06179-x.
3. Sen, M. Honavar, SG. Circumscribed choroidal hemangioma: an overview of clinical manifestation, diagnosis and management. Indian J Ophthalmol. 2019. Accessed on 27 Jan 2024. https://doi.org/10.4103/ijo.IJO_2036_19.

Case 83

83

Clinical History

A 25-year-old man presented with a history of progressive painless swelling of the right buccal cheek of 8 years duration.

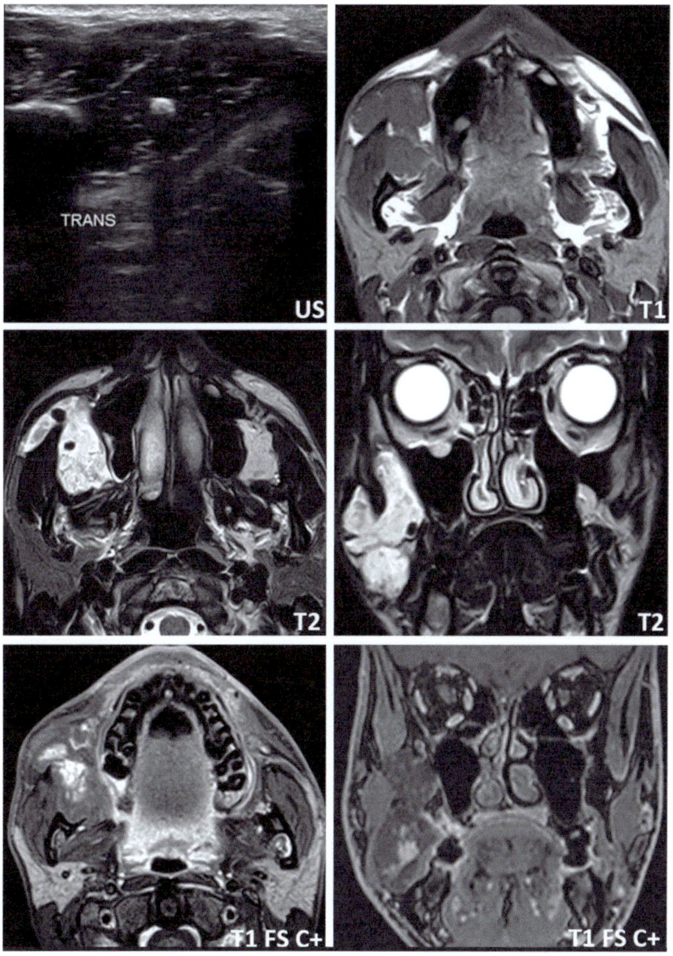

A. Haouimi et al., *Head and Neck Radiology Spot Diagnosis*,
https://doi.org/10.1007/978-3-032-14553-6_83

Findings

Heterogeneous hypoechoic mass in the cheek containing cystic spaces and calcification (phleboliths) on ultrasound. On MRI, the buccal space lesion is isointense to the muscles on T1, markedly hyperintense on T2 with foci of calcification (phleboliths). Progressive enhancement with partial filling on delayed images.

Diagnosis

Hemangioma of the buccal space.

Discussion

Anatomically, the buccal or buccinator space is a pyramidal, fat-filled, incomplete space interposed between the platysma and buccinator muscle. It is medial to the masseter, anterior to the medial pterygoid and mandibular ramus, and posterior to the orbicularis oris muscle. There is no real boundary between the buccal and submandibular spaces. This space contains no buccal mucosa and contains the distal Stensen's duct, minor salivary glands, a few lymph nodes, buccal branches of the facial and mandibular nerves as well as facial artery and facial veins. Buccal space lesions have potential to extend into the infratemporal, parapharyngeal, and pterygomandibular spaces.

On MR imaging, the hemangioma shows low signal on T1 and high signal on T2 with T1 enhancement. The primary purpose of imaging is to determine the site of origin and extent of the lesions. A sound knowledge of the expected CT and MR findings of the contents of buccal space is very helpful for the radiologist to reach a specific diagnosis.

Common Differential Diagnosis

- Arteriovenous malformation: serpiginous flow voids.
- Lymphangioma: low signal on T1 and high signal on T2, septated, fluid–fluid levels.
- Accessory parotid gland: along anterior margin of masseter, isosignal to parotid gland.

Management Options

The main purpose of treatment is to reduce symptoms and minimize functional and esthetic impairment. Small asymptomatic lesions are "do not touch" lesions. Management depends on size, location, and age. Options include beta-blockers, oral steroids, sclerotherapy, and surgical excision.

References and Further Reading

1. Haouimi A. Haemangioma – buccal space. "Radiopaedia.org". 2024. Accessed on 27 Jan 2024. https://doi.org/10.53347/rID-71055.
2. Hassani A et al. Hemangioma of the buccal fat pad. Contemp Clin Dent. 2014. Accessed on 25 Dec 2024. https://doi.org/10.4103/0976-237X.132368. PMID: 24963256; PMCID: PMC4067793.
3. Kim HC et al. MR imaging of the buccal space: normal anatomy and abnormalities. Korean J Radiol. 2005. Accessed on 10 June 2024:https://doi.org/10.3348/kjr.2005.6.1.22.

Case 84

84

Clinical History

A 15-year-old boy presented with a painless swelling of the right parotid region. “Wattle sign” on clinical examination.

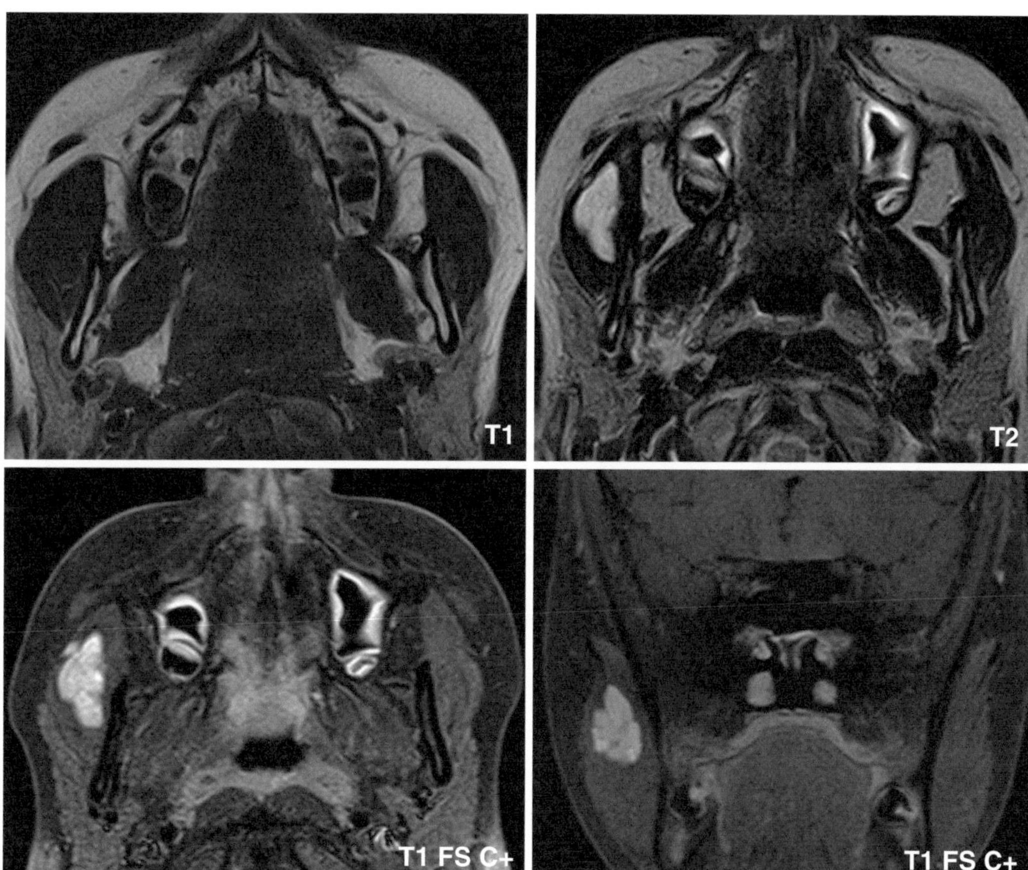

A. Haouimi et al., *Head and Neck Radiology Spot Diagnosis*,
https://doi.org/10.1007/978-3-032-14553-6_84

Findings

A small lobulated soft tissue mass within the right masseter muscle. It is isointense to the muscle on T1, markedly hyperintense on T2 with progressive enhancement on dynamic images (not shown). Complete fill-in on delayed postcontrast axial and coronal images.

Diagnosis

Intramuscular hemangioma of masseter muscle.

Discussion

About 15% of all intramuscular hemangiomas are found in the head and neck regions. The masseter muscle is the most common site. They are believed to arise from abnormal embryonic sequestrations, like congenital arteriovenous malformations. Trauma and hormonal factors have also been suspected as a triggering factor.

Clinically, the patient presents with a painless cheek swelling that increases in size with teeth-clenching or depending on head positioning. This pathognomonic clinical finding is the "wattle sign" where the lesion enlarges when the head is positioned such that the mass is in the dependent position and arises due to vascular engorgement within the lesion, which impedes venous return. The lesions are often cystic or echoic and heterogeneous with posterior acoustic shadows due to phleboliths. On CT, the lesions appear as a well-defined isodense mass containing phleboliths with enhancement. MRI shows the lesion as a well-defined, low-signal lobulated soft tissue mass on T1 and high signal on T2 with progressive enhancement and complete fill-in on delayed postcontrast sequences. No restricted diffusion is seen on dMRI.

Common Differential Diagnosis

- Sialocele of Stensen's duct: clinical, often traumatic, negative "wattle sign."
- Facial nerve schwannoma: signs of facial neuropathy, linear, nonprogressive enhancement.
- Lymphangiomas: multilocular, fluid–fluid level, septations may enhance.
- Masseter abscess: clinical, painful, dental infection +, ring enhancement.

Management Options

The treatment options are individualized depending on the clinical status of the patients.

References and Further Reading

1. Alami B. Presumptive intramuscular hemangioma of the masseter muscle. Am J Case Rep. 2015. Accessed on 27 Jan 2024. https://doi.org/10.12659/AJCR.890776.
2. Haouimi A. Intramuscular haemangioma – masseter muscle. "Radiopaedia.org". 2024. Accessed on 27 Jan 2024. https://doi.org/10.53347/rID-67796.
3. Koltsidopoulos P. et al. 2015. Intramuscular hemangioma with turkey wattle sign. CMAJ. Accessed on 27 Jan 2024. https://doi.org/10.1503/cmaj.140364

Case 85

85

Clinical History

A 15-year-old boy presented with a history of right nasal obstruction.

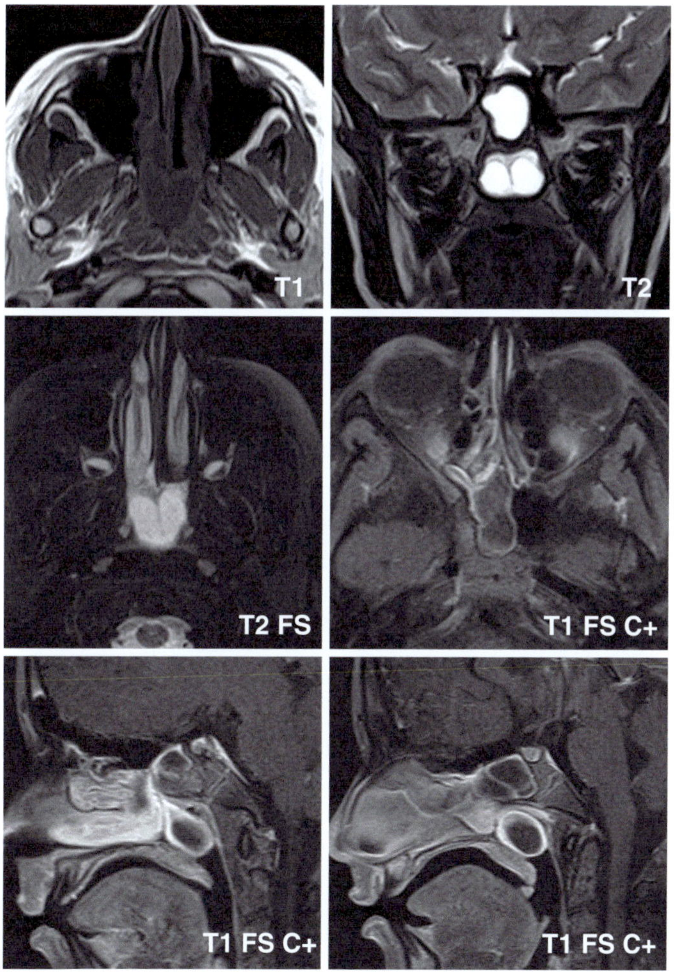

A. Haouimi et al., *Head and Neck Radiology Spot Diagnosis*,
https://doi.org/10.1007/978-3-032-14553-6_85

Findings

A well-defined pedunculated polypoid lesion arising from the sphenoid sinus, extending through the sphenoethmoidal recess to the nasopharynx, exiting through sphenoid sinusostium. It is obstructing both choanae. The lesion shows a low signal intensity on T1, high signal intensity on T2 with peripheral enhancement on postcontrast images. Clear maxillary sinuses.

Diagnosis

Sphenochoanal polyp.

Discussion

Nasal polyps that extend to the posterior nasal aperture are known as choanal polyps. Isolated sphenochoanal polyp is relatively uncommon. It is believed that sphenochoanal polyps arise from a precursor intramural cyst in the anterior mucosal wall of sphenoid sinus. Lesions are pedunculated, they exit the sphenoid sinus through the ostium and reach the choana through sphenoethmoidal recess. Most isolated sphenochoanal polyps do not reach the middle meatus. That is why they do not cause maxillary sinusitis. Isolated unilateral choanal lesion without any maxillary sinusitis should always raise the suspicion of sphenochoanal polyp.

Unilateral nasal obstruction, rhinorrhea, snoring, and headache are the most common clinical features.

Both CT and MRI are very important for diagnosis and for adequate preoperative evaluation. Both modalities help to identify the intrasinusal origin, detect ostial and extrasinusal components, and precisely specify the anatomical extent and relations to adjacent structures.

Common Differential Diagnosis

- Antrochoanal polyp: maxillary sinus origin passing through maxillary ostium.
- Nasopharyngeal angiofibroma: Holman-Miller sign + (anterior bulge of the posterior maxillary sinus wall), pterygopalatine epicenter, intralesional signal voids, intense enhancement.
- Inverted papilloma: striated cerebriform appearance on T2 or on postcontrast T1.

Management Options

Endoscopic sinus surgery and ostial widening need to be considered after adequate evaluation.

References and Further Reading

1. Haouimi A. Spheno-choanal polyp. “Radiopaedia.org”. 2024. Accessed on 30 Jan 2024. https://doi.org/10.53347/rID-65840.
2. Kumral TL, Yildirim G, Uyar Y. Sphenochoanal polyps and the optic nerve. Clin Pract. 2012. Accessed on 30 Jan 2024. https://doi.org/10.4081/cp.2012.e10. PMID: 24765409; PMCID: PMC3981331.

Case 86

86

Clinical History

A 55-year-old man presented with a history of hard swelling of the left cheek.

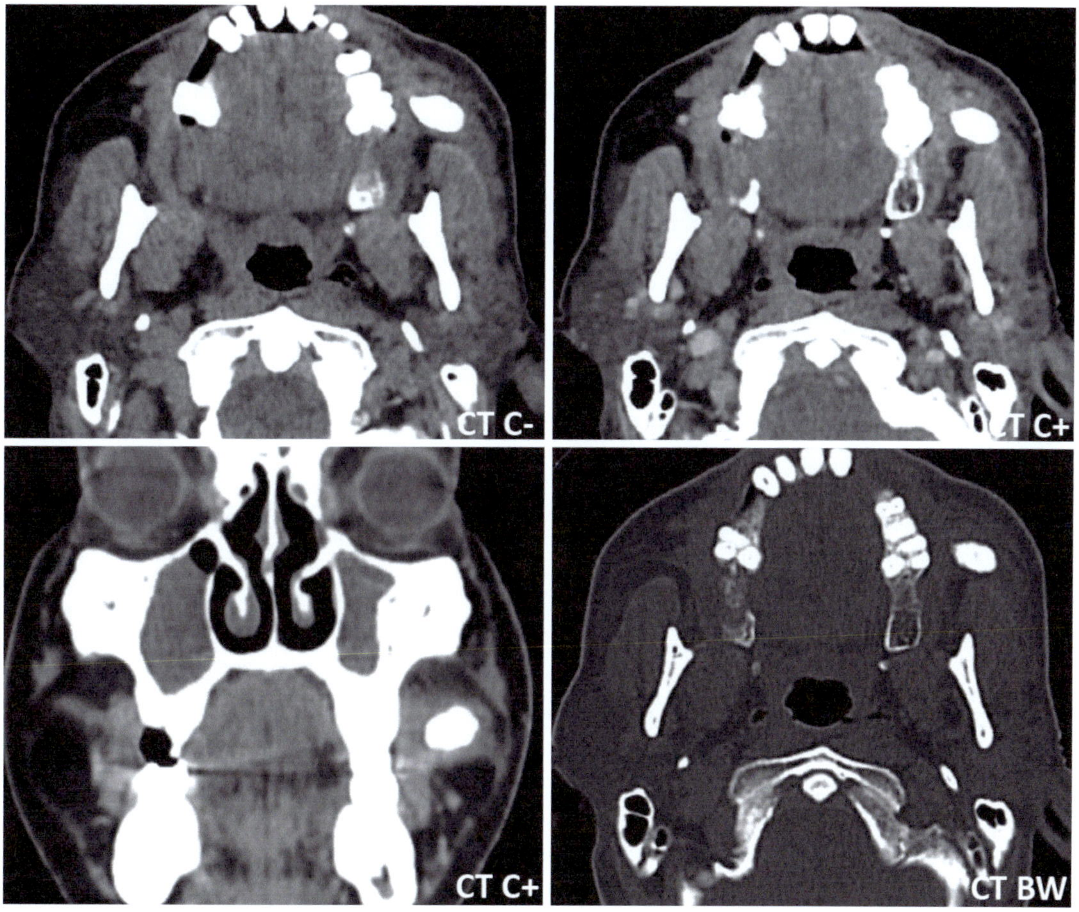

A. Haouimi et al., *Head and Neck Radiology Spot Diagnosis*,
https://doi.org/10.1007/978-3-032-14553-6_86

Findings

A calcification within the left Stensen's duct along the anterior edge of left masseter, at the level of second upper molar tooth. Induration of neighboring buccal space fat plane with strandings. Mild contrast enhancement of the ipsilateral parotid gland. Incidental bilateral chronic maxillary sinusitis.

Diagnosis

Sialolithiasis and chronic sialadenitis of the parotid gland.

Discussion

Sialolithiasis is a benign condition due to the presence of stones within salivary ducts, most frequently seen in Wharton's (up to about 80%) and Stensen's ducts (up to about 80%). It causes obstruction of the duct, leading to obstructive sialadenitis. Ductal stenosis and increased salivary calcium content are believed to be a risk of stone formation. Multiple internal microcalculi within salivary gland secretory granules act as a nidus for the formation of larger-sized sialoliths. Retrograde flow of food debris from the oral cavity can also be a potential pathophysiological factor in the development of sialolithiasis.

Due to off-and-on blockage of the duct, the patients complain of intermittent pain, especially worsening during eating, "salivary colic." In long-standing cases, the salivary gland may stop producing saliva, become firm and atrophic resulting in chronic sialadenitis.

Enhanced CT shows enlarged unilateral salivary gland with intraductal stone +/− and dilatation of proximal duct in acute cases. In chronic cases, the salivary gland appears atrophic.

Common Differential Diagnosis

- Small pleomorphic tumor: smoothly marginated, enhancing intraparotid lesion, no stone.
- Warthin tumor: history, intraparotid, no calcification, enhancement with mural nodule +/−.
- Sjögren syndrome: bilateral, no stone.

Management Options

Mostly conservative with anti-inflammatories and antibiotics, expecting spontaneous regression. Distal stones in Wharton's ducts are considered for marsupialization in selected cases.

References and Further Reading

1. Hammett JT, Walker C. Sialolithiasis. Stat Pearls Publishing. 2024. Accessed on 30 Jan 2024. https://www.ncbi.nlm.nih.gov/books/NBK549845/.
2. Haouimi A. Sialolithiasis – parotid. "Radiopaedia.org". 2024. Accessed on 30 Jan 2024. https://doi.org/10.53347/rID-71613.
3. Orlandi MA, Pistorio V, Guerra PA. Ultrasound in sialadenitis. J Ultrasound. 2013. Accessed on 14 Sept 2025: https://doi.org/10.1007/s40477-013-0002-4. PMID: 24046793; PMCID: PMC3774898.

Case 87

87

Clinical History

A 45-year-old man presented with a 2-year history of nasal obstruction.

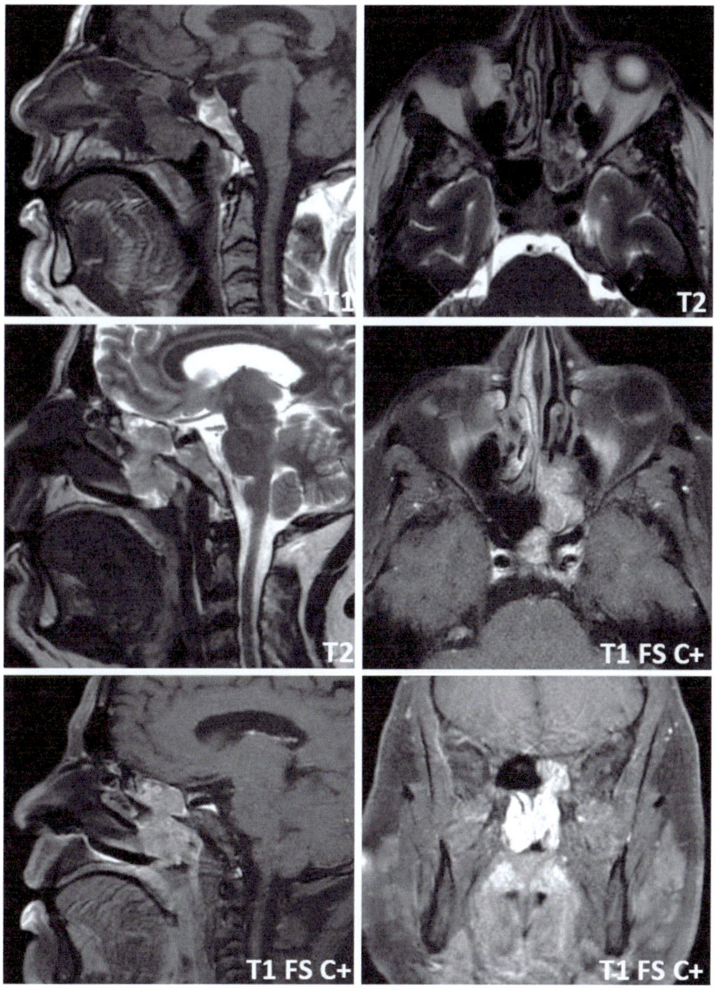

A. Haouimi et al., *Head and Neck Radiology Spot Diagnosis*,
https://doi.org/10.1007/978-3-032-14553-6_87

Findings

A well-defined soft tissue mass arising from the sphenoid sinus. It extends through the floor of the sphenoid sinus into the nasopharynx, obstructing both choanae (mainly the left). It is of intermediate signal on T1, inhomogeneously high signal on T2 with marked heterogeneous enhancement.

Diagnosis

Schneiderian papilloma.

Discussion

Schneiderian papillomas, or sinonasal papillomas, are uncommon benign epithelial neoplasms arising from ectodermally derived pseudostratified ciliated epithelial lining of the nasal cavity and the sinonasal tract. It affects mostly middle-aged men. The lesions have a tendency to recur, are locally aggressive, and have the potential to develop squamous cell carcinoma. Histologically, three different types have been identified: (a) fungiform, (b) oncocytic, and (c) inverted. The inverted type has the most malignant potential.

The etiology is unknown but there appears to be a strong association with human papillomavirus.

Clinically, the patients can remain asymptomatic for some time. While seeking medical attention, they have signs of chronic rhinosinusitis, nasal obstruction, epistaxis, postnasal dribbling, and anosmia.

Radiologically, most of the lesions appear as a soft tissue density/intensity "septate, striated" appearance along the nasal septum with/without evidence of septal erosion. Findings are nonspecific and need histological confirmation.

Common Differential Diagnosis

- Juvenile nasopharyngeal angiofibroma: sphenopalatine epicenter in male.
- Esthesioneuroblastoma: cribriform plate epicenter, figure of eight lesion.

Management Options

Surgical removal is the best primary option.

References and Further Reading

1. Bishop JA et al. An update on sinonasal (Schneiderian) papillomas. Head Neck Pathol. 2017. Accessed on 30 Jan 2024. https://doi.org/10.1007/s12105-017-0799-9. Epub 2017 Mar 20. PMID: 28321771; PMCID: PMC5550400.
2. Clarke SR, Amedee RG. Schneiderian papilloma. J La State Med Soc. 1997. Accessed on 30 Jan 2024. PMID: 9316345. https://pubmed.ncbi.nlm.nih.gov/9316345/.
3. Haouimi A. Schneiderian papilloma. "Radiopaedia. org". 2024. Accessed on 30 Jan 2024. https://doi.org/10.53347/rID-67059.

Case 88

88

Clinical History

A 20-year-old woman presented with dyspnea. History of road traffic accident, admitted in ICU, intubated for 6 months, then discharged with a Montgomery tracheal tube.

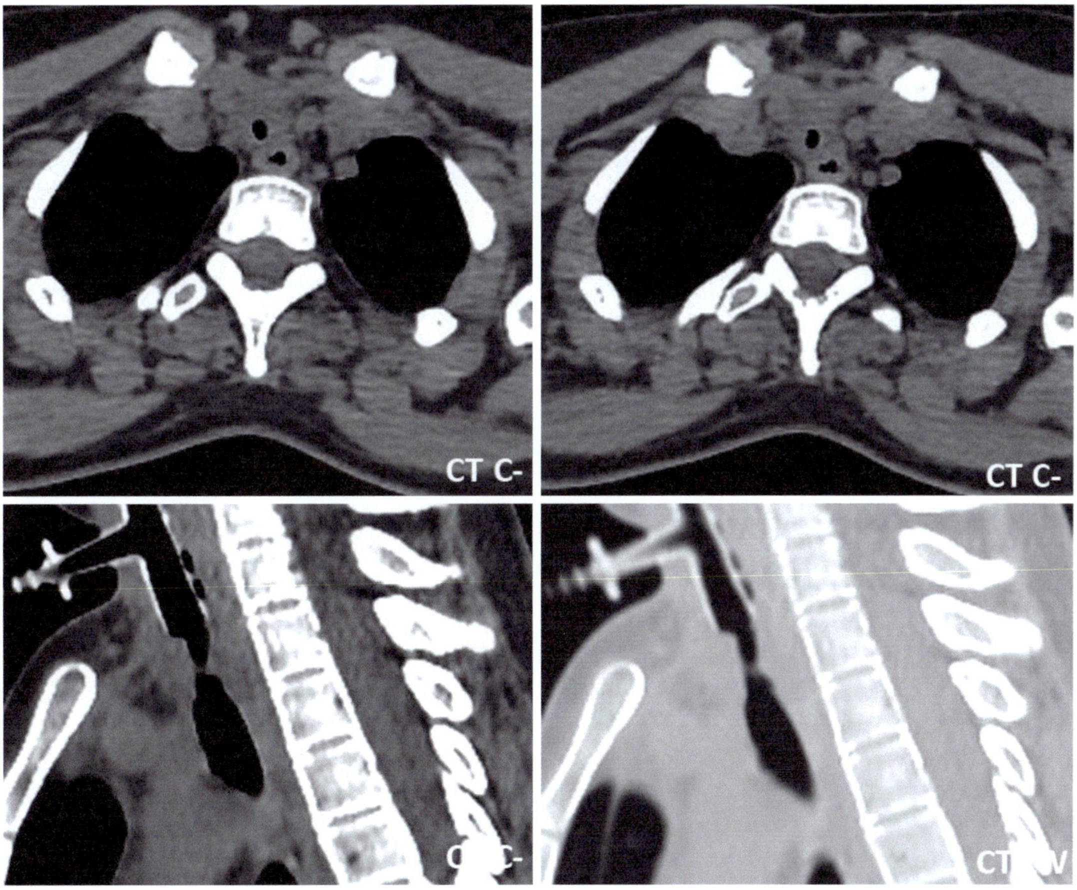

A. Haouimi et al., *Head and Neck Radiology Spot Diagnosis*,
https://doi.org/10.1007/978-3-032-14553-6_88

Findings

Narrowing of tracheal lumen for about 1.5 cm in length in the mid-trachea, well visualized on the sagittal reconstruction.

Diagnosis

Postintubation tracheal stenosis.

Discussion

Tracheal stenosis is mostly a complication of intubation or tracheostomy. Congenital causes are infrequent. Other less common causes are trauma, tumor and postradiation following cancer treatment. Acute postintubation narrowing is due to mucosal edema. Tracheal stenosis typically occurs weeks to months after extubation. High cuff pressure on the endotracheal or tracheostomy tube compresses the tracheal mucosa. Inflammation and constant pressure on the tracheal mucosa led to ischemia to necrosis, and fibrosis. A longer duration of intubation is associated with a greater risk of tracheal stenosis. Stenosis usually extends for several centimeters and typically involves the subglottic region and the site of the cuff above the level of the thoracic inlet. Posttracheostomy stenosis usually starts about 1 cm below the inferior margin of the tracheostomy.

The clinical issues are progressive shortness of breath, stridor and wheezing associated with persistent cough and recurrent respiratory tract infection.

Plain X-rays show narrowing of the intratracheal air column. CT shows eccentric or concentric narrowing of the tracheal lumen due to soft tissue thickening of tracheal mucosa. CT can identify the site and the degree of stenosis. No change of tracheal diameter is observed during inspiration and expiration.

Common Differential Diagnosis

- Diagnosis is straight forward in an appropriate clinical history.

Management Options

Mild cases are managed conservatively with anti-inflammatory drugs and antibiotics. Other options are endoscopic and surgical intervention.

References and Further Reading

1. Haouimi A. Tracheal stenosis: postintubation. Case study, Radiopaedia.org. Accessed on 07 Dec 2024. https://doi.org/10.53347/rID-68011.
2. Radswiki T, Walizai T, Ranchod A, et al. Tracheal stenosis. Reference article, Radiopaedia.org. Accessed on 12 Dec 2024. https://doi.org/10.53347/rID-15607.

Case 89

89

Clinical History

A 25-year-old man presented with a history of left mucopurulent nasal discharge and headaches.

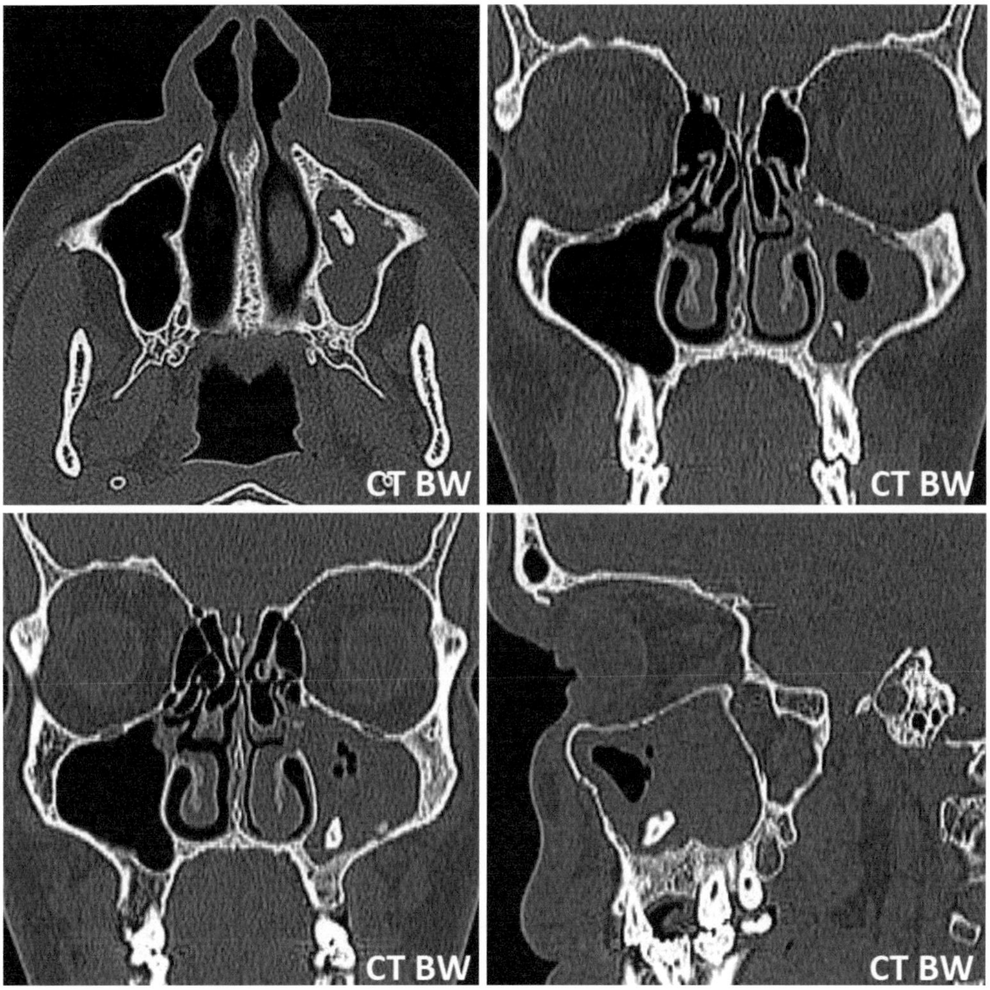

A. Haouimi et al., *Head and Neck Radiology Spot Diagnosis*,
https://doi.org/10.1007/978-3-032-14553-6_89

Findings

A dentiform radiopaque structure within the left maxillary antrum. Peripheral mucosal thickening of left maxillary sinus walls without an air-fluid level. Complete obstruction of left maxillary ostium. No bony defect of the orbital roof or floor.

Diagnosis

Ectopic intramaxillary molar tooth and chronic left maxillary sinusitis.

Discussion

Ectopic teeth refer to the presence of a tooth in any abnormal location. They are found at many sites, including the mandible, nasal septum, maxillary antrum, and maxillary sinus, due to abnormal interaction between oral epithelium and the underlying mesenchymal tissue during odontogenesis. The etiology remains poorly understood. Genetic predisposition, early loss of primary teeth, trauma, infection, and supernumerary teeth are all considered as risk factors.

Clinically, most ectopic teeth appear in the second or third decade of life with no symptoms. Intramaxillary ectopic tooth may cause signs of chronic sinusitis and occasional purulent discharge. Any atypical pain, swelling, and discharge in maxillofacial region should raise the possibility of an ectopic tooth.

Due to their radiopaque nature, ectopic tooth can be diagnosed by both plain film and panoramic radiograph. CT is the gold standard to determine the precise location, morphology, root inclination, and its relation to the underlying structures for optimized surgical planning.

Common Differential Diagnosis

- Rhinolith: round or oval shape, intranasal, normal dentition, normal dental arch.
- Intramaxillary osteoma: attached to bony maxillary wall.
- Chronic sinusitis: mucosal thickening, no dentiform intramaxillary radiopaque structure.

Management Options

Intramaxillary ectopic tooth is usually removed surgically. They tend to form a cyst or tumor and/or complications like chronic maxillary sinusitis and occasional perforation of the floor of the orbit.

References and Further Reading

1. Akbas M, Karabıyık Z, Varol A. Ectopic tooth in mandibular canal, maxillarysinus, and mandibular condyle. Case Rep Dent. Accessed on 06 Feb 2024. https://doi.org/10.1155/2022/3118998. PMID: 35103105; PMCID: PMC8800632.
2. Haouimi A. Ectopic tooth in maxillary antrum with secondary chronic sinusitis. "Radiopaedia.org". 2024. Accessed on 06 Feb 06, 2024. https://doi.org/10.53347/rID-180460.

Case 90

90

Clinical History

A 55-year-old man presented with a painless swelling of the right parietal region.

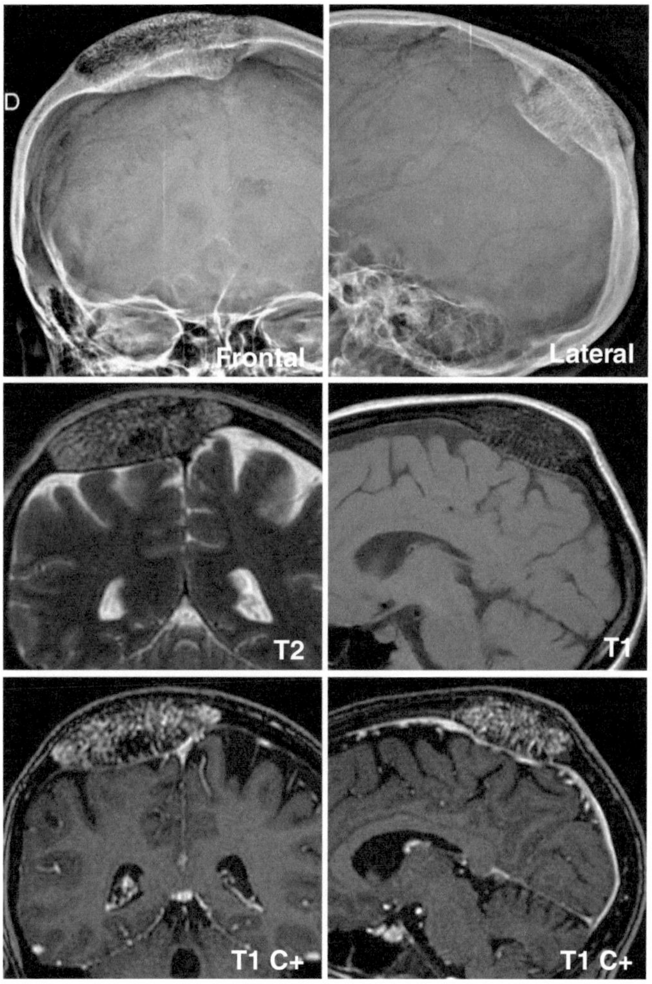

A. Haouimi et al., *Head and Neck Radiology Spot Diagnosis*,
https://doi.org/10.1007/978-3-032-14553-6_90

Findings

A well-circumscribed expansile lytic lesion of the right parietal bone with a sclerotic rim on X-ray. It is composed of thick and dense radiating spicules from the center, creating a classic "sunburst appearance." On MRI, it is nonhomogeneously hypointense on T1 and hyperintense on T2 with nonhomogeneous enhancement. There is a mass effect on the adjacent brain parenchyma and the superior sagittal sinus, which remains patent.

Diagnosis

Calvarial hemangioma.

Discussion

Calvarial hemangiomas are benign vascular tumors that arise from the diploic space. They primarily affect the parietal and frontal bones and are commonly observed in women between the fourth and fifth decades of life. These benign, slow-growing vascular lesions are typically asymptomatic and are discovered incidentally. Occasionally, they can raise cosmetic concerns. Histologically, these hamartomatous lesions may contain fatty and/or fibrous tissue and smooth muscle.

Plain X-rays classically demonstrate an expansile lytic lesion with a sclerotic rim. The lesions have well-defined borders with a characteristic "sunburst" or "wagon wheel" appearance. On CT, the lesions are sharply marginated intradiploic expansile masses with radiating spicules of bone, potentially causing thinning of the inner and outer tables. Thickened bony trabeculae extending beyond the cortical bone may produce a pseudo "hair-on-end" appearance. On MRI, the lesions appear as sharply demarcated T2 high-signal lesions with a typical "bunch of grapes" appearance and variable T1 signal depending on the fatty and vascular components and homogeneous enhancement.

Common Differential Diagnosis

- Fibrous dysplasia: ground glass appearance.
- Osteoma: osteosclerosis.
- Paget disease: "cotton wool" appearance.

Management Options

Skull vault hemangiomas are considered "do not touch" lesions. Rare cases may need intralesional ethanol injection, surgical resection, and radiation.

References and Further Reading

1. Haouimi A. Skull vault haemangioma. "Radiopaedia.org". 2024. Accessed on 06 Feb 2024. https://doi.org/10.53347/rID-180127.
2. Kirmani AR et al. A unique case of calvarial hemangioma. Surg Neurol Int. 2016. Accessed on 06 Feb 2024. https:/doi.org/10.4103/2152-7806.183498.
3. Prasad K et al. Calvarial hemangiomas: series of 6 cases & review of literature. World Neurosurg. 2024. Accessed on 30 Dec 2024. https://doi.org/10.1016/j.wnsx.2024.100297.

Case 91

91

Clinical History

A 60-year-old woman had a decompressive craniotomy for Chiari 1 malformation 1 year prior. Follow-up MRI was requested.

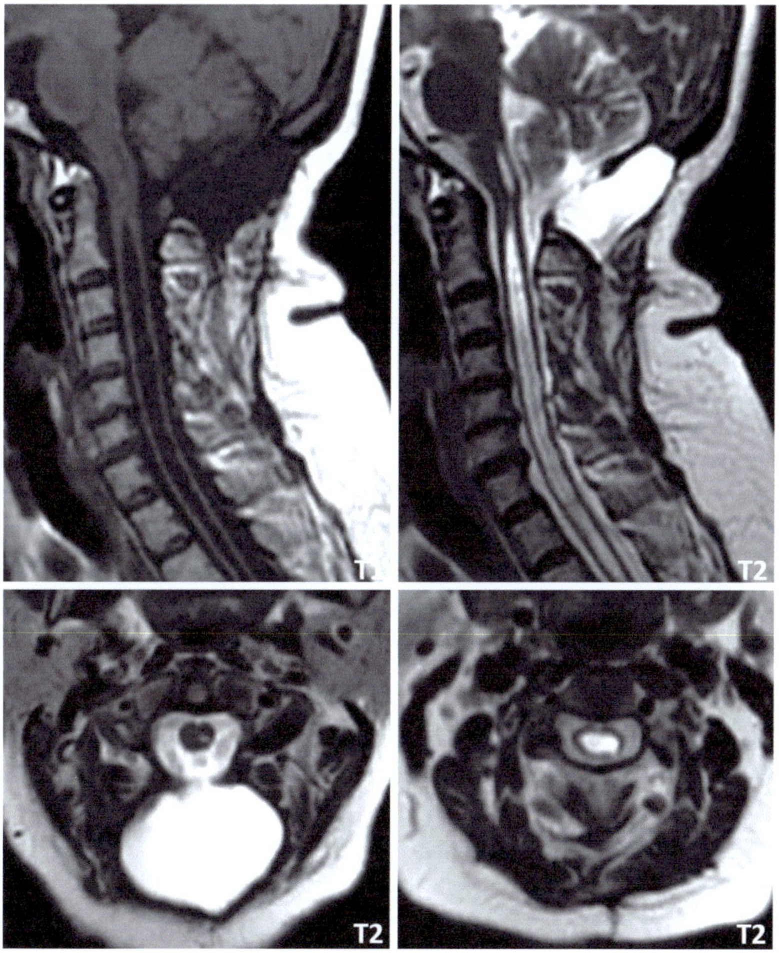

A. Haouimi et al., *Head and Neck Radiology Spot Diagnosis*,
https://doi.org/10.1007/978-3-032-14553-6_91

Findings

Extradural fluid collection of CSF signal intensity overlying the occipital craniotomy defect. It communicates with the adjacent CSF spaces and extends posteriorly to subcutaneous tissues of the neck. Medullary syrinx showing low signal on T1, high signal on T2 extending from the bulbomedullary junction to the distal spinal cord (the distal end is not shown). Normal CSF flow surrounding the cervicomedullary junction on CSF flow studies.

Diagnosis

Pseudomeningocele.

Discussion

Pseudomeningocele is the extravasation of CSF through a meningeal defect. They are seen as a consequence of posterior fossa decompression surgery or spinal surgery such as laminectomy and discectomy. They can also be of posttraumatic origin following nerve root avulsion.

A pseudomeningocele is not contained by dura. The cellular proliferation following trauma may result in closure of the dural tear within days. The transmitted CSF pulsations result in gradual enlargement of the sac. The CSF leakage (extradural collection) ultimately becomes encapsulated in a loculated pouch (fibrous sac), forming pseudomeningocele.

The diagnosis is made based on appropriate clinical context. On CT, a pseudomeningocele appears as a hypodense lesion (isodense to CSF) extending to the dura and may have faint peripheral enhancement. Occasionally, a jet of T2 signal loss may represent a communication with the subarachnoid space. The content of the sac appears isointense to CSF on all sequences.

Common Differential Diagnosis

- Epidural hematoma: T1 high signal, extrinsic compression on thecal sac.
- Postoperative abscess: no CSF communication, peripheral thick regular enhancement, restricted diffusion.
- Postoperative infection: T1 low-signal collection different from CSF, bony involvement.

Management Options

Pseudomeningoceles are managed with bed rest, lumbar drainage, and epidural blood patch. For those with unfavorable response and larger defects, surgical options may be considered.

References and Further Reading

1. Arora A. et al. Traumatic pseudomeningocele ESR case 8478. 2010. Accessed on 10 Feb 2024. https://www.eurorad.org/case/8478.
2. Haouimi A. Pseudomeningocele. "Radiopaedia.org". 2024. Accessed on 10 Feb 2024. https://doi.org/10.53347/rID-154453.
3. Radcliff K et al. Distinguishing pseudomeningocele, epidural hematoma, and postoperative infection on postoperative MRI. Clin Spine Surg. 2016. Accessed on 10 Feb 2024. https://doi.org/10.1097/BSD.0b013e31828f9203. PMID: 27755204.

Case 92

92

Clinical History

A 25-year-old man presented with a painless swelling of the hard palate on the right side.

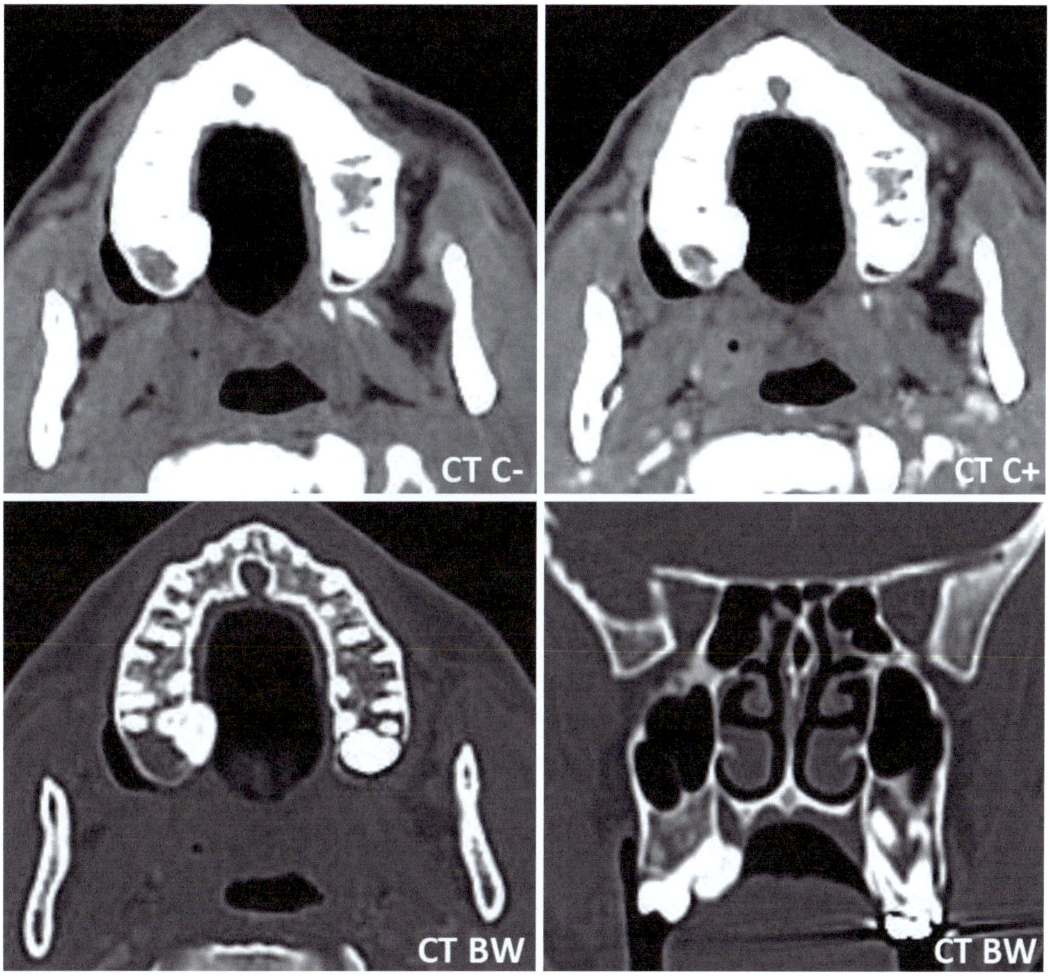

A. Haouimi et al., *Head and Neck Radiology Spot Diagnosis*,
https://doi.org/10.1007/978-3-032-14553-6_92

Findings

A well-defined radiodense exophytic lesion with a convex medial margin arising from the junction of the lateral aspect of the hard palate and the inferomedial aspect of the right maxillary bone. No adjacent bony destruction or soft tissue component.

Diagnosis

Peripheral osteoma of the hard palate.

Discussion

Osteomas are nonaggressive, benign osteogenic, slow-growing tumors with limited expansile growth. The central osteomas developing from endosteum are termed central osteomas, whereas those developing from periosteum are peripheral osteomas. Extraskeletal osteomas develop from muscles. The etiology remains unknown. However, developmental, infectious, endocrine, and traumatic origins have been postulated. Multiple osteomas may be a component of Gardner's syndrome.

Most of the osteomas in the palate are asymptomatic and secondary to minor remote and forgotten trauma. Patients report a protuberant, painless, hard swelling. Occasionally, the osteomas in the hard palate can cause speaking and eating impairments.

Peripheral "ivory osteomas" appear as sessile radiopaque, well-circumscribed, broad-based, oval lesions or may remain attached by a pedicle to the affected bone (cancellous type) on plain X-ray. CT scan does not reveal any perilesional soft tissue invasion.

Common Differential Diagnosis

- Fibrous dysplasia: ground-glass appearance.
- Osteoid osteoma: radiolucent nidus, pain response to aspirin.
- Gardner's syndrome: multiple colonic polyps, extra tooth +/−.

Management Options

Surgical option is considered only for clinically concerning cases.

References and Further Reading

1. Haouimi A. Peripheral osteoma of the hard palate. "Radiopaedia.org". 2024. Accessed on 10 Feb 2024. https://doi.org/10.53347/rID-99669.
2. Maksoud C et al. Peripheral osteoma: a report of a case in the anterior mandibular region. Cureus. 2023. Accessed on 10 Feb 2024.https:/doi.org/10.7759/cureus.48310. PMID: 37933320; PMCID: PMC10625802.
3. Prabhuji ML et al. Peripheral osteoma of the hard palate. J Indian Soc Periodontol. 2012. Accessed on February 10, 2024. https:/doi.org/10.4103/0972-124X.94623. PMID: 22628981; PMCID: PMC3357024.

Case 93

93

Clinical History

A 20-year-old man presented with a hard swelling in the right supraorbital region.

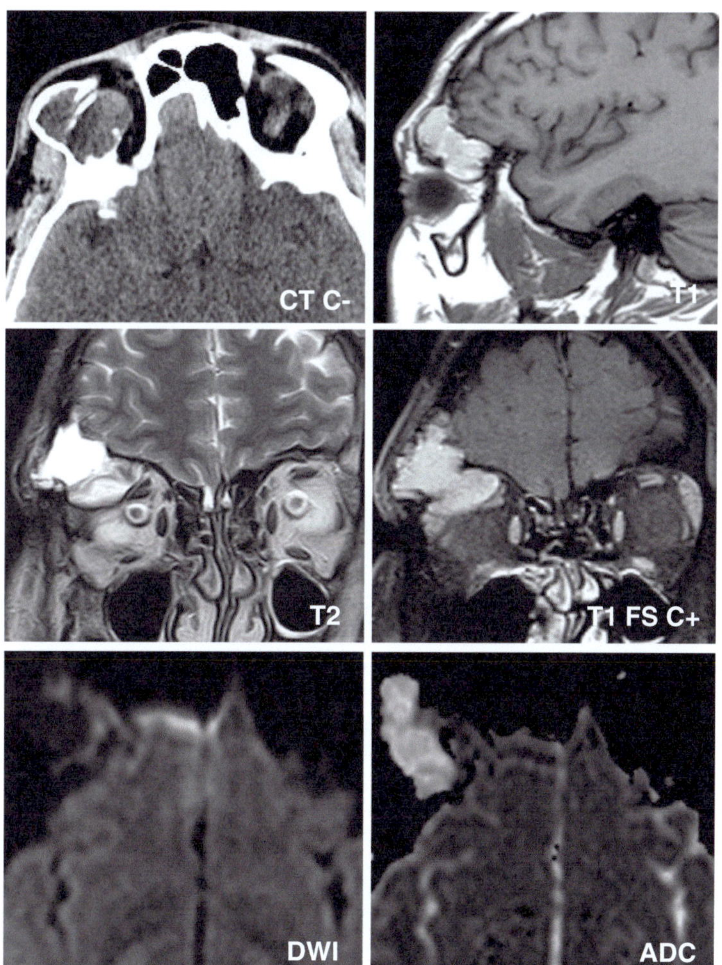

A. Haouimi et al., *Head and Neck Radiology Spot Diagnosis*,
https://doi.org/10.1007/978-3-032-14553-6_93

Findings

An expansile homogeneous intradiploic lytic lesion involving the right supraorbital region. Cortical defect on CT scan, having intraorbital component. On MRI, the lesion shows a homogeneous high signal on T1 and T2. No restricted diffusion and no enhancement. The extrinsic compression on the globe causes displacement of the lacrimal gland and the superior rectus muscle.

Diagnosis

Supraorbital white epidermoid cyst.

Discussion

Epidermoid cysts are benign, slow-growing lesions originating from ectodermal epithelial rests that become trapped during embryogenesis between the third and fifth weeks of gestation or from epithelial implantation following trauma or orbital surgery. The incidence of white epidermoid is less than 3%. Histologically, white epidermoids are lined by stratified squamous epithelium and filled with keratinized whitish material, giving them their characteristic appearance.

Clinically, patients present with a gradual onset of a painless orbital mass. Diplopia and proptosis are late presentations. Unless infected, symptoms usually do not indicate inflammation. Larger cysts can lead to restricted eye movement and cosmetic concerns.

On CT, classical epidermoid appears as well-defined nonenhancing hypodense lesions and may show calcification in approximately 25% of cases. On MRI, white epidermoid cysts appear hyperintense on T1 due to proteinaceous lipid and hemorrhagic contents. Black epidermoids are hypointense on T1 and isointense to cerebrospinal fluid (CSF) on T2 but can be differentiated by restricted diffusion.

Common Differential Diagnosis

- Dermoid cyst: restricted diffusion, calcification +/−.
- Lacrimal gland pleomorphic adenoma: lacrimal gland epicenter, well-circumscribed, lobulated, bony scalloping, isosignal on T1 and T2, mild enhancement +.

Management Options

Surgical resection with +/− orbital wall reconstruction to prevent pulsatile enophthalmos.

References and Further Reading

1. Ahmed RA et al. Orbital epidermoid cysts: a diagnosis to consider. J Ophthalmol. 2014. Accessed on 10 Feb 2024. https://doi.org/10.1155/2014/508425. Epub 2014 Sep 8. PMID: 25276416; PMCID: PMC4172983.
2. Haouimi A. Supraorbital white epidermoid cyst. "Radiopaedia.org". 2024. Accessed 10 Feb 2024. https://doi.org/10.53347/rID-90037.

Case 94

94

Clinical History

A 17-year-old boy presented with a history of motorcycle accident 2 weeks prior.

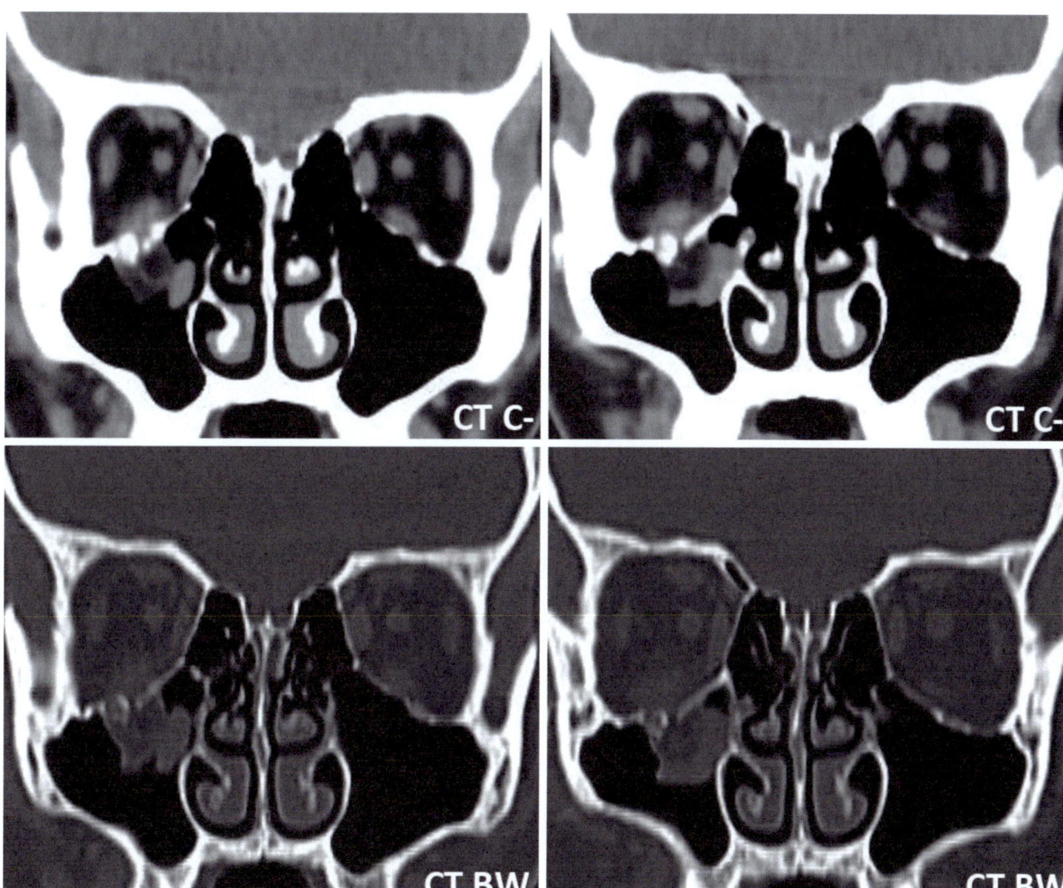

A. Haouimi et al., *Head and Neck Radiology Spot Diagnosis*,
https://doi.org/10.1007/978-3-032-14553-6_94

Findings

Prolapsed orbital soft tissue component including inferior rectus muscle into the right maxillary sinus—"trap door component" through the nondisplaced fracture gap. Normal appearance of the other extraocular muscles and optic nerve. Normal aeration of maxillary and ethmoid sinuses.

Diagnosis

Orbital blow-out fracture or trapdoor fracture.

Discussion

Orbital floor blow-out fractures are often secondary to blunt facial trauma and are almost exclusively seen in children and young adults. A direct blow to the orbit causes a sudden increase in intraorbital tension. Both "hydraulic" and "buckling" theories explain the mechanism of injury. Nondisplaced incomplete linear orbital floor fracture causes herniation and entrapment of orbital neuromuscular tissues "trap door component." Continued prolonged progressive bony pressure on herniated component causes ischemia and necrosis of entrapped component, leading to gaze restriction. The entrapment of intraorbital soft tissue, including the inferior rectus muscle, must be considered as a true emergency and warrants immediate ophthalmologic consultation. Failure of a timely, appropriate decision can lead to permanent limitation of extraocular motility and difficult-to-correct diplopia.

Patients often complain of postmidfacial trauma diplopia and/or pain with vertical movements of the eyes. Radiologically, many patients with inferior rectus herniation may not have clinical signs of entrapment, whereas many patients with evidence of simple orbital fat herniation with intact inferior rectus may have severe dysmotility. Hence, entrapment is a clinical diagnosis, not radiologic.

Common Differential Diagnosis

- No valid differential condition in appropriate clinical context.

Management Options

Treatment is mostly surgical.

References and Further Reading

1. Gowda, AU et al. Resolution of vertical gaze followinga delayed presentation of orbital floor fracture with inferior rectus entrapment. Craniomaxillofac Trauma Reconstr. 2020. Accessed on 10 Feb 2024. https://doi.org/10.1177/1943387520965804. Epub 2020 Nov 18. PMID: 33456696; PMCID: PMC7797985.
2. Haouimi A. Orbital blow-out fracture with inferior rectus muscle entrapment. "Radiopaedia.org". 2024. Accessed on 10 Feb 10 2024. https://doi.org/10.53347/rID-152157.

Case 95

95

Clinical History

An 85-year-old man presented with a history of vertigo. Incidental finding on CT.

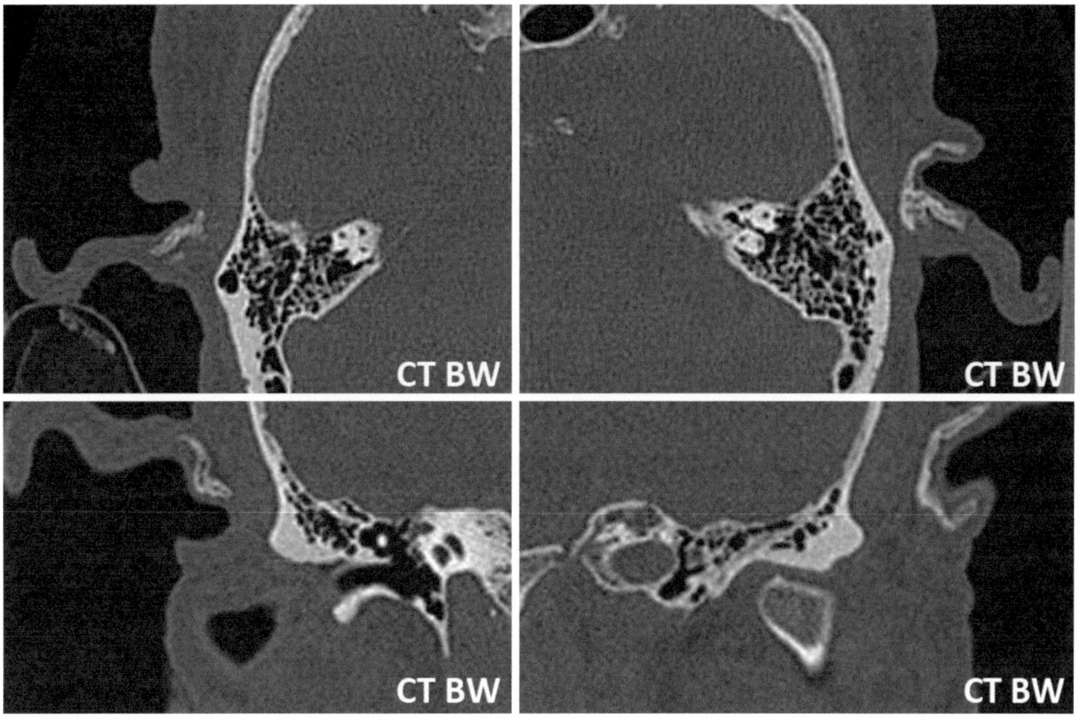

A. Haouimi et al., *Head and Neck Radiology Spot Diagnosis*,
https://doi.org/10.1007/978-3-032-14553-6_95

Findings

Bilateral ossification of the auricular cartilage seen as high-density areas of both auricles with radiolucent areas within. Both EACs and the middle and inner ears were normal. Normal pneumatization of the mastoid air cells.

Diagnosis

Ossification of the external ear.

Discussion

The external ear is primarily composed of elastic cartilage, which remains flexible throughout life. In certain conditions, this cartilage can undergo calcification or ossification, resulting in the hardening of the auricle. This process is uncommon and is most frequently observed in older men, often after the age of 60. It was first described by Dr. Bochdalek in 1866 and was first reported as an X-ray finding in 1899 by Dr. Wassmund. It may be triggered by local trauma, frostbite, chronic inflammation, endocrine disorders such as Addison's disease, or metabolic disturbances.

When ossification occurs, the ear becomes rigid, brittle, and less pliable, a condition sometimes referred to as "petrified ear."

On plain radiographs and CT, the pinna shows linear or diffuse dense opacities conforming to its contour, consistent with calcification or ossification. MRI demonstrates areas of signal void within the auricular cartilage, confirming the loss of normal elastic tissue and replacement by mineralized tissue.

Common Differential Diagnosis

- Diagnosis is straightforward.

Management Options

Auricular ossificans is an irreversible condition. There is no specific treatment. Treatment is focused on symptomatic relief.

References and Further Reading

1. Haouimi A. Ossification of the external ear (auricular cartilage). "Radiopaedia.org". 2024. Accessed on 10 Feb 2024. https://doi.org/10.53347/rID-99223.
2. Kim SY et al. A case of auricular ossification. Ann Dermatol. 2011. Accessed on 10 Feb 2024. https://doi.org/10.5021/ad.2011.23.S2.S261. Epub2011Oct 31. PMID: 22148066; PMCID: PMC3229081.
3. Mastronikolis NS et al. Bilateral ossification of the auricles: anunusual entityandreview of the literature. Head Face Med. 2009. Accessed on 10 Feb 2024. https://doi.org/10.1186/1746-160X-5-17.

Case 96

96

Clinical History

An 11-year-old girl presented with a history of painless left facial swelling near the parotid region.

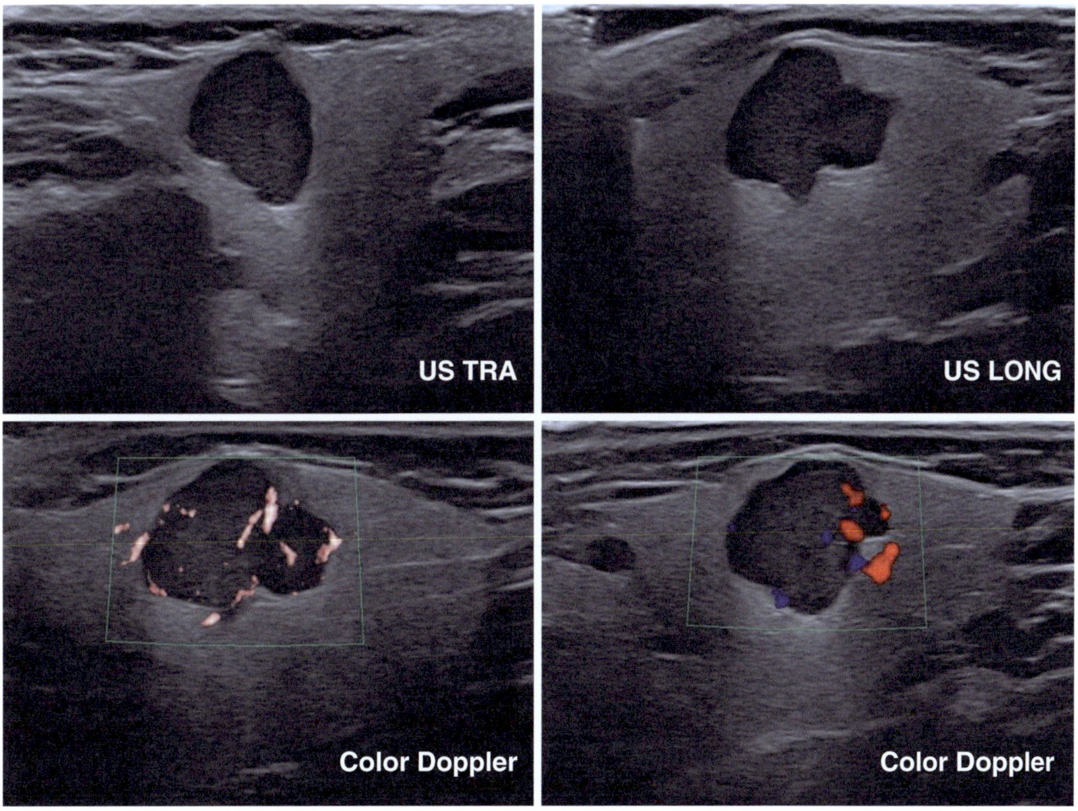

A. Haouimi et al., *Head and Neck Radiology Spot Diagnosis*,
https://doi.org/10.1007/978-3-032-14553-6_96

Findings

A well-defined lobulated homogeneously hypoechoic lesion with posterior acoustic enhancement within the superficial lobe of the left parotid gland. The lesion is well vascularized on color Doppler.

Diagnosis

Pleomorphic adenoma of the parotid gland.

Discussion

Pleomorphic adenomas, also known as benign mixed tumors, constitute up to two-thirds of all salivary gland tumors, having both epithelial and myoepithelial elements with a remote malignant potential. The lesions can occur at any age but are more common between the third and sixth decades with a female predominance (2:1). The etiology remains unknown. Oncogenic simian virus (SV40) and radiation exposure may play a role at the onset or during progression.

Clinically, the patients present with long-standing mobile, solitary, painless swelling. The symptoms depend on size and location. The larger lesions rarely cause facial nerve neuropathy. Deep lobe pleomorphic adenomas may present as a retro-tonsillar or para-pharyngeal mass.

On ultrasound, the lesions appear hypoechoic and may show posterior acoustic enhancement. On CT, the larger lesions appear heterogeneous due to areas of dystrophic calcifications and pockets of necrosis, whereas the smaller lesions are solid and homogeneously enhancing.

On T1, smaller lesions are ovoid and homogeneously enhancing and larger lesions are lobulated and heterogeneous. On T2, smaller lesions are isointense and bigger lesions are heterogeneously hyperintense. The lesions are more conspicuous on STIR sequences.

Common Differential Diagnosis

- Warthin's tumor: multicentric, bilateral, no calcification.
- Primary parotid carcinoma: heterogeneous, ill-defined infiltrating, perineural extension.
- Kutner's tumor: mostly affecting submandibular gland, associated sialolithiasis.

Management Options

Surgical resection.

References and Further Reading

1. Bokhari MR, Greene J. Pleomorphic Adenoma. Stat Pearls Publishing. 2023. Accessed on 27 Feb 2024. https://www.ncbi.nlm.nih.gov/books/NBK430829/.
2. Borner Urs et al. Pleomorphic adenoma of the parotid gland. Am J Med. 2015. Accessed on 27 Feb 2024. https://doi.org/10.1016/j.amjmed.2015.08.014.
3. Haouimi A. Pleomorphic adenoma - paediatric. "Radiopaedia.org". 2024. Accessed on 27 Feb 2024. https://doi.org/10.53347/rID-147291.

Case 97

97

Clinical History

A 25-year-old woman presented with progressive dysphagia to solid foods and weight loss. The laboratory investigations revealed iron deficiency anemia.

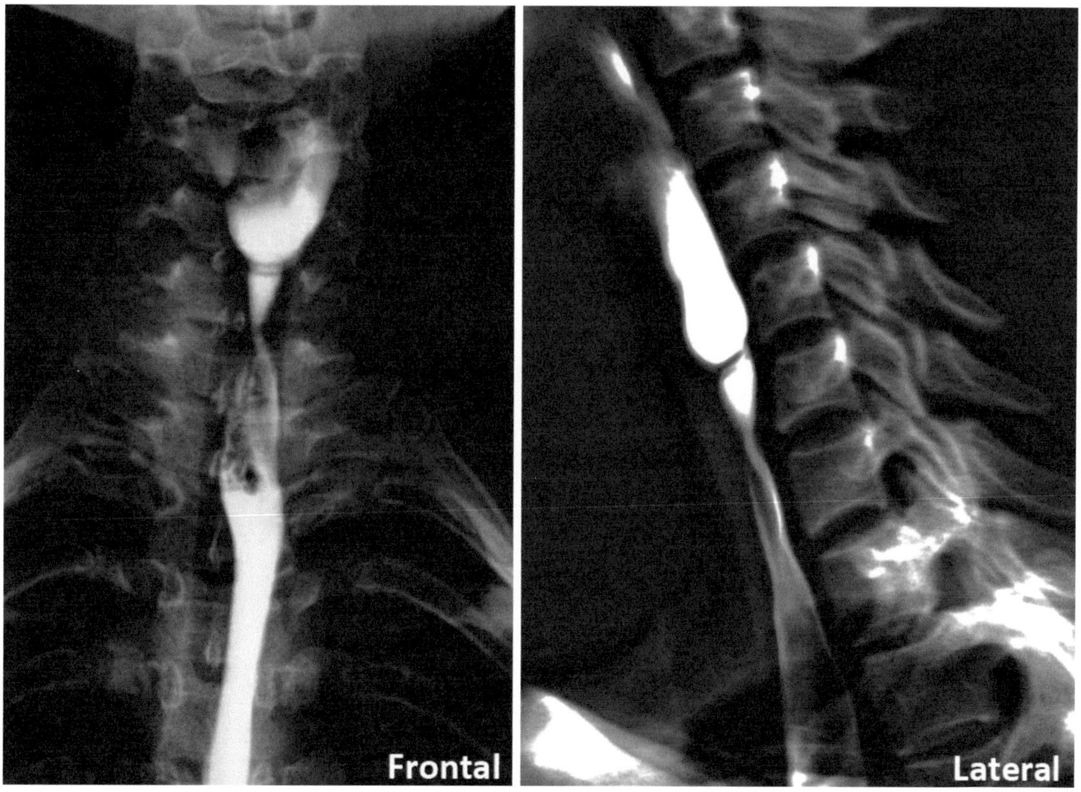

A. Haouimi et al., *Head and Neck Radiology Spot Diagnosis*,
https://doi.org/10.1007/978-3-032-14553-6_97

Findings

The barium swallow shows a short, smooth concentric narrowing of the proximal esophagus, well-demonstrated on both frontal and lateral views, suggestive of an esophageal web.

Diagnosis

Plummer–Vinson syndrome.

Discussion

Plummer–Vinson syndrome refers to the classic triad of postcricoid dysphagia, iron-deficiency anemia, and esophageal web. Plummer–Vinson syndrome is a rare condition of unknown etiology, more common in middle-aged women. Clinically, patients present with loss of weight and progressive intermittent dysphagia over the years, limited to solid foods. Patients are prone to develop squamous cell carcinoma of the pharynx and proximal esophagus if left untreated.

Chronic iron deficiency causes iron-dependent enzyme dysfunction. Dysfunctional iron-dependent oxidative enzymes lead to myasthenic changes of the esophageal muscles. Repeated epithelial injury leads to mucosal atrophy and degradation of pharyngeal muscles and the development of esophageal web, a thin mucous membrane composed of squamous cell epithelium.

Radiologically, esophageal webs can be documented by swallowing barium bolus during video fluoroscopy. They appear as a thin noncircumferential transverse filling defect perpendicular to the anterior esophageal wall. High-volume barium esophagogram can be seen when fully distended. "Jet effect" of contrast can be seen as it passes distal to the web. Esophagogastroscopy can be both diagnostic and therapeutic.

Common Differential Diagnosis

- Prominent cricopharyngeus: at C5–C6, broader persistent defect, normal serum iron.
- Esophageal stricture: circumferential involvement, delayed emptying.
- Gastroesophageal reflux: involves distal esophagus.

Management Options

Treatment options are endoscopic bougienage and balloon dilatation, as well as iron therapy.

References and Further Reading

1. Haouimi A. Plummer-Vinson syndrome. "Radiopaedia.org". 2024. Accessed on 27 Feb 2024. https://doi.org/10.53347/rID-179649.
2. Novacek G. Plummer-Vinson syndrome. Orphanet J Rare Dis. 2006. Accessed on 27 Feb 2024. https://doi.org/10.1186/1750-1172-1-36. PMID: 16978405; PMCID:
3. Verma S, Mukherjee S. Plummer-Vinson Syndrome. Stat Pearls Publishing. 2023. Accessed on 27 Feb 2024. https://www.ncbi.nlm.nih.gov/books/NBK538306/.

Case 98

98

Clinical History

A 60-year-old man presented with a nasopharyngeal mass on ENT examination.

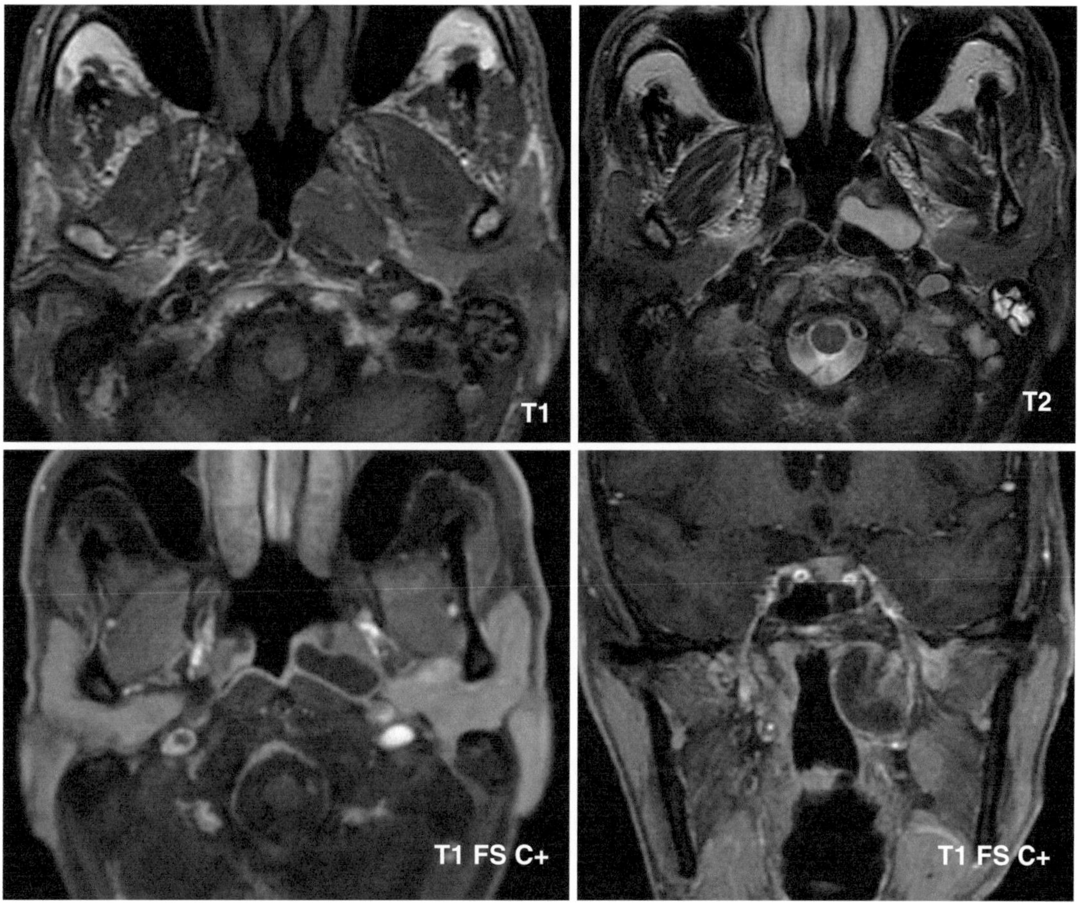

A. Haouimi et al., *Head and Neck Radiology Spot Diagnosis*,
https://doi.org/10.1007/978-3-032-14553-6_98

Findings

A well-defined submucosal pear-shaped cyst of the left fossa of Rosenmüller, bulging into the nasopharyngeal lumen. It shows homogeneous fluid content having low signal on T1 and high signal on T2 with no enhancement. Normal nasopharynx.

Diagnosis

Retention cyst of the fossa of Rosenmüller.

Discussion

Retention cyst within the fossa of Rosenmüller is an asymptomatic, benign, incidental lesion seen during routine CT and MRI. They are caused by the accumulation of secretions within a dilated mucus gland. Larger lesions can occasionally cause symptoms such as hearing deficit, tinnitus, unilateral fullness of the ear, odynophagia, and dysphonia.

On CT scan, the lesions appear as low-density cysts without perilesional invasion or contrast enhancement. Faint peripheral enhancement may be seen if infected. MRI signals are variable depending on cystic content. T2 axial and coronal images make the diagnosis easier. The shape of the lesion is very suggestive, being "pear shaped" or "light bulb shaped." The narrow portion is limited by the fossa itself, and the wider portion represents unrestricted expansion in the nasopharyngeal territory.

Common Differential Diagnosis

- Branchial cleft cyst: more lateral but medial to the carotid artery.
- Tornwaldt cyst: midline cyst, deep to pharyngobasilar fascia.
- Rathke's pouch cyst: very rare, midline lesion, signs of endocrinopathy +/−.
- Benign mixed tumor: solid, homogeneously enhancing lesion.
- Nasopharyngeal carcinoma: unilateral, invasive lesions involving perilesional fat plane.

Management Options

Retention cysts of fossa of Rosenmüller are "do not touch" lesions. The options for bigger lesions include aspiration, sclerotherapy, incision, drainage, and marsupialization.

References and Further Reading

1. Haouimi A. Retention cyst of Rosenmüller fossa. "Radiopaedia.org". 2024. Accessed on 27 Feb 2024. https://doi.org/10.53347/rID-153870.
2. Lloyd SK et al. Cysts of the fossa of Rosenmüller: report of two cases. Ear Nose Throat J. 2010. Accessed on 12 Apr 2024. https://doi.org/10.1177/014556131008900805. PMID: 20737363.
3. Peters B, De Cuyper K, Vanhoenacker FM. Pear-shaped lesion of the Fossa of Rosenmüller. J Belg Soc Radiol. 2016. Accessed on 27 Feb 2024. https://doi.org/10.5334/jbr-btr.921.

Case 99

99

Clinical History

A 6-year-old boy presented with a left-sided abducens nerve palsy and ipsilateral retro-orbital pain.

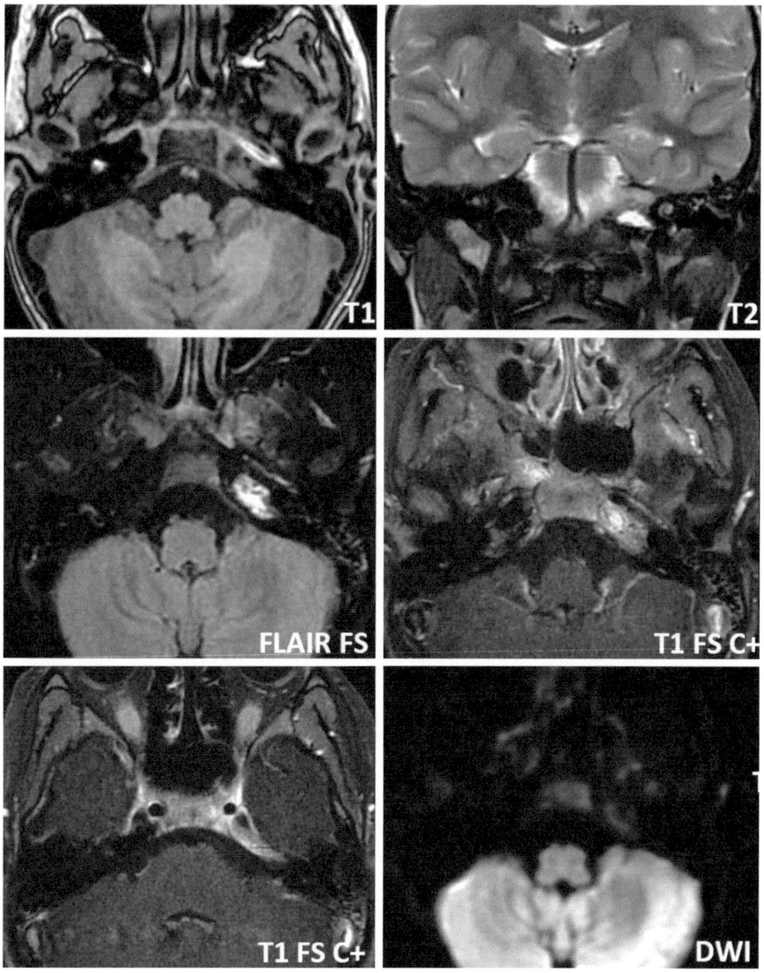

A. Haouimi et al., *Head and Neck Radiology Spot Diagnosis*,
https://doi.org/10.1007/978-3-032-14553-6_99

Findings

Abnormal signal of the left petrous apex showing an intermediate to low signal on T1, high signal on T2, FLAIR fat sat, and DWI with peripheral enhancement. Associated middle ear fluid and partial opacification of the mastoid air cells as well as dural thickening of the ipsilateral Meckel's cave and cavernous sinus.

Diagnosis

Petrous apicitis.

Discussion

Petrous apicitis is the consequence of chronic suppurative otitis media spreading to the petrous apex by contiguity. The common pathogens are *Pseudomonas* and *Enterococcus*. The clinical symptoms include nonspecific headache, fever, and otalgia. It can also present as a component of Gradenigo syndrome when associated with cranial nerve deficits (affecting V2, VI, and VII). The symptoms of Gradenigo syndrome highlight the potential risk of untreated ear infections. Secondary complications may include meningitis, cavernous sinus thrombosis, subdural empyema, and cerebral abscesses. A high index of suspicion for petrous apicitis always exists in patients presenting with otalgia combined with other associated neurological signs.

CT scans can reveal bony erosion with poorly defined bony edges. Opacification of mastoid air cells and/or middle ear often coexists. MRI shows low signal on T1 and high signal on T2 with peripheral enhancement. The intracranial complications are better depicted on MRI.

Common Differential Diagnosis

- Cholesterol granuloma: T1 high signal cannot be suppressed on fat sat, no enhancement.
- Congenital cholesteatoma: T1 low signal, brighter than CSF on T2, no FLAIR attenuation.
- Chordoma: bilateral, irregular intratumoral calcifications, blooming on SWI.

Management Options

Treatment generally involves high-dose intravenous antibiotics. In cases where there is an abscess, surgical intervention may be considered as an option to drain the affected area.

References and Further Reading

1. Haouimi A. Petrous apicitis. “Radiopaedia.org”. 2024. Accessed on 29 Feb 2024. https://doi.org/10.53347/rID-184900.
2. Murakami T et al. Gradenigo’s syndrome: CT and MRI findings. Pediatr Radiol. 1996. Accessed on 29 Feb 2024. https://doi.org/10.1007/BF01356837. PMID: 8781114.
3. Valles JM et al. Gradenigo syndrome: unusual consequence of otitis media. Case Rep Neurol. 2014. Accessed on 29 Feb 2024. https://doi.org/10.1159/000365843. PMID: 25232331; PMCID: PMC4164058.

Case 100

100

Clinical History

A 60-year-old man presented with a painless left facial swelling.

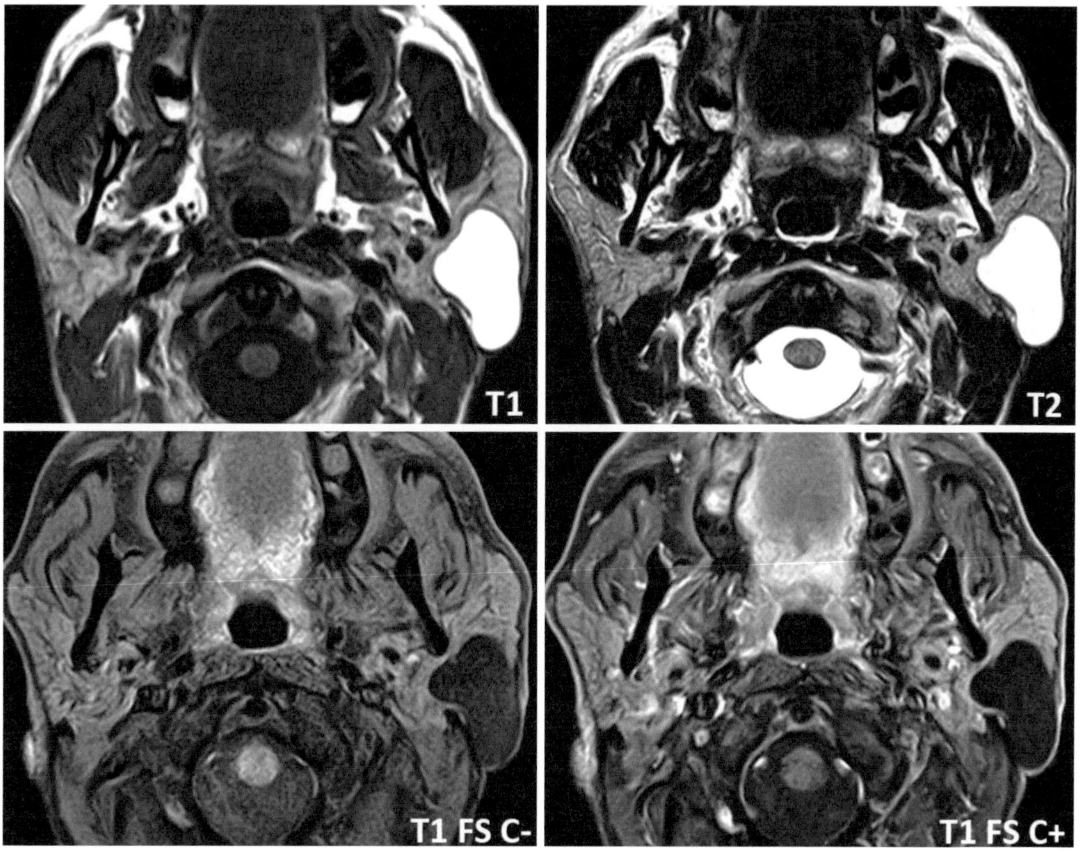

A. Haouimi et al., *Head and Neck Radiology Spot Diagnosis*,
https://doi.org/10.1007/978-3-032-14553-6_100

Findings

A well-defined intraparenchymal lobulated mass of high signal on T1 and T2 of the left parotid gland. The lesion signal suppresses with fat saturation with no contrast enhancement.

Diagnosis

Parotid lipoma.

Discussion

Lipomas are well-defined, slow-growing, benign tumors, and about one-fifth of all lipomas are seen in the head and neck region. The parotid lipomas are mostly involving the superficial lobe, and the peak incidence is seen in middle-aged adults between 40 and 60 years with near-zero malignant potential.

Clinically, they present as a unilateral, mobile, indolent, soft tissue, painless mass that may cause facial contour deformity. However, the involvement of the facial nerve is highly suggestive of malignant transformation of pleomorphic adenoma.

On ultrasound, the parotid lipomas appear as well-defined iso- or hypoechoic solid masses with parallel linear intralesional echogenic bands. On CT, the lipomas are seen as a well-circumscribed, low-density, homogeneous mass, and the lesions do not enhance. MRI is very helpful for tissue characterization and is the modality of choice to diagnose lipomas. On MRI, the lesions appear as well-defined high signal on both T1 and T2. The fat-suppression sequence allows complete suppression of the fatty signal and helps to reach a near-histologic diagnosis.

Common Differential Diagnosis

- Pseudolipoma: history of trauma.
- Mixed parotid tumor: lobulated, homo/heterogeneous, enhancement, calcification +/-.
- Liposarcoma: enhancing lesion, locoregional invasion, thick septations.

Management Options

Both enucleation and partial or complete parotidectomy are the options available, depending on the size, site, and clinical concerns.

References and Further Reading

1. Haouimi A. Parotid lipoma. 2024. Radiopaedia.org. https://doi.org/10.53347/rID-184951. Accessed on 29 Feb 2024
2. Paparo F Massarelli M Giuliani G. A rare case of parotid gland lipoma arising from the deep lobe of the parotid gland. Ann Maxillofac Surg. 2016. https://doi.org/10.4103/2231-0746.200335. Accessed on 29 Feb 2024. PMID: 28299278; PMCID.
3. Tong KN, Seltzer S, Castle JT. Lipoma of the parotid gland. Head Neck Pathol. 2020. https://doi.org/10.1007/s12105-019-01023-3. Accessed on 29 Feb 2024. Epub 2019 Mar 19. PMID: 30888640; PMCID: PMC7021912.

Case 101

101

Clinical History

A 45-year-old woman presented with a slowly progressive left occipital swelling and signs of increased intracranial pressure.

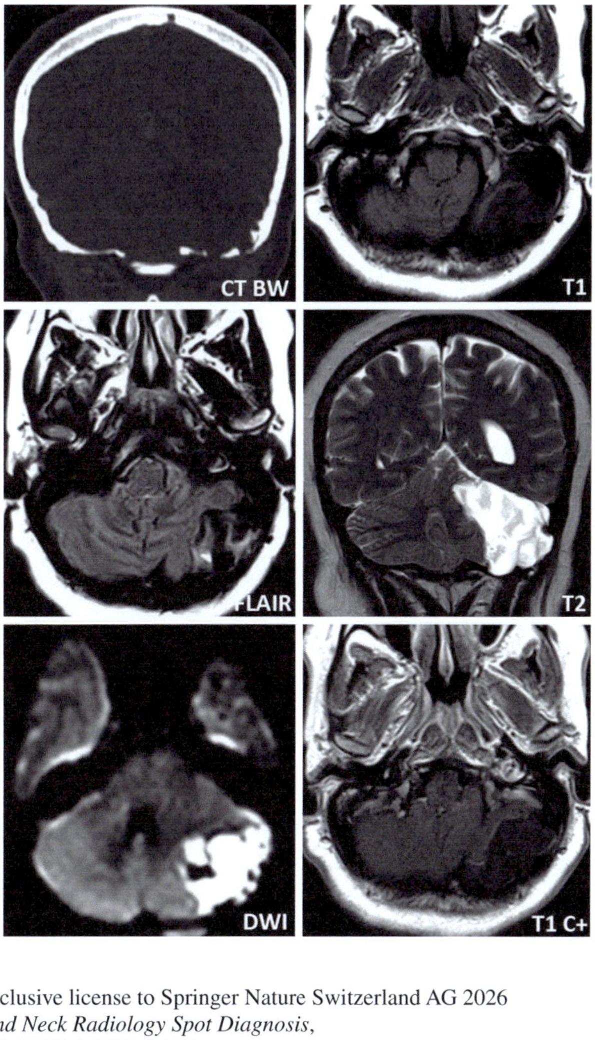

A. Haouimi et al., *Head and Neck Radiology Spot Diagnosis*,
https://doi.org/10.1007/978-3-032-14553-6_101

Findings

CT scan in bone window reveals an expansile osteolytic lesion with scalloping of the occipital bone on the left side. On MRI, this intradiploic lesion appears as low signal on T1, heterogeneous on FLAIR, and high signal on T2 with restricted diffusion. No enhancement after gadolinium. Extrinsic compression on adjacent vermis and cerebellar hemisphere causing slight dilatation of the ventricular system and mild tonsillar herniation. No associated brain edema.

Diagnosis

Intradiploic epidermoid cyst.

Discussion

Intradiploic epidermoid cysts are rare, benign, slow growing lesions with a diploic space epicenter. They are mostly congenital, arising from trapped ectodermal embryonal remnants during closure of the neural tube between the third and fifth gestational weeks. Acquired cases are posttraumatic. Pathologically, the lesions are filled with keratin and lined by stratified squamous epithelium. The frontal, parietal, and occipital bones are the commonest sites.

Clinically, the patients are asymptomatic. Some cases may present local pain and tenderness. The bigger lesions can cause cosmetic concern and can produce neurologic symptoms.

Intradiploic lesions with erosion of both the inner and outer tables can be seen on CT. The appearance varies depending on the proportion of keratin lamellae and cholesterol clefts within the cyst. A characteristic pattern of low signal intensity on T1-weighted images, high signal on T2-weighted images, and restricted diffusion, together with an expansile lytic skull lesion, is highly suggestive of an epidermoid cyst. The presence of diffusion restriction on MRI and the absence of marked T1 hyperintensity help distinguish it from a dermoid tumor.

Common Differential Diagnosis

- Dermoid cyst: T1 hyperintensity, no restricted diffusion.
- Fibrous dysplasia: "ground glass" expansile appearance.
- Skull bone hemangioma: fluid–fluid level on MRI.

Management Options

Symptomatic and "wait and see" approach. Surgical excision is the treatment of choice.

References and Further Reading

1. Farag AA, et al. An atypical intradiploic epidermoid cyst, radiological findings, and surgical management. Surg Neurol Int. 2025. https://doi.org/10.25259/SNI_170_2025. Accessed on 21 Sept 2025. PMID: 40469342; PMCID: PMC12134849.
2. Haouimi A. Intradiploic epidermoid cyst. 2023. Radiopaedia.org. https://doi.org/10.53347/rID-168467. Accessed on 07 Dec 2024.

Case 102

102

Clinical History

A 50-year-old man presented with bilateral proptosis.

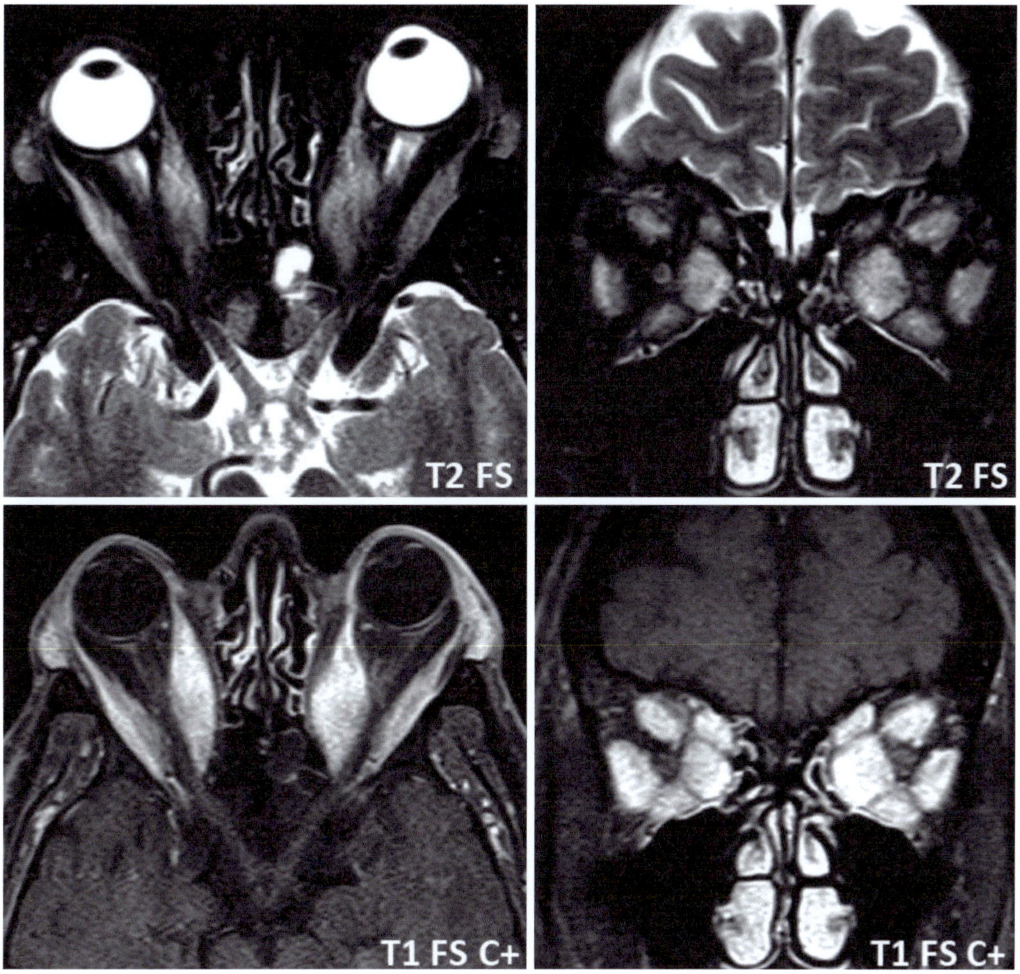

A. Haouimi et al., *Head and Neck Radiology Spot Diagnosis*,
https://doi.org/10.1007/978-3-032-14553-6_102

Findings

Bilateral symmetrically thickened bellies of the extraocular muscles, sparing the tendinous insertions, resembling a "Coca-Cola bottle" on axial images. Homogeneous high-signal extraocular muscles on T2 fat sat with enhancement. Bilateral proptosis causing stretching of the optic nerves.

Diagnosis

Graves' disease.

Discussion

Graves' disease is an autoimmune disorder involving extraocular muscles and neighboring connective tissue due to infiltration with inflammatory cells. It is 5–10 times more common in women, mostly seen between the ages of 30 and 60 years. The typical distribution in order of preference is the inferior rectus muscle, medial rectus, superior rectus, and then finally lateral rectus. The understanding of the pathogenesis is incomplete. Antibodies to thyroid-stimulating hormone are believed to cross-react with antigens, resulting in infiltration by activated T lymphocytes and subsequent release of inflammatory mediators.

Clinically, due to elevated T3 and T4, patients present with fatigue, heat intolerance, palpitations, anxiety, polydipsia, and sweating.

Both CT and MRI show markedly thickened isodense/isointense extraocular muscle belly, sparing the tendons. Crowding of enlarged extraocular muscles causes compression on optic nerves.

Common Differential Diagnosis

- Orbital pseudotumor: painful ophthalmoplegia, involving the tendinous segment.
- Orbital lymphoma: unilateral, restricted diffusion, normal extraocular muscles.
- Sarcoidosis: scleral nodule, thickened optic nerve and sheath, brain involvement.

Management Options

Most cases are managed by medical treatment.

References and Further Reading

1. Haouimi A. 2021. Thyroid orbitopathy. Radiopaedia.org. https://doi.org/10.53347/rID-94394. Accessed on 20 July 2023.
2. Hutchings KR, et al. Graves' eye disease: clinical and radiological diagnosis. 2023. Biomedicines. https://doi.org/10.3390/biomedicines11020312. Accessed on 19 July 2025. PMID: 36830848; PMCID: PMC9953404.
3. Pokhrel B, Bhusal K. Graves disease. "StatPearls Publishing". 2023. https://www.ncbi.nlm.nih.gov/books/NBK448195/. Accessed on 21 Dec 2024.

Case 103

103

Clinical History

A 40-year-old woman. Incidental finding.

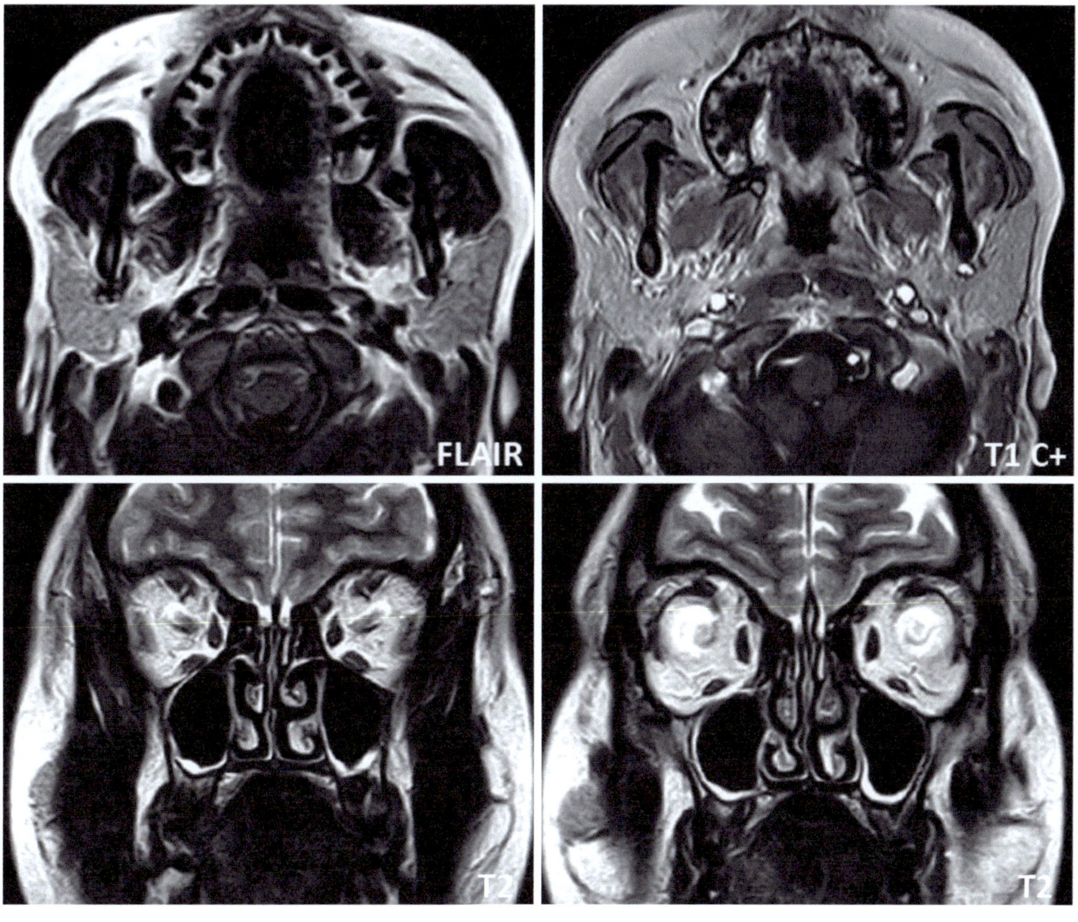

A. Haouimi et al., *Head and Neck Radiology Spot Diagnosis*,
https://doi.org/10.1007/978-3-032-14553-6_103

Findings

A small, well-defined soft-tissue area lateral to the right masseter muscle completely separated from the parotid gland. It shows isosignal to the normal parotid gland on all sequences.

Diagnosis

Accessory parotid gland.

Discussion

Accessory parotid gland is a separate focus of parotid tissue lying on or above the Stensen's duct. Anatomically, the accessory parotid gland is small lobulated salivary tissue lying over the masseter muscle. Although completely detached, the accessory parotid gland has one or more tributaries emptying into the main parotid duct and thus is indirectly connected to the main parotid gland. They have their own blood supply from the transverse facial artery. Anatomically, it is located anterior to the parotid gland, lateral to masseter muscle, and on or above the Stensen's duct. This is a very common anatomical variant and can be seen in up to 55% of normal individuals. Because of the high incidence, it is mandatory to identify this gland before performing parotidectomy, as it will reduce the recurrence rate.

Accessory parotid gland can be affected by parotitis. Surprisingly, the incidence of parotid neoplasm is higher in the accessory gland than in the main parotid gland itself.

The accessory parotid gland has the same echotexture as the main parotid gland on ultrasound. The structure appears isodense/isointense on CT and MRI.

Common Differential Diagnosis

Facial process of parotid gland: parenchymal continuity with parotid gland.

Management Options

The accessory salivary gland is a normal variant. This has preoperative surgical importance.

References and Further Reading

1. Ahn D, et al. The accessory parotid gland and facial process of the parotid gland on computed tomography. PLoS One. 2017. https://doi.org/10.1371/journal.pone.0184633. Accessed on 20 June 2025. PMID: 28915265; PMCID: PMC5600370.
2. Atikuzzaman K. Warthin's tumour in accessory parotid gland. Bangladesh J Otorhinolaryngology. 2015;20(1):43–5. https://doi.org/10.3329/bjo.v20i1.22017.
3. Haouimi A. 2021. Accessory parotid gland. Radiopaedia.org. https://doi.org/10.53347/rID-92173. Accessed on 20 June 2025.

Case 104

104

Clinical History

A 17-year-old adolescent with a right ear fullness. CT to rule out a nasopharyngeal tumor.

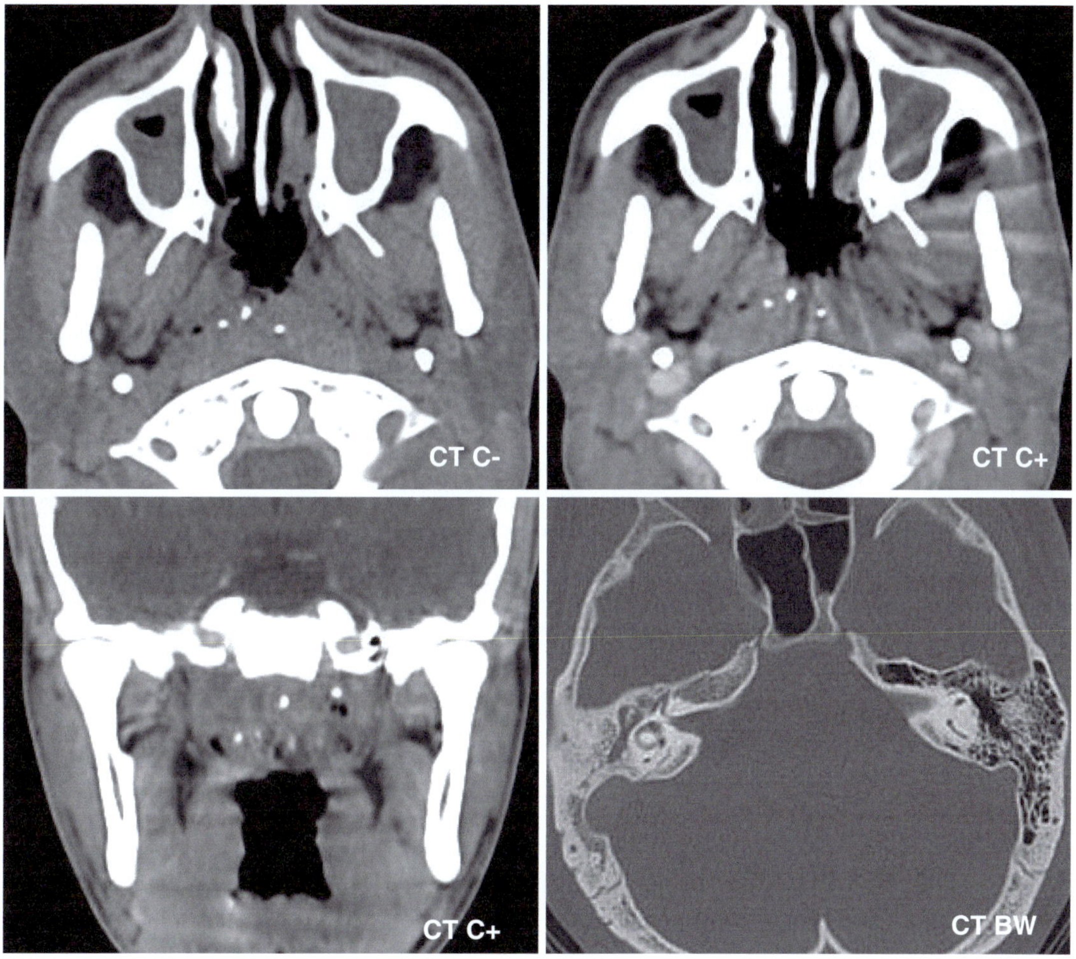

A. Haouimi et al., *Head and Neck Radiology Spot Diagnosis*,
https://doi.org/10.1007/978-3-032-14553-6_104

Findings

Thickened adenoid tonsils with numerous small (<3 mm) calculi within the cryptic folds of adenoids. Normal mucosal enhancement of the nasopharynx. Opacified right mastoid air cells and middle ear cavities, confirming otomastoiditis. Incidental bilateral chronic maxillary sinusitis.

Diagnosis

Adenoid stones within hypertrophied adenoid tonsils.

Discussion

Adenoliths or tonsillar stones are found in the cryptic tonsillar folds. This is formed due to bacterial aggregation in chronically inflamed caseous tonsillitis. The stones are described as biofilms of aerobic and anaerobic bacteria, which calcify over time.

Streptococcal and viral infections (EBV, adenovirus, and rhinovirus) are the common causes. In fact, any tonsillitis (bacterial, viral, or fungal) can initiate the calcification process, which is attributed to the stasis of saliva. Though the pharyngeal tonsils are the commonest site, stones can also be seen anywhere in the lymphoid tissue of the Waldeyer's ring. Histologically, they are composed of densely packed polymicrobial bacteria, held together by extracellular matrix.

Adenoliths may remain clinically silent. A few patients can complain of chronic sore throat, metallic taste, dysphagia, and halitosis due to volatile sulfur molecules. Advanced cases may cause otalgia and hearing deficit due to blockage of the Eustachian tubes.

Millimetric adenoliths are frequently detected on CT as foci of calcification.

Common Differential Diagnosis

- Calcified kissing carotids: linear and tortuous calcification, not punctiform
- Foreign bodies: clinical history
- Phlebolith: really challenging, concentric layers, "bull's eye" or "targetoid appearance"
- Eagle syndrome: bilateral, more lateral, and shows continuity with styloid process

Management Options

Good oral hygiene is recommended for asymptomatic cases. Warm saline, chlorhexidine, and cetylpyridinium chloride (CPC) gurgling may relieve the symptoms. Partial or complete tonsillectomy is a surgical option depending on clinical judgment.

References and Further Reading

1. Haouimi A. Adenoid stones within hypertrophied adenoid tonsils. 2021. Radiopaedia.org. https://doi.org/10.53347/rID-90528. Accessed on 12 July 2025.
2. Sakano H, et al. Adenoid stones -adenoliths. J Otol Rhinol. 2015. https://doi.org/10.4172/2324-8785.1000240. Accessed on 12 July 2025. Epub 2015 Jul 13. PMID: 26798664.

Case 105

105

Clinical History

A 50-year-old woman with a history of progressive midline swelling of the neck.

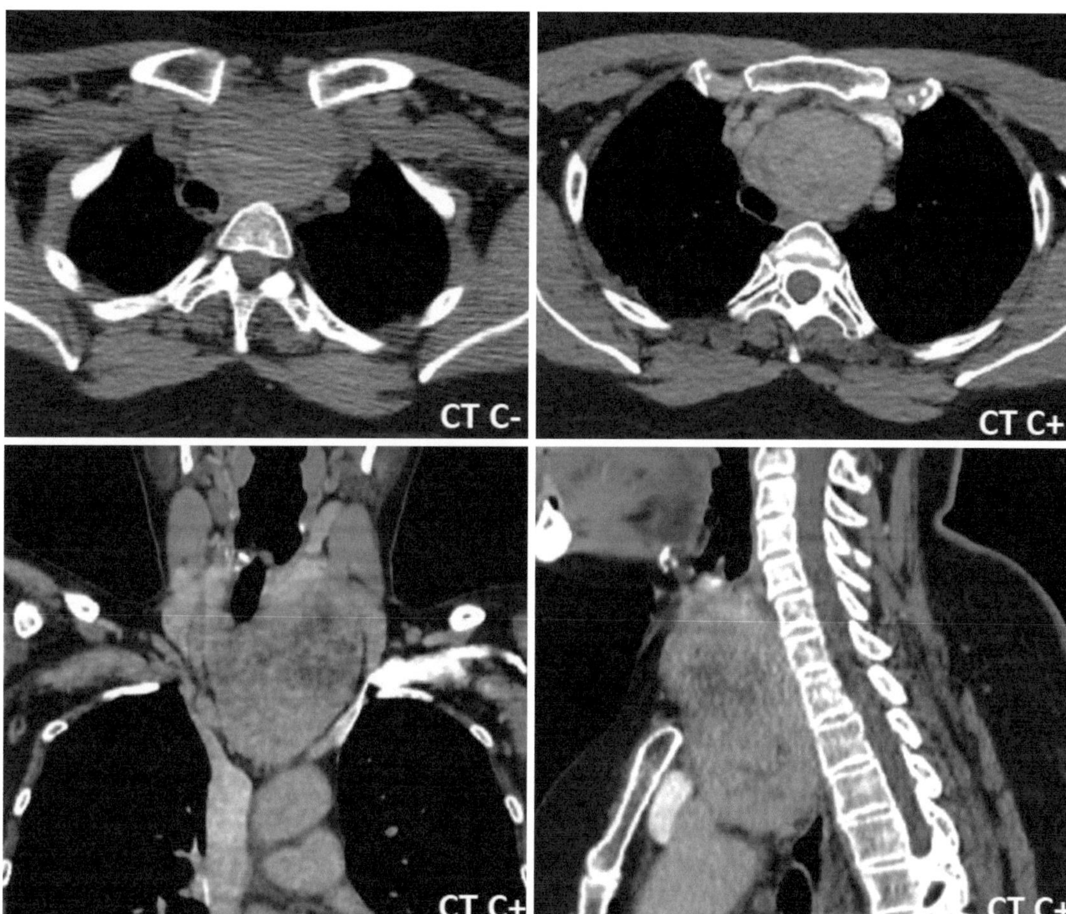

A. Haouimi et al., *Head and Neck Radiology Spot Diagnosis*,
https://doi.org/10.1007/978-3-032-14553-6_105

Findings

Heterogeneously enhancing enlarged left thyroid lobe with intrathoracic extension. It displaces the adjacent mediastinal vascular structures with tracheal shift to the right.

Diagnosis

Substernal goiter.

Discussion

Substernal or retrosternal goiter is the descent of cervical goiter through the thoracic inlet to reach the level of the chest. The incidence may range up to 45% and is more frequent after the age of 50. It is four times more common in females than in males.

The lesion develops slowly over time and the symptoms are due to the compressive nature on the adjacent structures. The patients are often asymptomatic and are discovered incidentally. A few patients may complain of midline or minimally off-midline neck swelling and dysphagia. Due to intimate relation to vital structures, FNA biopsy must be avoided in retrosternal areas.

Though ultrasound is the modality of choice at the cervical region, CT is preferred to explore the retrosternal goiter. CT can detect the extent of the prolongation of the thyroid mass, its size, morphology, and anatomic relationships. CT also allows assessment of the tracheal deviation and quantification of tracheal compression. Occasionally, the continuity with the cervical thyroid tissue is lost and it is connected to a cervical goiter via a fascial extension.

Common Differential Diagnosis

- Teratoma: mostly cystic with foci of fat and calcification without thyroid continuity
- Thymic cyst: typical location, water density without perceptible wall
- Lymphoma: FDG avid structure, encasement, and compression of mediastinal veins

Management Options

Treatment of symptomatic retrosternal goiter is often surgical.

References and Further Reading

1. Can AS, Nagalli S. Substernal Goiter. Stat Pearls Publishing. 2024. https://www.ncbi.nlm.nih.gov/books/NBK557416/. Accessed on 20 July 2025.
2. Haouimi A. Substernal goitre. Radiopaedia.org. 2020. https://doi.org/10.53347/rID-76358. Accessed on 20July 2025.
3. Mercante G, et al. CT cross-sectional imaging classification system for substernal goiter based on risk factors for an extracervical surgical approach. Head Neck. 2010. https://doi.org/10.1002/hed.21539. Accessed on 10 Apr 2024. Epub 2010 Aug 24. PMID: 20737483.

Case 106

106

Clinical History

A 10-year-old girl with a history of right ear fullness.

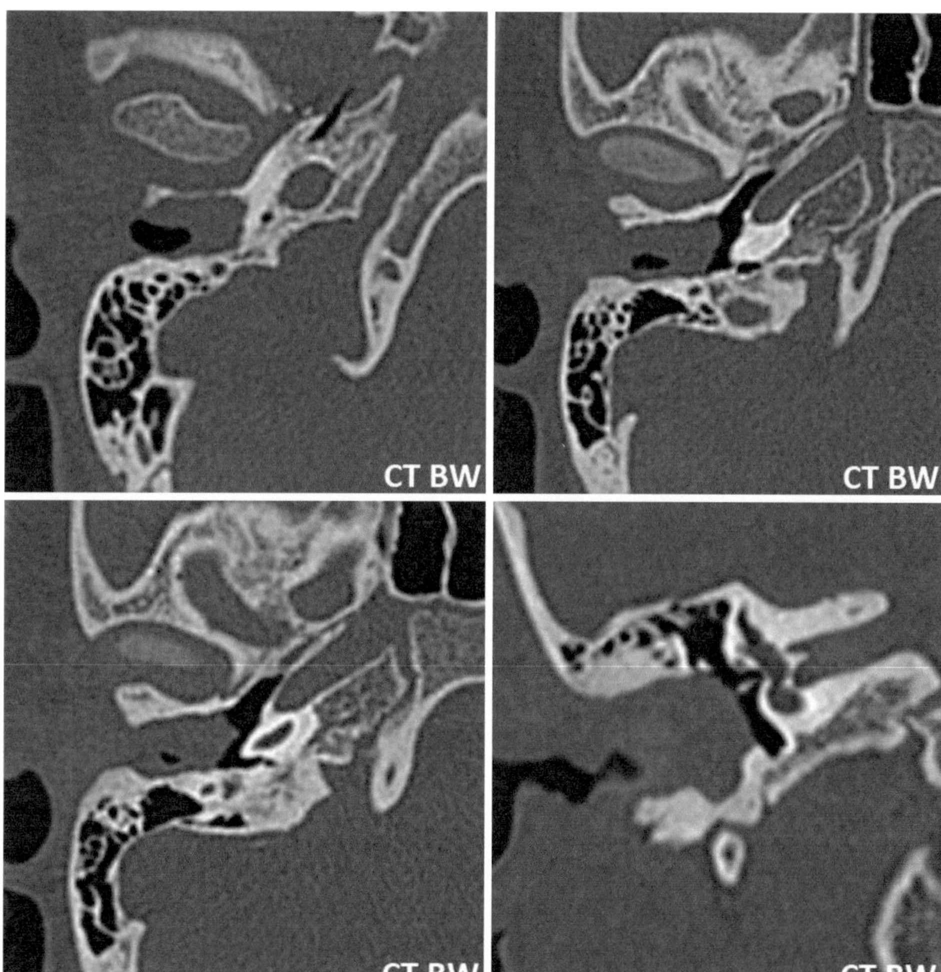

A. Haouimi et al., *Head and Neck Radiology Spot Diagnosis*,
https://doi.org/10.1007/978-3-032-14553-6_106

Findings

Soft-tissue mass filling the external auditory canal (EAC) with erosion of its posterior wall and partial destruction of the tympanic part of the temporal bone. Intact tympanic membrane with no extension into the middle ear.

Diagnosis

External auditory canal cholesteatoma.

Discussion

Cholesteatoma can be either congenital or acquired, most often affecting the middle ear. The external auditory canal involvement is extremely rare, representing <1% of cases. The lesions are composed of keratinizing stratified squamous epithelium capable of causing bone erosion and may extend into the middle ear, mastoid air cells, or facial canal. The lesions may extend locoregionally in the middle ear cavity, mastoid air cells, and facial canal.

The exact etiology is not clear. Prior surgery, external ear stenosis, and repeated trauma from cotton swabs/hearing aids are considered as predisposing factors. In a normal individual, epithelial migration clears keratin debris from the tympanic membrane, and disruption of this process is believed to contribute to external auditory canal cholesteatoma formation.

Most of the patients present with dull otalgia, otorrhea, and sometimes hearing loss. A soft-tissue mass with small bone fragments and erosion, mainly along the posterior and inferior walls of the external auditory canal, can be seen on CT.

Common Differential Diagnosis

- Keratosis obturans: no bony erosion, mildly enlarged canal.
- Necrotizing otitis externa: phlegmonous, diabetic, and immunosuppressed patients.
- Medial canal fibrosis: no bony change, lesion abuts at tympanic membrane.

Management Options

Conservative management includes regular cleaning, analgesics, and topical antibiotics. Untreated lesions may continue to grow. Smaller lesions are approached endoscopically, whereas larger lesions may need surgery.

References and Further Reading

1. Haouimi A. External auditory canal cholesteatoma. “Radiopaedia.org”. 2020. https://doi.org/10.53347/rID-84619. Accessed on 13 June 2024.
2. Heilbrun ME, et al. External auditory canal cholesteatoma: clinical and imaging spectrum. AJNR Am J Neuroradiol”. 2003. https://pubmed.ncbi.nlm.nih.gov/12695217/. Accessed on 13 June 2025. PMID: 12695217; PMCID: PMC8148678.

107 Case 107

Clinical History

An 85-year-old man presented with poor vision without any history of trauma.

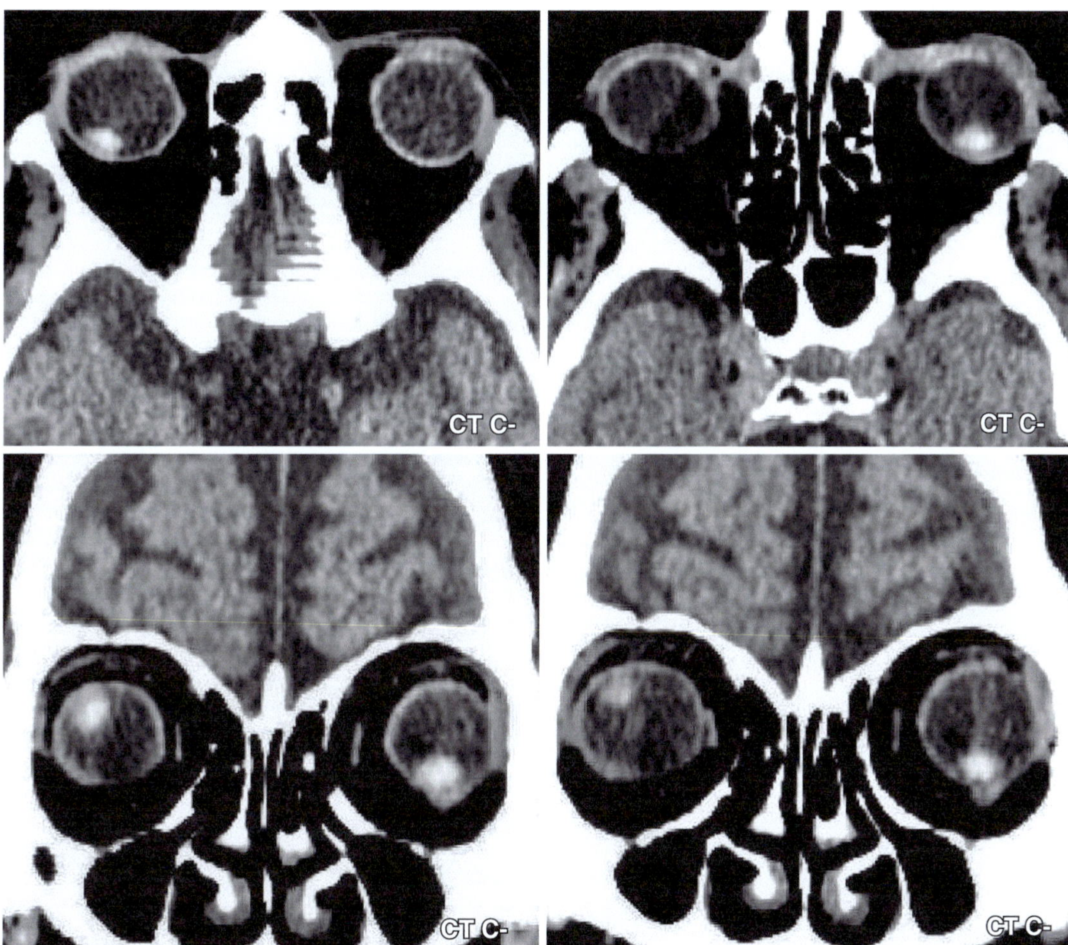

A. Haouimi et al., *Head and Neck Radiology Spot Diagnosis*,
https://doi.org/10.1007/978-3-032-14553-6_107

Findings

Bilateral posterior dislocation of the lens lying within the vitreous humor. On coronal MPR, the right lens is located anteriorly, whereas the left one is posteriorly.

Diagnosis

Bilateral ectopia lentis.

Discussion

Lenticular dislocation or subluxation is known as ectopia lentis. The lens is considered dislocated when it lies outside the hyaloid fossa, floating freely in the vitreous anteriorly, or lies directly on the retina. The lens is considered subluxed when it is partially displaced but remains within the lens space. Ectopia lentis is mostly traumatic. The condition may also be hereditary without (isolated) or with syndromic disorders such as Marfan syndrome, Ehlers–Danlos syndrome, phacomatosis.

Ultrasound can differentiate between lenticular subluxation and dislocation. With subluxation, there is unilateral posterior lenticular displacement into the anechoic vitreous. However, the contralateral margin remains attached to the iris. With lenticular dislocation, the lens occupies the most dependent position in vitreous and shows free mobility. CT has the advantage of identifying additional injuries in traumatic context.

Common Differential Diagnosis

- Marfan syndrome: additional cardiovascular involvement.
- Postsurgical complication in cataract surgery: clinical history.
- Pseudo-exfoliation open-angle glaucoma: unique characteristics and physical findings.

Management Options

Progressive noncomplicated ectopia can be managed with refractive correction. Complicated cases may need lensectomy/vitrectomy along with optical rehabilitation.

References and Further Reading

1. Haouimi A.Bilateral ectopia lentis. Radiopaedia.org. 2021. https://doi.org/10.53347/rID-89889. Accessed on 12 Apr 2023.
2. Kaur K, Gurnani B. Ectopia lentis. Stat Pearls Publishing. 2023. https://www.ncbi.nlm.nih.gov/books/NBK578193/. Accessed on 12 Apr 2023.
3. Leonard BN et al. Ectopia lentis. Surv Ophthalmol. 1982. https://www.sciencedirect.com/science/article/abs/pii/0039625782900698. Accessed on 12 Apr 2023.

Case 108

108

Clinical History

A 25-year-old woman complaining of nasal congestion. No history of trauma, surgery, or chronic inflammatory conditions of the paranasal sinuses.

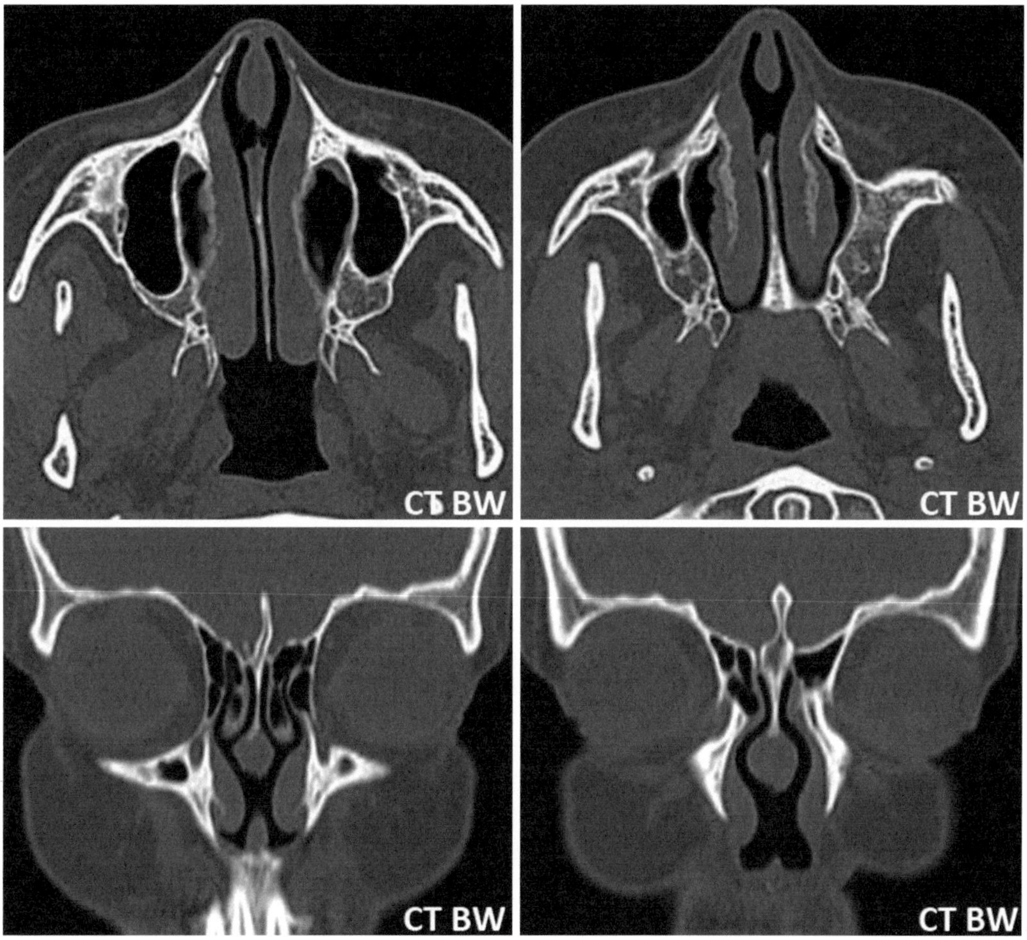

A. Haouimi et al., *Head and Neck Radiology Spot Diagnosis*,
https://doi.org/10.1007/978-3-032-14553-6_108

Findings

Focal defect of the nasal septum involving the anterior cartilaginous segment. Moderate hypertrophy of the inferior nasal turbinates. Bilateral concha bullosa. Normal pneumatization of the paranasal sinuses.

Diagnosis

Nasal septal perforation.

Discussion

The nasal septum is composed of three layers. The structural foundation is formed by the quadrangular cartilage, the perpendicular plate of the ethmoid bone, and the vomer, which are covered by bilateral mucoperichondrial leaflets. Vascular compromise to the nasal septum predisposes to septal perforation due to ischemia and necrosis. Multiple etiologic factors include trauma, infection, neoplasm, recreational drug abuse, self-manipulation (nose picking), repeated post-cauterization, and post-septoplasty. Septal perforation most commonly involves the anterior cartilaginous segment.

The turbulence of laminar airflow following septal perforation leads to mucosal dryness, crusting, epistaxis, subjective nasal obstruction, and even audible whistling.

CT can identify the nasal septal defect involving mostly the anterior cartilaginous portion. It can also evaluate the preoperative assessment of the size of perforation. Once diagnosed, the possibility of aggressive fungal sinusitis, granulomatosis with polyangiitis, sarcoidosis, lymphoma, squamous cell carcinoma, and nasosinusal melanomas needs to be ruled out.

Common Differential Diagnosis

- Diagnosis is anatomical and straightforward.

Management Options

Diligent humidification by nasal gels and emollients to minimize discomfort, crusting, and epistaxis. Formal repair and septal prostheses are the surgical options.

References and Further Reading

1. Downs BW, et al. Septal perforation. Stat Pearls Publishing. 2024. https://www.ncbi.nlm.nih.gov/books/NBK537208/. Accessed on 22 June 2025.
2. Gold M, et al. Imaging prevalence of nasal septal perforation in an urban population. Clin Imaging. 2017. https://doi.org/10.1016/j.clinimag.2017.02.002. Accessed on 22 June 2024. Epub 2017 Feb 20. PMID: 28242555.
3. Haouimi A. Nasal septal perforation. Radiopaedia.org. 2021. https://doi.org/10.53347/rID-88726. Accessed on 22 June 2025.

Case 109

Clinical History

A 30-year-old man complaining of right orbital pain with exophthalmos and extensive orbital and periorbital edema.

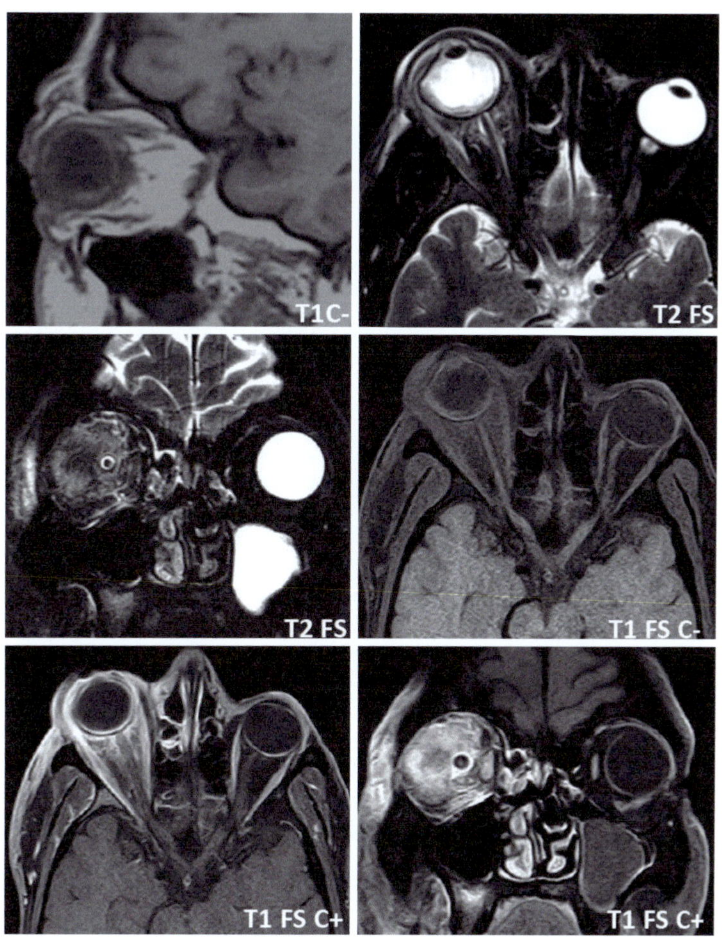

A. Haouimi et al., *Head and Neck Radiology Spot Diagnosis*,
https://doi.org/10.1007/978-3-032-14553-6_109

Findings

Slightly deformed right orbital contour with grade 3 proptosis and vitreous exudate. Thickened periorbital and preseptal soft tissues with enhancement. Haziness and enhancement of the postseptal intraconal retro-orbital soft tissues. Diffuse smooth uveal/scleral thickening with enhancement. Swelling with enhancement of the right orbital muscles with edema. Incidental left maxillary sinus retention cyst and bilateral ethmoid sinusitis, more on the right side.

Diagnosis

Orbital infection or panophthalmitis.

Discussion

Orbital infection is a serious medical emergency. It is a complex clinical entity composed of (a) periorbital cellulitis, (b) orbital cellulitis, and (c) endophthalmitis. Periorbital cellulitis is anterior to the orbital septum, whereas orbital cellulitis (also known as postseptal cellulitis) extends posterior to the septum. There is a risk of intraorbital abscess formation in orbital cellulitis. Intraocular extension of the infection is known as endophthalmitis.

Pre- or periorbital cellulitis is the extension of facial infection by contiguity. On the other hand, orbital or postseptal cellulitis is due to extension of adjacent paranasal sinusitis, and in particular, the ethmoid sinus. Endophthalmitis is often post-surgical or due to penetrating injury.

Common Differential Diagnosis

- Tolosa–Hunt syndrome: cavernous sinus involvement, ophthalmoplegia.
- Thyroid orbitopathy: hormonal abnormality; involves the belly of recti muscles.
- Orbital lymphoma: gradual onset, does not respond to antibiotics and steroids.
- Orbital sarcoidosis: systemic involvement.

Management Options

Panophthalmitis is treated with antibiotics. Surgery is also considered for subperiosteal abscess, to repair open globe injuries and/or removal of intraocular foreign bodies.

References and Further Reading

1. Danishyar A, Sergent SR. Orbital cellulitis. Stat Pearls Publishing. 2024. https://www.ncbi.nlm.nih.gov/books/NBK507901/. Accessed on 01 July 2025
2. Haouimi A. Orbital infection. Radiopaedia.org. 2022. https://doi.org/10.53347/rID-151960. Accessed on 22 July 2025.
3. Rodriguez A, et al. Orbital cellulitis with panophthalmitis and scleral necrosis – a case report. BMC Ophthalmol. 2023. https://doi.org/10.1186/s12886-023-03193-9. Accessed on 22 April 2024. PMID: 37957590; PMCID: PMC10641989.

Case 110

110

Clinical History

A 70-year-old woman complaining of chronic headache with right proptosis.

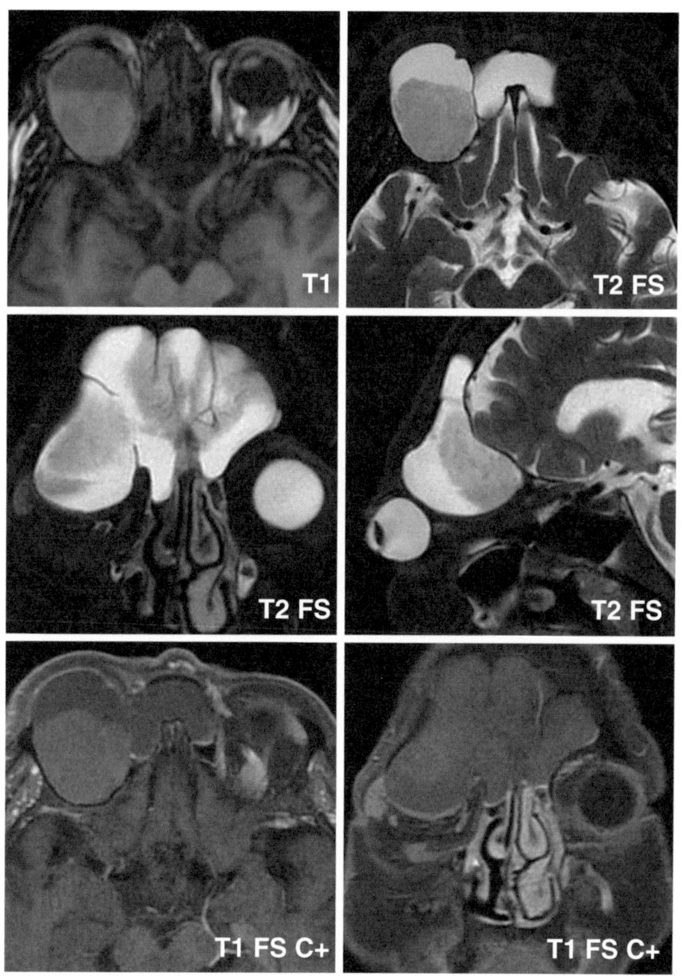

A. Haouimi et al., *Head and Neck Radiology Spot Diagnosis*,
https://doi.org/10.1007/978-3-032-14553-6_110

Findings

Right frontal sinus expansile fluid-filled cyst with smooth, scalloped bony margins. It contains areas of high signal on T1 and low signal on T2 (protein-rich content) with mild peripheral enhancement. Right eye grade III proptosis.

Diagnosis

Frontal mucocele.

Discussion

A mucocele of the frontal sinus is a mucus-filled cyst due to inflammation and blockage of the fronto-nasal duct. Intralesional buildup of mucus leads to enlargement of the size of the lesion and bony wall expansion. This finding is a sine qua non of this entity. Prostaglandins and collagenases allow the mass to grow further and lead to bony remodeling and erosion. Histologically, the lesions have the features of respiratory mucosa with cystic walls made of single-layered, pseudostratified ciliated columnar epithelium.

The onset of a mucocele can be insidious, initially remaining asymptomatic. Patients may present with headache, supraorbital swelling, and even signs of orbital cellulitis with a gradual increase in size. Larger lesions may present with proptosis and diplopia.

On CT, mucoceles are homogenously hypodense, expansile intrasinusal nonenhancing masses. There is associated bony thinning, remodeling, and occasionally osteolysis of the sinus wall. MRI signal depends on the viscosity of the cystic content. In most of the cases, they show a low signal on T1 and a high signal on T2. However, high signal on T1 and low signal on T2 can be seen due to high proteinaceous content.

Common Differential Diagnosis

- Retention cyst: no bony expansion, aeration of sinus.
- Fibrous dysplasia: "ground glass" appearance.
- Allergic fungal sinusitis: hyperdense central area, no bony expansion, multiple polyps +.

Management Options

Surgical excision is the management of choice to prevent visual complications.

References and Further Reading

1. Capra GG, et al. Paranasal sinus mucocele. Head Neck Pathol. 2012. https://doi.org/10.1007/s12105-012-0359-2. Accessed on 12 May 2024. Epub 2012 May 24. PMID: 22623085; PMCID: PMC3422585.
2. Haouimi A. Frontal mucocele. Radiopaedia.org. 2022. https://doi.org/10.53347/rID-97574. Accessed on 12 May 2024.
3. Van Tassel P, et al. Mucoceles of the paranasal sinuses: MR imaging with CT correlation. AJR Am J Roentgenol. 1989. https://doi.org/10.2214/ajr.153.2.407. Accessed on 16 Sept 2024. PMID: 2750628.

Case 111

111

Clinical History

A 45-year-old woman complaining of painful swelling of the left medial canthus.

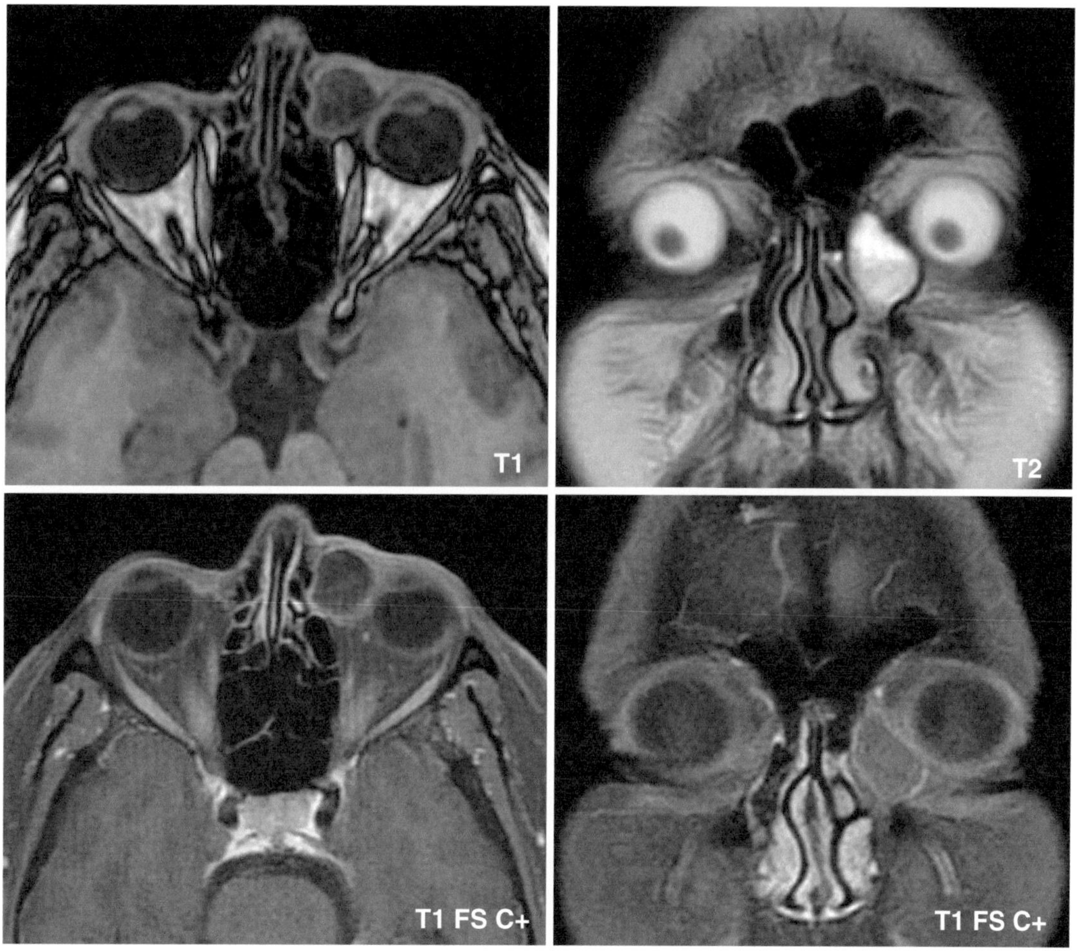

A. Haouimi et al., *Head and Neck Radiology Spot Diagnosis*,
https://doi.org/10.1007/978-3-032-14553-6_111

Findings

A thin-walled cystic mass at the left medial canthus with tapered upper and lower margins. The content shows low signal on T1 and high signal on T2, with thin peripheral wall enhancement.

Diagnosis

Dacryocystocele.

Discussion

Dacryocystocele means dilatation of the lacrimal sac in contiguity with the nasolacrimal duct. Morphologically, they appear as round or ovoid medial canthal masses due to proximal or distal obstruction of the lacrimal drainage system. Lesions can be both uni- and bilateral. Congenital dacryocystocele is mostly found in newborn babies. The congenital form is mostly associated with intranasal cysts obstructing the ductal passage. Women are more prone to dacryocystocele (3:1) as they have narrower nasal ducts. Trauma, previous surgery, chronic infection, tumors, and mucoceles are the main causes of acquired dacryocystocele.

Clinically, the patients present with epiphora, eyelid crusting, and swelling of the medial canthus. Congenital cases present as a tense, bluish grey mass during the perinatal period.

On ultrasound, the lesions are anechoic and cystic. CT is the modality of choice. The lesions are expansile, nonenhancing, thin-walled, hypodense round or ovoid masses at the medial canthus communicating with the dilated nasolacrimal duct. Cysts neighboring the distal duct may cause deviation of the inferior meatus and nasal septum. On MR, they appear as low signal on T1 and high signal on T2. However, the signal depends on the protein content. Faint peripheral enhancement can be seen, whereas a thick peripheral enhancement suggests acute dacryocystitis.

Common Differential Diagnosis

- Naso-orbital encephalocele: communication with intracranial contents.
- Dermoid cyst: heterogeneous, more at the lateral canthus, intralesional fat density/intensity.
- Ethmoid mucocele: expansile lesion, bony remodeling.

Management Options

Manual massage and prophylactic antibiotics. Most lesions regress spontaneously by one year of age. Probing, resection with marsupialization may be needed in a small percentage of cases.

References and Further Reading

1. Anwar M, et al. Idiopathic acquired dacryocystocele presenting only with epiphora: a very rare case report. Cureus. 2017. https://doi.org/10.7759/cureus.1653. Accessed on 21 June 2024. PMID: 29142801; PMCID: PMC5669535.
2. Haouimi A. Infected dacryocystocele. Radiopaedia.org. 2023. https://doi.org/10.53347/rID-181357. Accessed on 21 June 2024.

Case 112

112

Clinical History

A 40-year-old woman presented with a painless swelling of the left submandibular region.

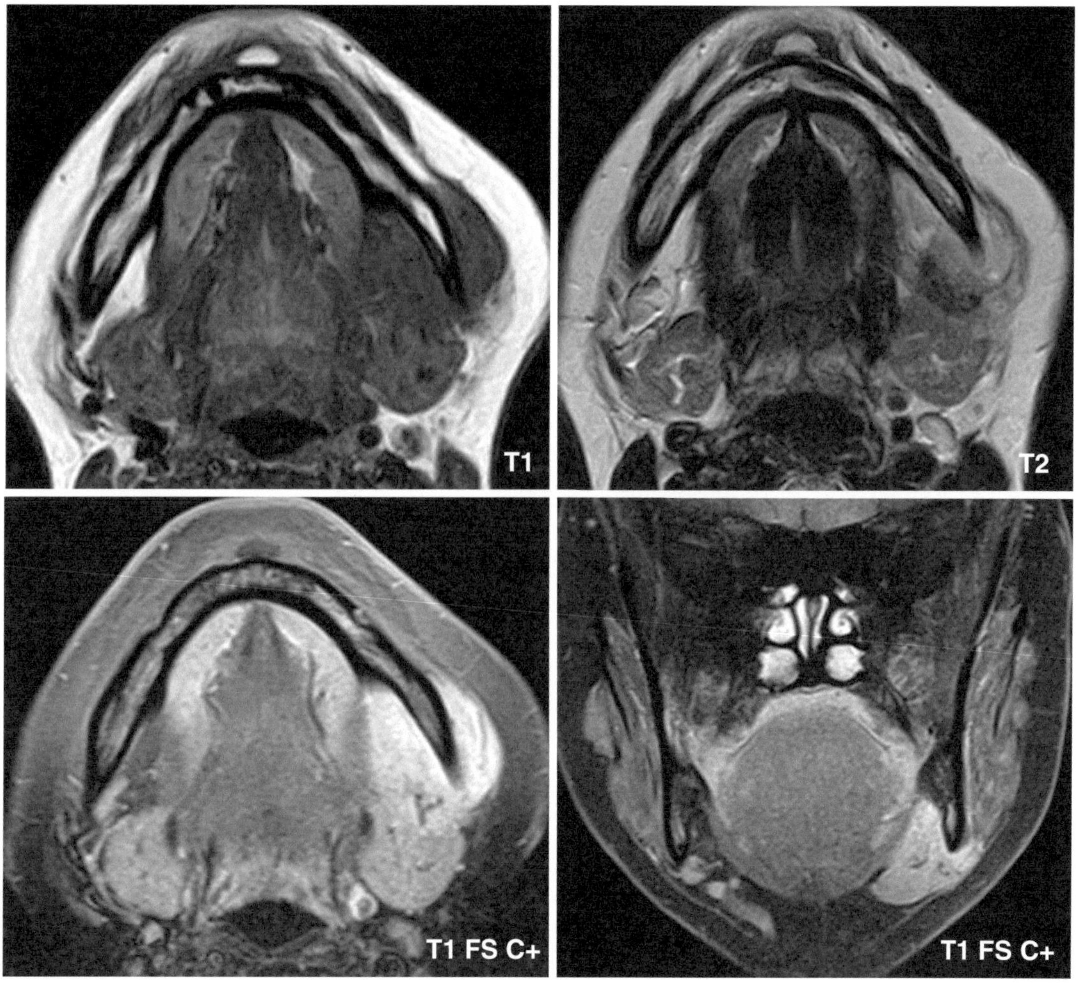

A. Haouimi et al., *Head and Neck Radiology Spot Diagnosis*,
https://doi.org/10.1007/978-3-032-14553-6_112

Findings

Left submandibular space ill-defined intraglandular soft tissue mass arising from the anterior aspect of the submandibular gland. It shows a low signal on T1, a high signal on T2 with enhancement. Pre- and retromandibular extension with displacement of the platysma and mylohyoid muscle and infiltration of the masseter.

Diagnosis

Adenoid cystic carcinoma of the submandibular gland.

Discussion

Adenoid cystic carcinoma (ACC) is a rare malignancy accounting for approximately 1% of all malignancies in the head and neck region but is the second most common tumor of the major salivary glands (up to 10% of all salivary gland tumors).

ACC presents as a painless, slow-growing swelling. Occasionally, patients may present with painful submandibular gland mass with or without paresthesia. Pathologically, the lesions arise from ductal epithelium and are locally aggressive. On CT, the smaller intraglandular lesions are seen as well-circumscribed ovoid enhancing lesions. The bigger lesions can be seen as a "beaking" exophytic enhancing mass with hazy invasive margin. On MRI, lesions appear as isointense on both T1 and T2 with homo- or heterogeneous enhancement. It is important to differentiate the lesion, whether intrinsic or extrinsic to the gland, after localizing the mass in the submandibular space.

Common Differential Diagnosis

- Sialadenitis: enlarged enhancing gland, ductal dilatation, stone +/-.
- Pleomorphic tumor: well-circumscribed, lobulated, normal fat plane, dystrophic calcification +/-.
- Malignant lymph node: clinical history, extraglandular.

Management Options

Complete resection of the tumor whenever possible is the mainstay of treatment, along with nodal dissection and postsurgical radiotherapy.

References and Further Reading

1. Ammad U, Din M, Shaikh H. Adenoid cystic cancer. Stat Pearls Publishing; 2024. https://www.ncbi.nlm.nih.gov/books/NBK557855/. Accessed on 15 June 2025
2. Coca-Pelaz A, et al. Adenoid cystic carcinoma of the head and neck–an update. Oral Oncol. 2015. https://doi.org/10.1016/j.oraloncology.2015.04.005. Accessed on 12 May 2025. Epub 2015 May 2. PMID: 25943783.
3. Haouimi A. Adenoid cystic carcinoma-submandibular gland. Radiopaedia.org. 2021. https://doi.org/10.53347/rID-93064. Accessed on 15 June 2025.

113 Case 113

Clinical History

A 35-year-old woman presented with a history of watery discharge from the right nose. Had a facial trauma a few months ago.

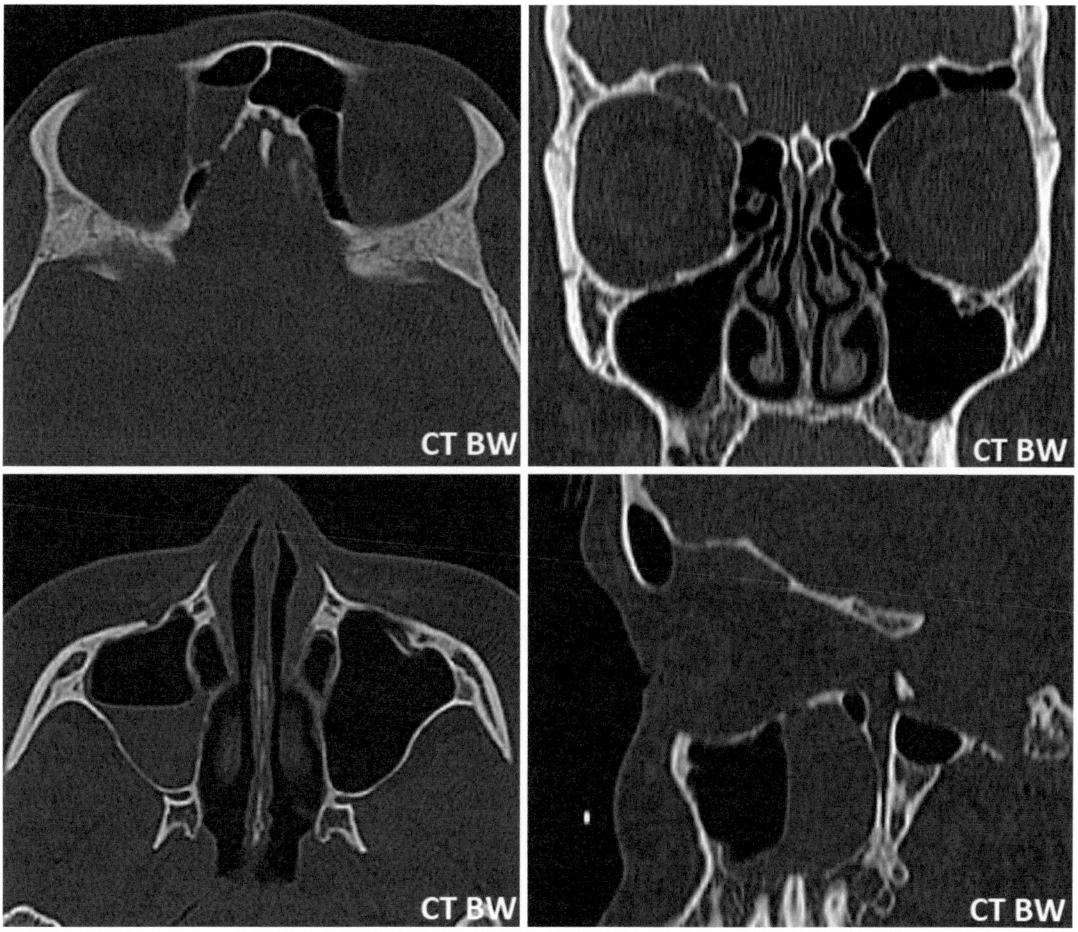

A. Haouimi et al., *Head and Neck Radiology Spot Diagnosis*,
https://doi.org/10.1007/978-3-032-14553-6_113

Findings

Bony defect of the posterior wall of the right frontal sinus with fluid accumulation within the ipsilateral frontal and maxillary sinuses. Normal mucosal thickening of paranasal sinuses.

Diagnosis

CSF rhinorrhea.

Discussion

Dural tear for any reason allows the cerebrospinal fluid to escape into the paranasal sinuses. The etiology can be: (a) spontaneous in idiopathic intracranial hypertension due to increased intracranial pressure, (b) post-traumatic and iatrogenic (as a complication of neurosurgery and endoscopic surgery), (c) certain aggressive intranasal lesions such as inverted papilloma and malignant tumors involving the anterior cranial fossa, and (d) congenital skull base defect. Obesity and obstructive sleep apnea, especially in female patients, are at increased risk of spontaneous rhinorrhea. The common sites of tear are at the cribriform plate of the ethmoid bone and perisellar region of the sphenoid sinus.

The patients present with intermittent positional discharge of clear fluid from the nose. The diagnosis is confirmed biochemically by detecting beta-2-transferrin in the fluid.

High-resolution CT can detect the larger defects. CT cisternography can detect the site of the leakage by observing a streak of contrast or pooling of contrast in the nasal cavity and paranasal sinuses. Presence of pneumoencephalus and air-fluid levels within the paranasal sinuses is an indirect sign of CSF tear in the appropriate clinical context.

Common Differential Diagnosis

- CSF otorrhea: leakage in temporal bone
- Allergic rhinitis: always bilateral
- Acute sinusitis: clinical history, purulent nasal discharge, mucosal wall thickening

Management Options

Spontaneous recovery is possible in the vast majority of small tears. Prophylactic antibiotics to prevent ascending meningitis. Surgical options include both intracranial and transnasal endoscopic repair after failure of conservative management and for patients with larger defects.

References and Further Reading

1. Haouimi A. CSF rhinorrhoea. Radiopaedia.org. 2021. https://doi.org/10.53347/rID-92102. Accessed on 25 June 2024.
2. Xie M, et al. Diagnosis and localization of cerebrospinal fluid rhinorrhea: a systematic review. Am J Rhinol Allergy. 2021. https://doi.org/10.1177/19458924211060918. Accessed on 10 Oct 2024. Epub 2021 Nov 30. PMID: 34846218.
3. Hirabayashi M, et al. Recurrent meningitis caused by idiopathic cerebrospinal fluid rhinorrhoea. BMJ Case Rep. 2018. https://doi.org/10.1136/bcr-2017-222296

Case 114

114

Clinical History

A 20-year-old woman presented with a painless swelling of the right mandibular region.

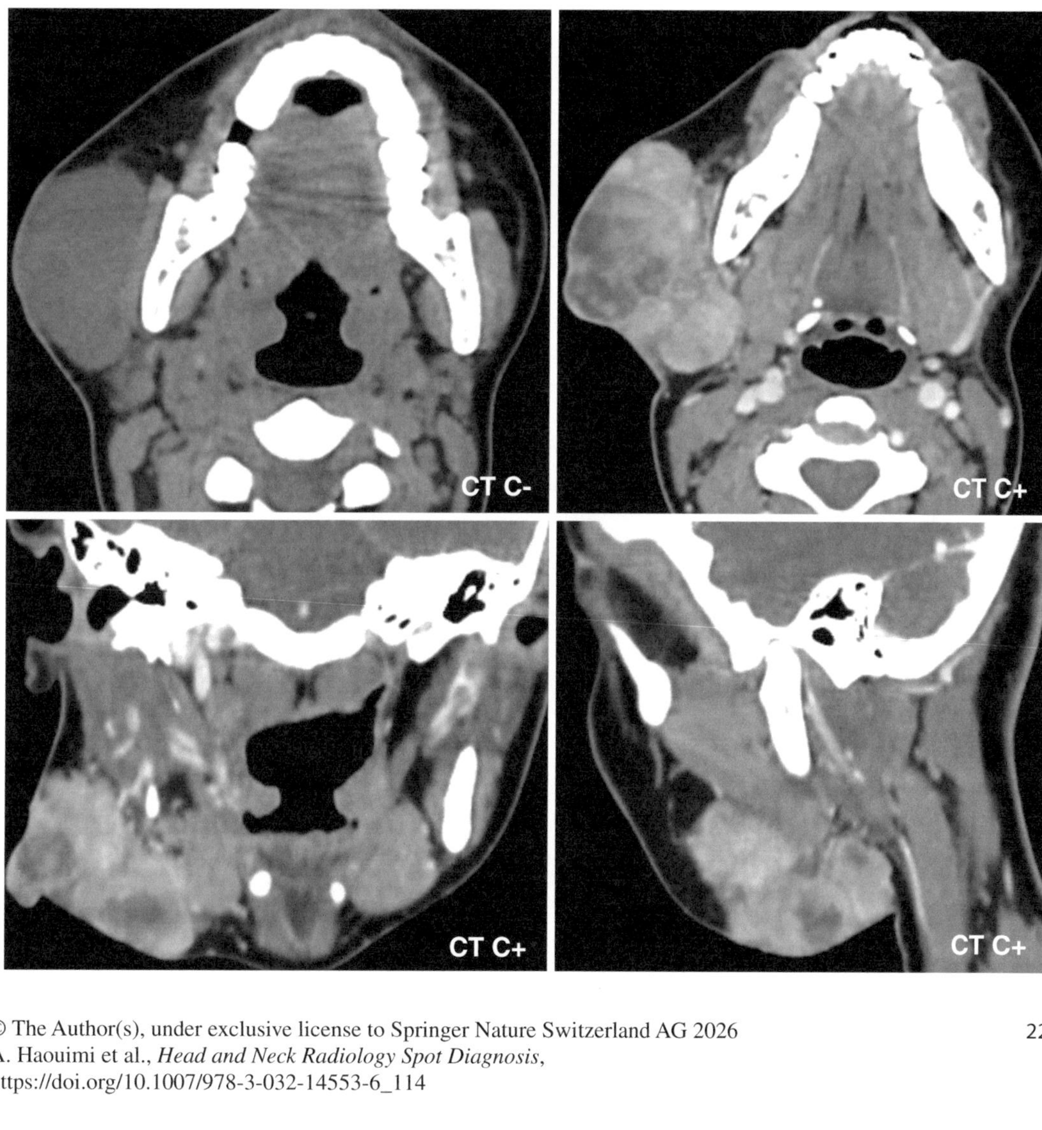

A. Haouimi et al., *Head and Neck Radiology Spot Diagnosis*,
https://doi.org/10.1007/978-3-032-14553-6_114

Findings

A large lobulated enhancing subcutaneous soft-tissue mass of the right pre-and submandibular regions with central necrotic foci. The mass contacts the adjacent masseter muscle and ipsilateral submandibular gland with infiltration of the skin. No cervical lymphadenopathy is seen.

Diagnosis

Facial myxofibrosarcoma.

Discussion

The incidence of head and neck myxofibrosarcoma (MFS) is rare. They are a connective tissue malignant neoplasm of fibroblastic origin set in myxoid matrix. It is the most common soft-tissue sarcoma of late adult life, peaking in the seventh decade with male predominance. The lesions are locoregionally aggressive, with a high risk of recurrence. The lesions grow underneath the skin. Both dermis and hypodermis are the preferential sites.

On MRI, the lesions are heterogeneous. The myxoid component shows low signal on T1 and high signal on T2 without enhancement, whereas the remaining soft-tissue component enhances. Enhancing linear/tapered extension of soft tissue along the fascial plane can give rise to a "fascial tail sign," which is suggestive of diagnosis, though not specific.

Common Differential Diagnosis

- Melanoma: high signal on T1 and low signal on T2.
- Liposarcoma: nonhomogeneous high signal on T1 and T2, can be suppressed on fat sat.
- Rhabdomyosarcoma: epicentered at muscles not dermal and subdermal preference.

Management Options

Management options are surgical: curettage, enucleation, and "en block" resection. Other options are radiotherapy and occasionally chemotherapy, depending on the histological grading.

References and Further Reading

1. Dell'Aversana O, et al. Head and neck myxofibrosarcoma: a case report and review of the literature. J Med Case Rep. 2014 https://doi.org/10.1186/1752-1947-8-468. Accessed on 12 Dec 2024. PMID: 25547541; PMCID: PMC4320505.
2. Haouimi A. Myxofibrosarcoma-facial. Radiopaedia.org. 2021. https://doi.org/10.53347/rID-94426. Accessed on 12 Dec 2024.
3. Vanni S, et al. Myxofibrosarcoma landscape: diagnostic pitfalls, clinical management and future perspectives. Ther Adv Med Oncol. 2022. https://doi.org/10.1177/17588359221093973. Accessed on 12 Dec 2024. PMID: 35782752; PMCID: PMC9244941.

Case 115

115

Clinical History

A 30-year-old woman presented with a painless hard left frontoparietal lump.

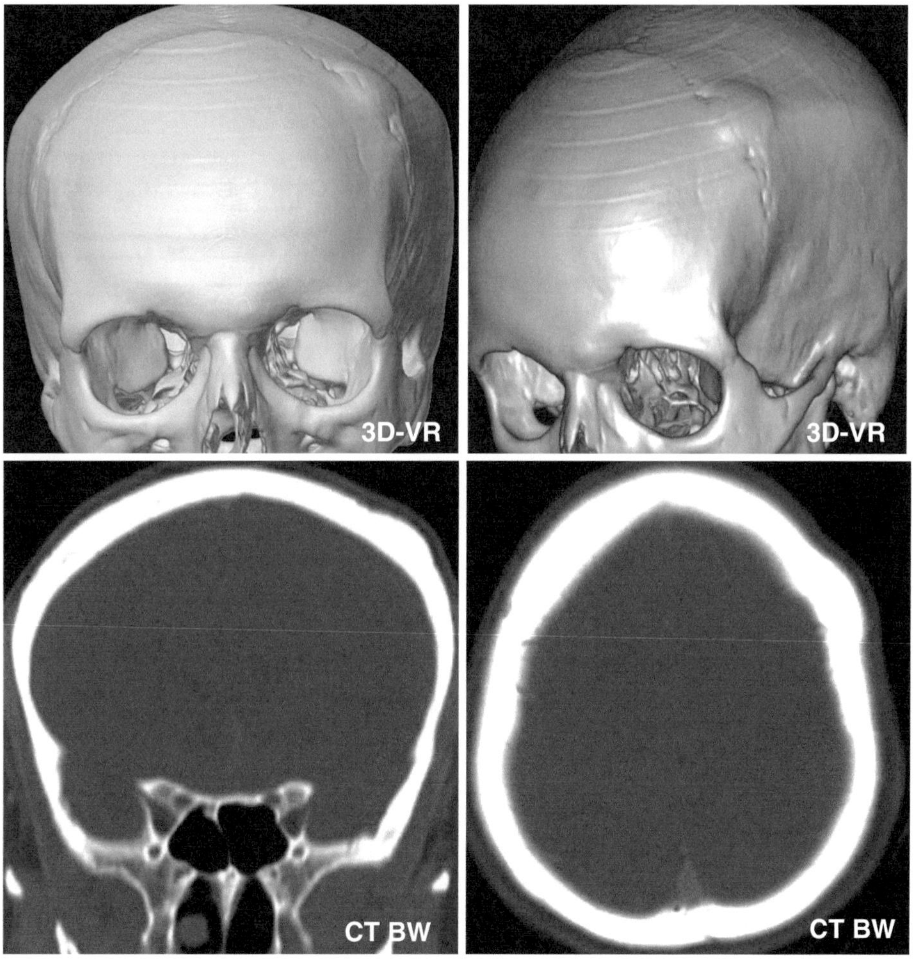

A. Haouimi et al., *Head and Neck Radiology Spot Diagnosis*,
https://doi.org/10.1007/978-3-032-14553-6_115

Findings

A broad-based dense lesion arising from the outer table of the left frontoparietal calvarium, overlapping the coronal suture with no adjacent soft-tissue abnormality.

Diagnosis

Osteoma of the cranial vault: "Button osteoma."

Discussion

Cranial vault osteomas, also known as "button osteoma" or "ivory exostosis," are usually an incidental finding. They are slow-growing, expansile, and benign lesions usually arising from both inner and outer tables of the skull vault, typically between 2 and 4 cm in maximal diameter. Osteomas are seen almost exclusively in the craniofacial region. The most frequent locations for skull vault osteomas are the parietal and frontal bones.

Histologically, osteomas are hamartomas without stromal cellular proliferation. They can be compact and bony, lacking Haversian systems (ivory osteoma), mature osteoma (osteoma spongiosum: normal trabecular bone often with the presence of marrow), and mixed type.

Clinically, osteomas are painless and asymptomatic. Occasionally, the extensive growth of the lesion may cause aesthetic or functional problems that vary according to location. Multifocal osteomas can be seen as part of Gardner syndrome associated with multiple colonic polyps.

Radiologically, osteomas are well-circumscribed hyperostotic lesions without any involvement of adjacent soft tissue. The ivory osteomas appear very dense, like the bony cortex, whereas mature osteomas may show central marrow.

Common Differential Diagnosis

- Paget's disease: "cotton wool" appearance.
- Fibrous dysplasia: homogeneous "ground glass" appearance in diploic space.
- Metastasis: usually involves diploic space, sclerotic and lytic components, clinical history.

Management Options

No treatment is needed for osteomas unless they are symptomatic. Larger osteomas need to be evaluated to rule out other diagnoses.

References and Further Reading

1. Eppley BL, et al. Large osteomas of the cranial vault. J Craniofac Surg. 2023. https://doi.org/10.1097/00001665-200301000-00018. Accessed on 18 June 2024. PMID:12544230.
2. Gundewar S, et al. Osteomas of the craniofacial region: a case series and review of literature. Indian J Plast Surg. 2013. https://doi.org/10.4103/0970-0358.121982. Accessed on 12 Jan 2024. PMID: 24459335; PMCID: PMC3897090.
3. Haouimi A. Osteoma of the cranial vault. Radiopaedia.org. 2019. https://doi.org/10.53347/rID-71620. Accessed on 03 July 2022.

Case 116

116

Clinical History

A 59-year-old woman presented to the emergency room with a 1-week history of increasing stridor. No other positive medical history.

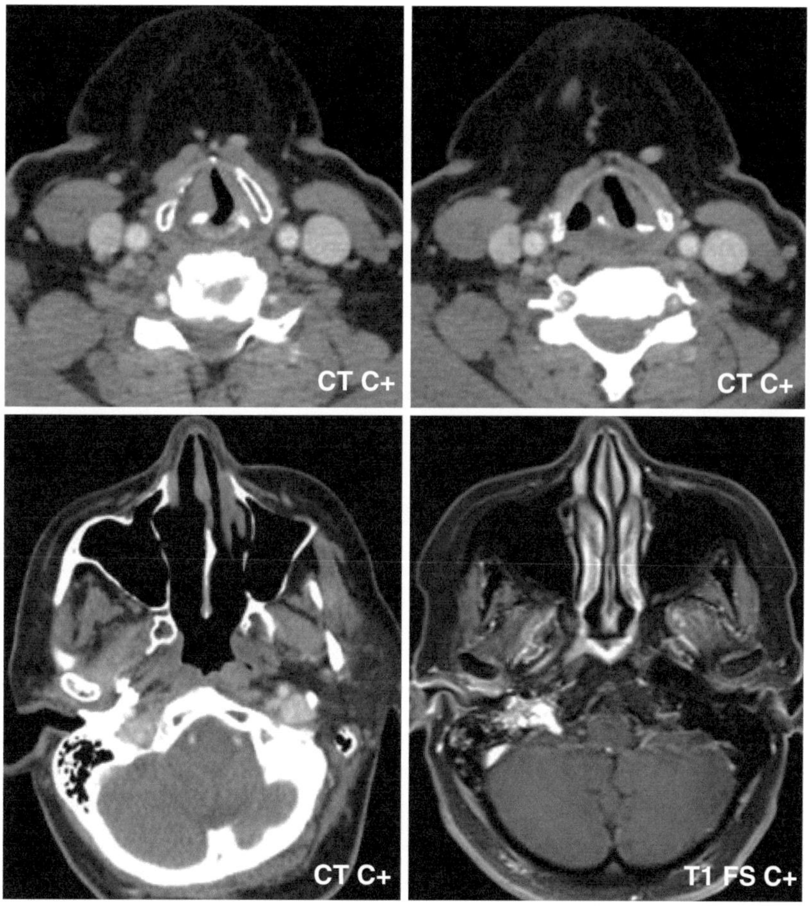

A. Haouimi et al., *Head and Neck Radiology Spot Diagnosis*,
https://doi.org/10.1007/978-3-032-14553-6_116

Findings

Enhanced CT scan of the neck shows asymmetric enlargement of the right piriform sinus. Thickened right aryepiglottic fold, rotation of the right arytenoid cartilage, and medialization/adduction with fullness of the right vocal cord. The CT of the neck at the skull base revealed an enhancing right jugular fossa mass, confirmed by an enhanced MRI.

Diagnosis

Right vocal cord paralysis (VCP).

Discussion

VCP can be unilateral or bilateral. Clinical presentation depends on whether paralysis is acute or chronic. Symptoms may impact voice, breathing and airway, or swallowing.

In about 40% of the cases, it is idiopathic with negative imaging findings. Iatrogenic causes may arise following thyroid, carotid, or skull base surgery. Other causes include stroke, demyelination, and amyotrophic lateral sclerosis. Tumoral compression on the nerve pathway from cancer of lung and thyroid, as well as skull base foramina, is potentially treatable cause. Viral causes include EBV and Ramsay Hunt syndrome.

CT helps to identify secondary lesions along the course of the vagus nerve and recurrent laryngeal nerves. Direct radiological signs include glottic asymmetry, thickened aryepiglottic fold, dilated ipsilateral piriform sinus, as well as medial rotation of arytenoid cartilage. Medialization of both vocal cords (no abduction during respiration), medial rotation of arytenoid cartilages, both sided piriform sinus dilatation and narrowing of glottic airway suggest bilateral VCP.

Common Differential Diagnosis

- Lateral medullary syndrome: acute onset, posterior fossa abnormality.
- Skull base tumors: gradual onset, enhancing lesions at skull base.
- Thyroid carcinoma: asymmetric thyroid with calcification, +/- infiltration.0

Management Options

The secondary causes would require specific targeted treatments (glomus tumors, thyroid masses). Conservative and supportive management is the treatment of choice for idiopathic cases.

References and Further Reading

1. Alwan M, Paddle PM. Vocal cord paralysis: pathophysiology, etiologies, and evaluation. Int J Head Neck Surg. 2022;12(4):153–60. https://doi.org/10.5005/jp-journals-10001-1515.
2. Bashir MH, et al. Revisiting CT signs of unilateral vocal fold paralysis: a single, blinded study. Am J Neuroradiol. 2022;43(4):592–6. https://doi.org/10.3174/ajnr.A7451.

Case 117

117

Clinical History

A 40-year-old woman presented with difficulty in mastication and right facial numbness.

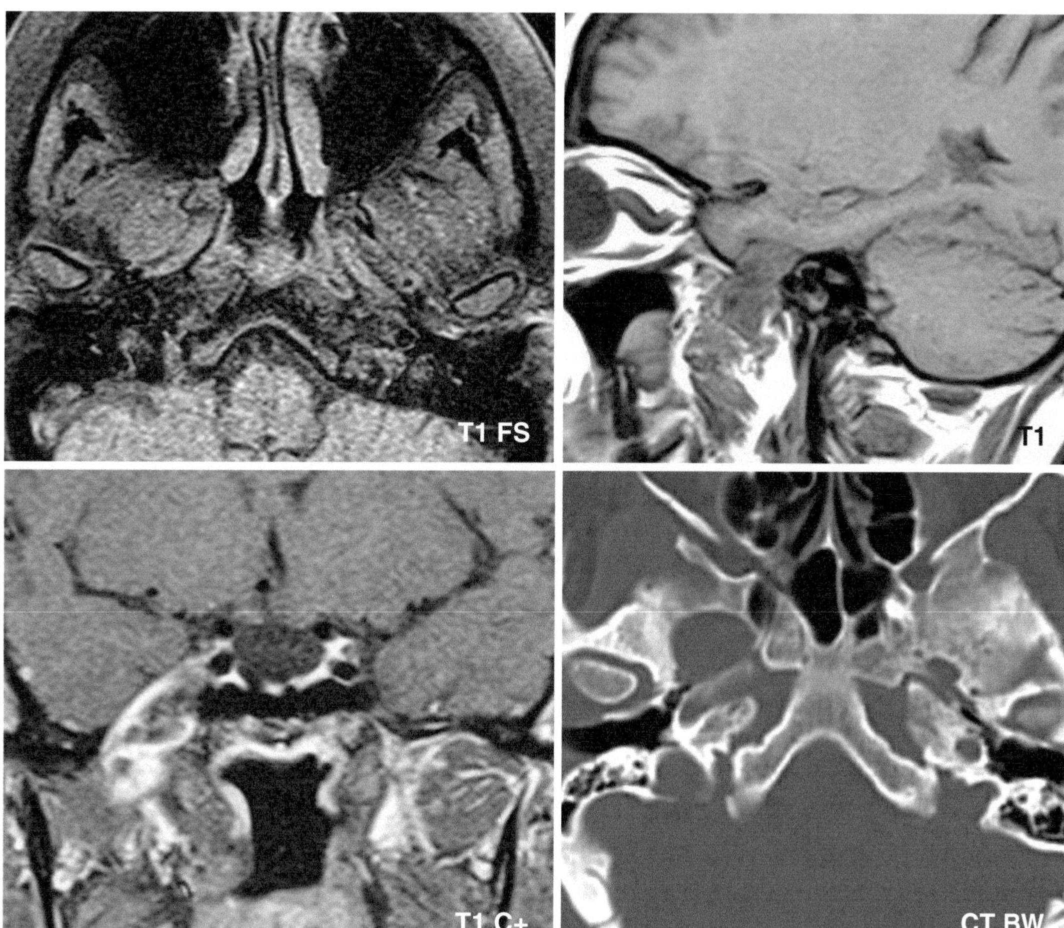

A. Haouimi et al., *Head and Neck Radiology Spot Diagnosis*,
https://doi.org/10.1007/978-3-032-14553-6_117

Findings

Tubular soft-tissue mass extending from the ipsilateral cavernous sinus through an enlarged foramen ovale. It appears hypointense on T1 with heterogeneous contrast enhancement. The bone window shows an enlarged right foramen ovale without erosion. Partially empty sella.

Diagnosis

Mandibular schwannoma.

Discussion

Mandibular schwannomas are indolent benign tumors arising from the perineural Schwann cells, mostly in the vicinity of foramen ovale. Schwannomas are more frequently seen in the second and third decades of life and probably with no gender predilection. Mandibular schwannomas can also be seen in the setting of neurofibromatosis. Hence, once a schwannoma is diagnosed, an additional lesion should be sought to rule out this possibility.

Clinically, mandibular schwannomas are asymptomatic and may slowly increase in size until they cause aesthetic deformities or difficulty with mastication.

On MRI, the lesions are iso/slightly hyperintense on T1 and high signal on T2 with marked enhancement after gadolinium. Calcification is rare. Masticator muscle atrophy can be seen in advanced cases. In the absence of any history of cancer, any tubular lesion passing through foramen ovale should be considered a schwannoma until proved otherwise.

Common Differential Diagnosis

- Skull base meningioma: do not follow nerve tract, may show calcification.
- Perineural extension: lesions are often identified in the cavernous sinus and/or masticator space.
- Non-Hodgkin lymphoma (NHL): usually not tubular.

Management Options

Treatment is surgical. Adjuvant radiosurgery for incomplete excision and for recurrent lesions.

References and Further Reading

1. Agrawal A, et al.Trigeminal schwannoma. Natl J Maxillofac Surg. 2017. https://doi.org/10.4103/njms.NJMS_82_14. Accessed on 20 May 2024. PMID: 29386819; PMCID: PMC5773990.
2. Haouimi A. Radiopaedia.org. 2022. https://doi.org/10.53347/rID-87850. Accessed on 20 May 2024.
3. Shetty SR, et al. J Neurosci Rural Pract. 2011. https://doi.org/10.4103/0976-3147.80108. Accessed on 20 May 2022.

Case 118

118

Clinical History

A 60-year-old man presented with a chronic headache.

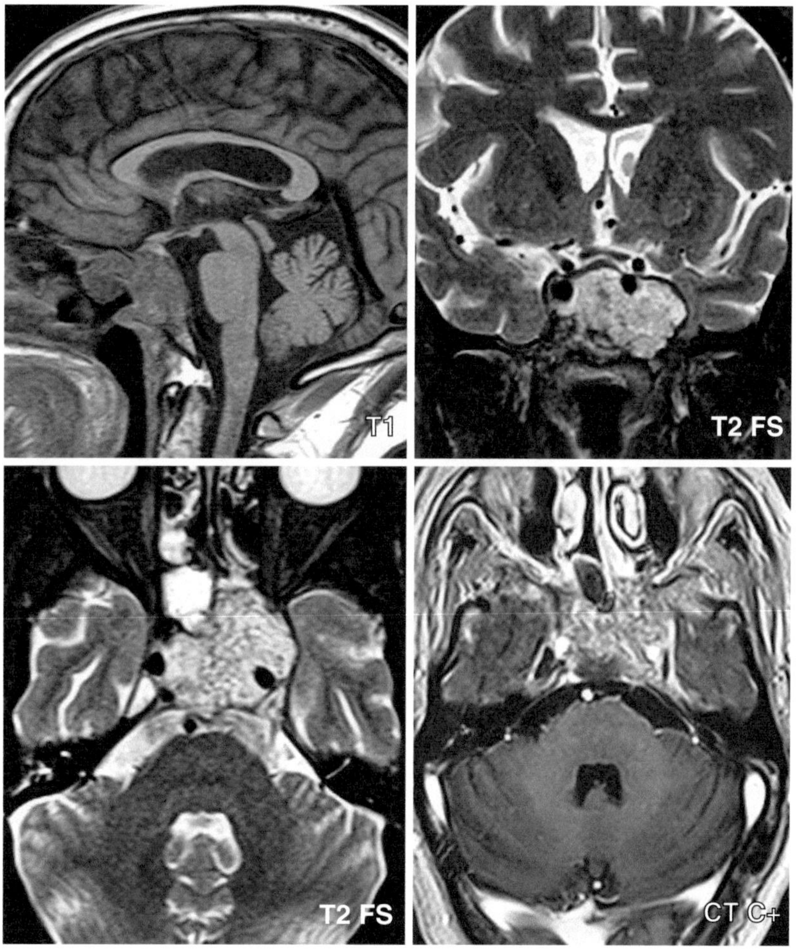

A. Haouimi et al., *Head and Neck Radiology Spot Diagnosis*,
https://doi.org/10.1007/978-3-032-14553-6_118

Findings

Well-circumscribed lesion centered on the clivus with extension to the sphenoid and cavernous sinuses, mainly on the left. Mass shows low signal on T1, nonhomogeneous high signal on T2 FS with moderate heterogeneous contrast enhancement.

Diagnosis

Chordoma.

Discussion

Chordomas are slow-growing midline tumors originating from notochordal remnants. Sacrococcygeal and spheno-occipital locations are the most common. They are mainly seen among middle-aged adults with no sexual predominance. Most cases are spontaneous. The lesions expand locoregionally and can lead to brainstem and hypothalamic compression and hydrocephalus.

Symptoms include headache, nausea, and visual disturbances. As the tumor grows, the patients show the signs of cranial nerve neuropathies.

The lesions are mostly solid on CT and MRI. Necrotic and hemorrhagic foci, calcifications, and bony sequestrations are responsible for signal nonhomogeneity. Any destructive heterogeneous mass with clival epicenter should always raise the suspicion of chordoma.

Common Differential Diagnosis

- Pituitary macroadenoma: intact clival fat.
- Chondroblastoma: mostly off-midline.
- Clival meningioma: often associated with “dural tail sign”.

Management Options

Chordomas are difficult to treat due to their central location and involvement of critical neurovascular structures. When symptomatic and feasible, surgical resection is preferred. Radiotherapy is considered for residual and recurrent cases.

References and Further Reading

1. Haouimi A. Radiopaedia.org. 2019. https://doi.org/10.53347/rID-65149. Accessed on 26 June 2022.
2. Khawaja A, et al. Pol J Radiol. 2017. https://doi.org/10.12659/PJR.902008. Accessed on 26 June 2022.
3. Tenny S, Varacallo M. Chordoma. Stat Pearls Publishing. 2023. https://www.ncbi.nlm.nih.gov/books/NBK430846/. Accessed on 10 Apr 2024.

Case 119

119

Clinical History

A 40-year-old woman presented with a cervicalgia and restricted neck movement.

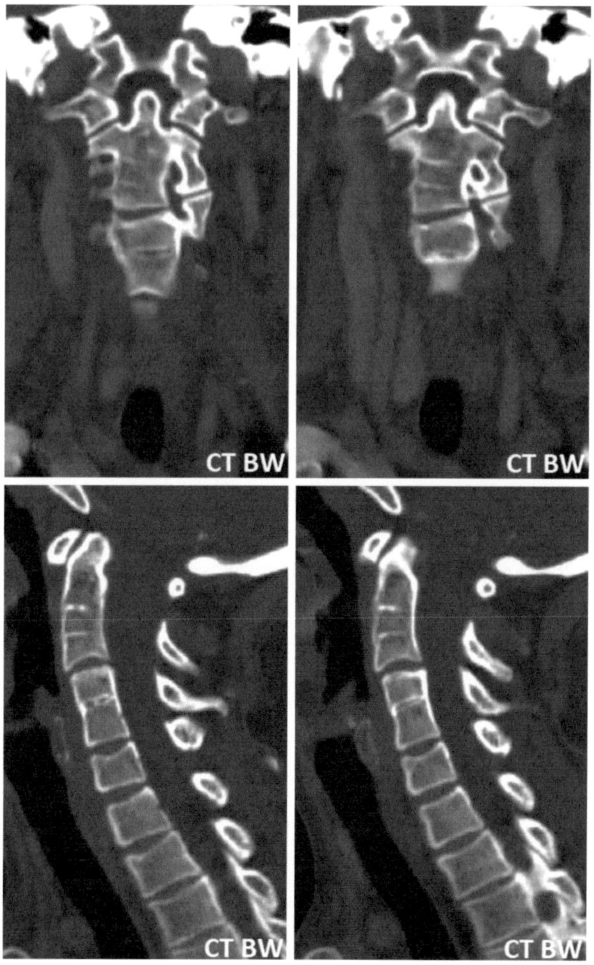

A. Haouimi et al., *Head and Neck Radiology Spot Diagnosis*,
https://doi.org/10.1007/978-3-032-14553-6_119

Findings

Fusion of multiple vertebral bodies with rudimentary discs and preservation of anteroposterior diameter of cervical canal. Slight cervical scoliosis of right-sided convexity. Normal pre- and paravertebral soft tissue.

Diagnosis

Klippel–Feil syndrome (KFS).

Discussion

Klippel–Feil syndrome (KFS), also known as cervical vertebral fusion syndrome, is a congenital disorder characterized by fusion of two or more cervical vertebrae. The syndrome is possibly due to genetic mutations in growth differentiation factor 6 and 3 (GDF6 and GDF3) and to failure of normal segmentation of the cervical somites during the 3rd to 8th weeks of gestation. The incidence is 1 in 42,000 births and 60% of cases are female. KFS can be associated with Sprengel shoulder deformity, scoliosis, urinary tract anomalies, and congenital heart disease.

KFS is frequently identified incidentally. Clinically, affected patients may be asymptomatic or present with characteristic features such as a short neck, restricted cervical mobility, reduced flexibility, facial asymmetry, torticollis, and a low posterior hairline. Nagib and colleagues proposed a clinical classification consisting of three types: Type I, characterized by two sets of fused vertebrae separated by mobile segments that may sublux progressively or following trauma; Type II, involving cranio-cervical anomalies such as occipitalization of the atlas and basilar invagination, which may result in foramen magnum encroachment; and Type III, defined by fusion at multiple spinal levels often associated with spinal canal stenosis.

Common Differential Diagnosis

- Ankylosing spondylitis: Romanus lesion or "shiny corner sign," "bamboo spine."
- Forestier's disease: ligamentous calcification of anterior longitudinal ligament, affect at least four contiguous vertebrae.

Management Options

Most patients are asymptomatic and treated nonoperatively. Surgical indication depends on the amount of deformity, spinal stability, location, and neurologic problems.

References and Further Reading

1. Haouimi A. Klippel-Feil syndrome. Radiopaedia.org. https://doi.org/10.53347/rID-79511. Accessed on 08 Dec 2024.
2. Menger RP, Rayi A, Notarianni C. Klippel Feil syndrome. Stat Pearls Publishing. 2024. https://www.ncbi.nlm.nih.gov/books/NBK493157/. Accessed on 08 Dec 2024. PMID: 29630209.

Case 120

Clinical History

A 60-year-old woman with a palpable right supraclavicular mass and radiculopathy of the right upper limb.

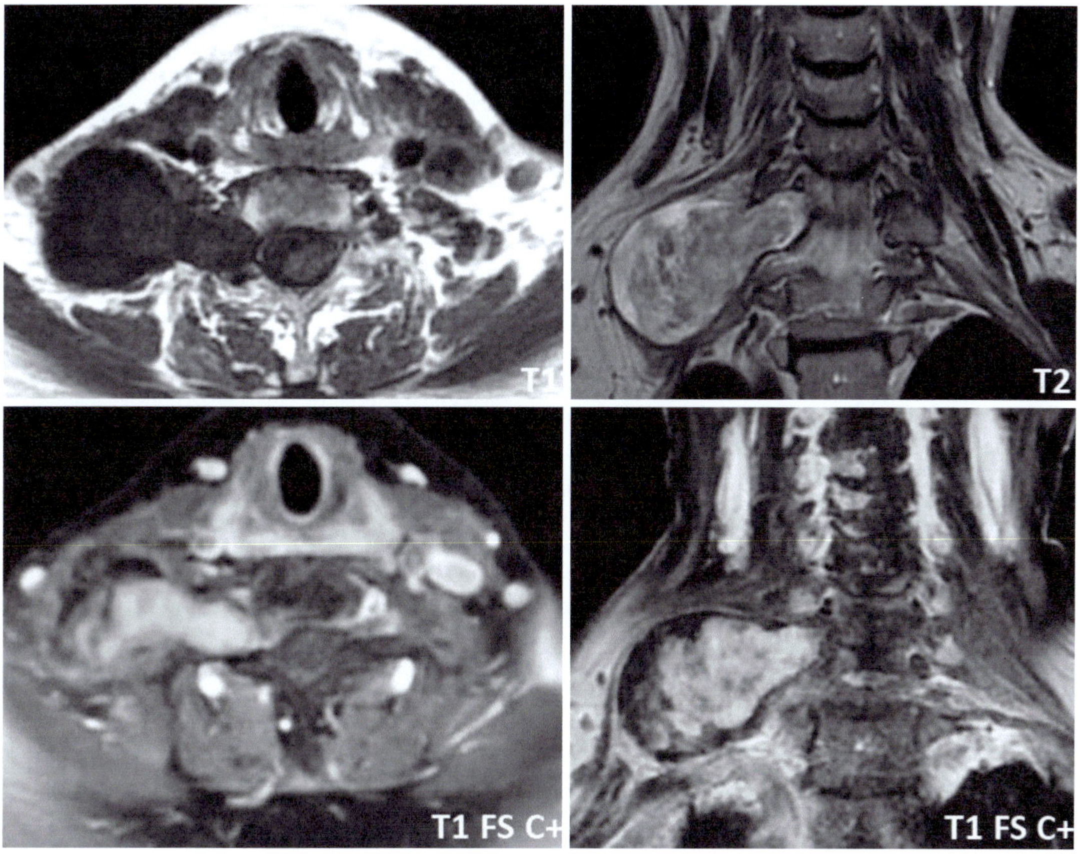

A. Haouimi et al., *Head and Neck Radiology Spot Diagnosis*,
https://doi.org/10.1007/978-3-032-14553-6_120

Findings

Well-circumscribed “dumbbell-shaped” soft tissue mass extending through an enlarged C6-C7 exit foramen, along the C7 nerve root with vertebral scalloping. It appears hypointense to the spinal cord on T1, inhomogeneously hyperintense on T2 with heterogeneous contrast enhancement.

Diagnosis

Brachial plexus schwannoma.

Discussion

Brachial plexus schwannomas are a benign neoplasm appearing as “fusiform” or “dumbbell-shaped” lesions along the course of the brachial plexus. The specific course of the lesion is key to the diagnosis. Anatomically, they are located between anterior and middle scalene muscles. The lesion may undergo cystic degeneration and may be hemorrhagic. Due to the slow-growing nature, most of the lesions are clinically silent but may have signs of lateral neck radiculopathy. The presence of pain raises suspicion for malignancy, though the incidence is extremely rare.

On MRI, brachial plexus schwannomas show spherical thickening of the nerves along the longitudinal course with no appreciable perilesional edema. Tumors usually show a "dumbbell configuration” with both intra and extraspinal components. Lesions are of low/isosignal on T1 and high on T2 with enhancement. The “fascicular sign” (multiple ring-like structures with peripheral hyperintensity on T2) is nonspecific for any neurogenic tumor.

Common Differential Diagnosis

- Perineural root sleeve cyst: low signal on T1, high signal on T2 with no enhancement.
- Paraspinal ganglioneuroma: homogeneously low intensity lesion, calcification +/-.
- Systemic nodal metastases: clinical history, not dumbbell-shaped, often multiple.

Management Options

Symptomatic cases need surgical excision with low chance of recurrence.

References and Further Reading

1. Haouimi A. Radiopaedia.org. 2023. https://doi.org/10.53347/rID-169077. Accessed on 23 May 2023.
2. Szaro P, et al. Magnetic resonance imaging of the brachial plexus. Part 2: Traumatic injuries. Eur J Radiol Open. 2022. https://doi.org/10.1016/j.ejro.2022.100397. Accessed on 17 Apr 2024. PMID: 35111891; PMCID: PMC8789590.
3. Vučemilo L, et al. Brachial plexus schwannoma – case report and literature review. Acta Clin Croat. 2018. https://doi.org/10.20471/acc.2018.57.02.19. PMID: 30431732.

Case 121

121

Clinical History

A 65-year-old man presented with signs of left facial nerve palsy.

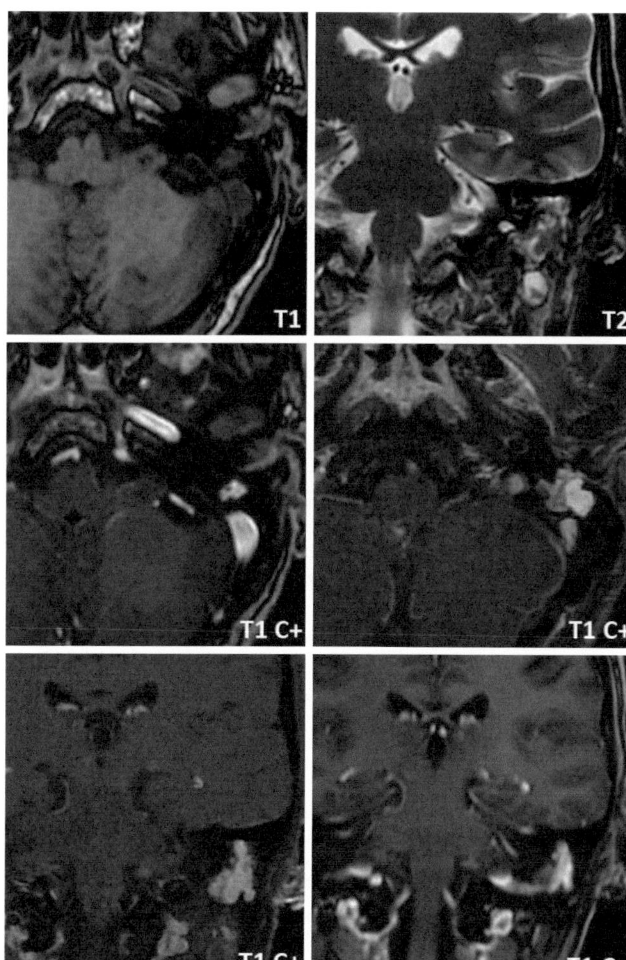

A. Haouimi et al., *Head and Neck Radiology Spot Diagnosis*,
https://doi.org/10.1007/978-3-032-14553-6_121

Findings

Thickened mastoid segment of left facial nerve. It shows an isosignal on T1, a heterogeneously high signal on T2 with linear contrast enhancement. The lesion is minimally lobulated with intraparotid extension along the branches of the facial nerve.

Diagnosis

Facial nerve schwannoma.

Discussion

Facial schwannomas are rare benign tumors arising from Schwann cells at the periphery of the nerve. Though they can involve any segments of the nerve, there is a strong predilection for the geniculate ganglion.

Clinically, facial nerve schwannomas present with a gradual onset of facial palsy. Hearing loss may occur due to mass effect on the vestibular nerve or bony ossicles. Clinically, Bell's palsy may have similar expression, but its mode of onset is always acute. The radiologist must be aware of normal perineurovascular enhancement of the facial nerve to avoid overdiagnosis, particularly in the absence of any clinical symptoms.

Common Differential Diagnosis

- Acute facial neuronitis: sudden onset, interval disappearance in about 3–6 months.
- Chemodectomas: positive "salt and pepper sign," conductive hearing loss.
- Congenital cholesteatoma: no enhancement.

Management Options

Tiny lesions need follow-up and symptomatic management. Surgical options include debulking with or without radiosurgery and stylomastoid foramen decompression.

References and Further Reading

1. Haouimi A. Radiopaedia.org. 2021. https://doi.org/10.53347/rID-94276. Accessed on 17 Nov 2023.
2. Mundada P, et al. Imaging of facial nerve schwannomas: diagnostic pearls and potential pitfalls. Diagn Interv Radiol. 2016. https://doi.org/10.5152/dir.2015.15060. Accessed on 17 Nov 2023. PMID: 26712680; PMCID: PMC4712896.
3. Skolnik AD, et al. Cranial nerve schwannomas: diagnostic imaging approach. Radiographics. 2016. https://doi.org/10.1148/rg.2016150199. Accessed on 12 June 2024. Epub 2016 Aug 19. PMID: 27541436.

Case 122

122

Clinical History

A 55-year-old man presented with a cervicalgia and numbness in the right hand.

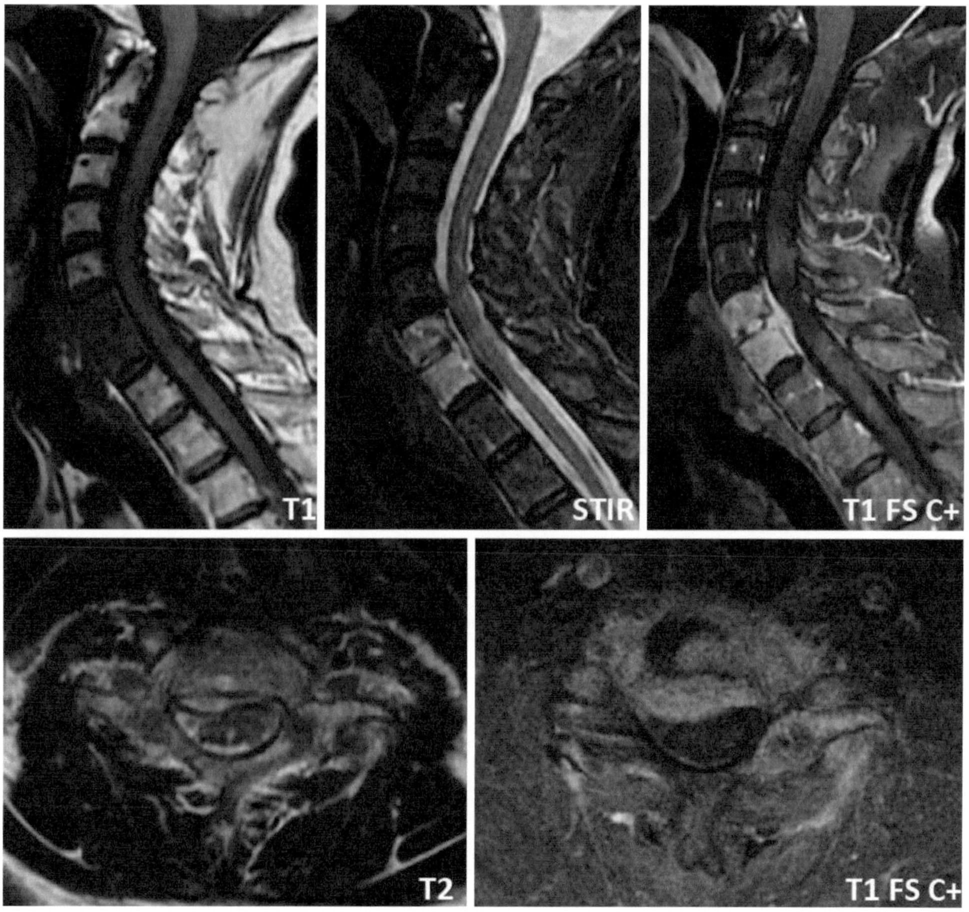

A. Haouimi et al., *Head and Neck Radiology Spot Diagnosis*,
https://doi.org/10.1007/978-3-032-14553-6_122

Findings

Subtle disk space narrowing at C6-C7 level with low signal from intervertebral disk and adjacent vertebral bodies on T1 and high signal on T2 with enhancement. Thickened prevertebral and epidural soft tissue showing isosignal on T1 and high signal on T2 with contrast enhancement.

Diagnosis

Cervical spondylodiscitis.

Discussion

Spondylodiscitis, also known as discitis, is an infectious process involving both vertebral bodies and intervertebral disk. The infection is often through the hematogenous route. Propagation by contiguity and direct inoculation is rare. The common etiologic agents are *Staphylococcus aureus*, *Streptococcus viridians*, *Escherichia coli*, and *Mycobacterium tuberculosis*.

Clinically, patients present with cervicalgia and/or backache and may or may not be associated with fever. Laboratory findings reveal elevated sedimentation rate and C-reactive proteins.

MRI is the investigation of choice. On T1, both the disk space and the adjacent vertebral bodies appear hypointense, and on T2 fat sat, they appear hyperintense. The lesion as well as the paravertebral soft tissue enhances after gadolinium. There may be restricted diffusion at the acute stage. Disk space narrowing, irregularities of vertebral end plates, and sclerotic changes are late findings and can be seen on CT and plain X-rays in the later stage.

Common Differential Diagnosis

- Vertebral metastasis: clinical history, multifocal, posterior bulge of vertebral bodies.
- Degenerative Modic 1 signal: no enhancement.
- SAPHO syndrome: erosion of anterior vertebral corners, involvement of sacroiliac and sterno-clavicular joints, paravertebral ossification.

Management Options

Most cases are managed with medical treatment including systemic antibiotics and rest. Some nonresponsive cases and cases with neurological compromise may need surgical intervention.

References and Further Reading

1. Haouimi A. Cervical spondylodiscitis. Radiopaedia.org. 2020. https://doi.org/10./rID-81362. Accessed on 08 Dec 2024.
2. Treffy RW, et al. Cervical spine spondylodiscitis: review of literature on current treatment strategies. Heliyon. 2023. https://doi.org/10.1016/j.heliyon.2023.e17875. Accessed on 15 June 2024. PMID: 37483708; PMCID.

Case 123

123

Clinical History

A 30-year-old man with a history of chronic cervicalgia.

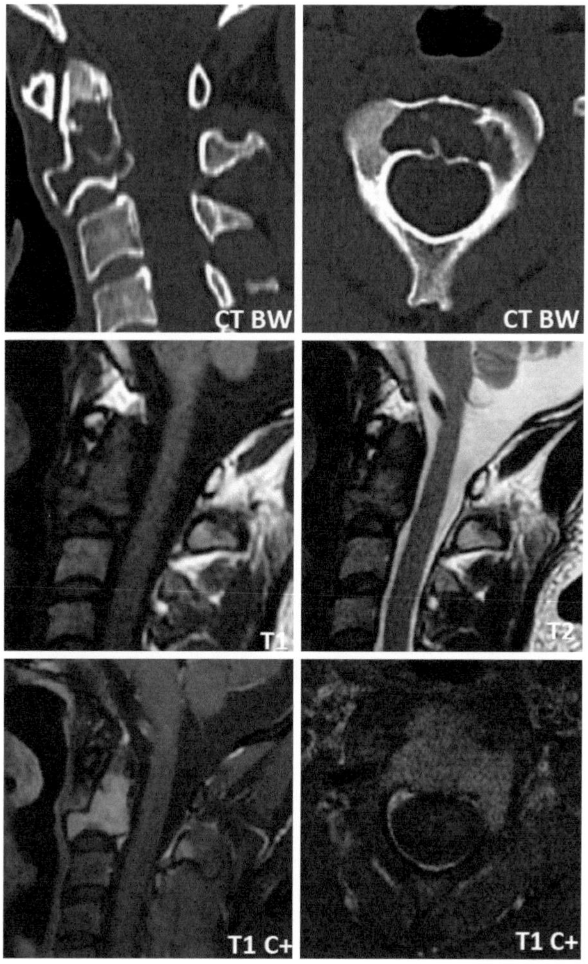

A. Haouimi et al., *Head and Neck Radiology Spot Diagnosis*,
https://doi.org/10.1007/978-3-032-14553-6_123

Findings

C2 corporeal lytic lesion with cortical interruption on CT. The lesion appears homogeneously isointense on both T1 and T2 with moderate enhancement following IV contrast. Normal pre-, peri-, and epidural soft tissues. Partial encasement of vertebral arteries. Normal spinal cord.

Diagnosis

Solitary bone plasmacytoma.

Discussion

Solitary bone plasmacytoma is a rare disease of unknown etiology characterized by a localized proliferation of neoplastic monoclonal plasma cells of bone marrow, without evidence of systemic disease. This pathology is considered as an early-stage plasma cell malignancy between monoclonal gammopathy of undetermined significance and multiple myeloma.

The symptoms depend on the size and location. C1 and C2 vertebrae have unique anatomical characteristics and biomechanical function. Lesions in this region mainly present with cervicalgia and cervical instability. As the lesions grow, spinal plasmacytomas may lead to myelo- and radiculopathy due to extrinsic compression.

On CT, the lesions appear as an expansile intraosseous lytic mass with nonsclerotic margins and locoregional extension. MRI shows intermediate signal on both T1 and T2 with homo/heterogeneous enhancement. Features may be identical to those of individual multiple myeloma. All suspected solitary bone plasmacytomas need further work-up to rule out multiple myeloma.

Common Differential Diagnosis

- Osteolytic metastasis: clinical history.
- Aneurysmal bone cyst: multiloculated, fluid–fluid level.
- Multiple myeloma: multifocal involvement.

Management Options

Patients are treated with radiation therapy as the first line of treatment due to high sensitivity. Some patients may need additional chemotherapy and adjuvant surgery. Up to 70% of patients with solitary bone plasmacytoma will develop multiple myeloma in 5–10 years on follow-up.

References and Further Reading

1. Haouimi A. Radiopaedia.org. 2020. https://doi.org/10.53347/rID-80189. Accessed on 09 May 2024.
2. Iqbal QUA, Majid HJ. Stat Pearls Publishing. 2023. https://www.ncbi.nlm.nih.gov/books/NBK573076/#. Accessed on 09 May 2024.

Case 124

124

Clinical History

A 50-year-old man presented with a left abducens nerve palsy.

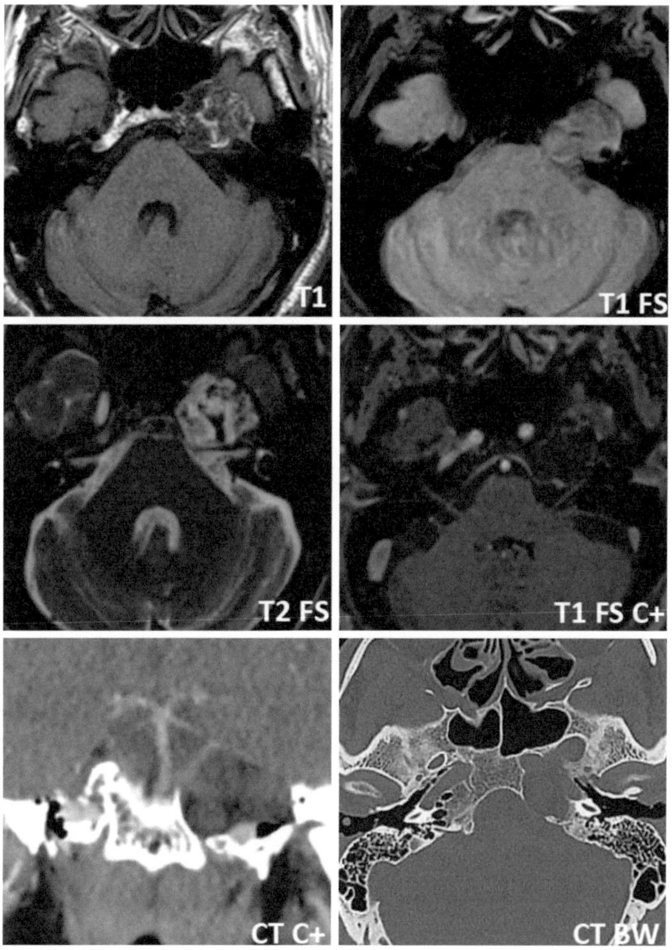

A. Haouimi et al., *Head and Neck Radiology Spot Diagnosis*,
https://doi.org/10.1007/978-3-032-14553-6_124

Findings

Left petrous bone lytic lesion showing low signal on T1, high signal on T2, containing fatty component of high T1, completely suppressed on T1 and T2 fat-sat images. Cortical breach of posterior wall of the petrous bone and carotid canal, best seen on CT. Thickening and displacement of the adjacent dura. Locoregional extension to cavernous sinus, causing medial displacement of intracavernous ICA.

Diagnosis

Petrous bone dermoid cyst.

Discussion

Dermoid cysts are rare developmental anomalies involving pluripotential embryonal cells that probably originate from ectodermal remnants. They are inclusion cysts. These congenital lesions originate during early embryogenesis, often contain fatty components, and are mostly found along the midline and in the infratentorial regions. Petrous apex location is extremely rare. The exact etiology is unknown, though theories include incomplete closure at lines of fusion or traumatic implantation of dermal elements.

Clinical presentations depend on location and the presence of lesion rupture. They may present with headaches, seizures, cranial neuropathies (CN V, VI, VII, VIII), and chemical meningitis.

On CT scan, the lesions appear iso- and hypodense (high lipid content). On MRI, dermoids are mostly iso- or hyperintense (high fatty content) on T1 and from hypo- to hyperintense on T2 (high fat content). In the absence of fatty component, the lesions may mimic epidermoid cysts and may be radiologically misdiagnosed.

Common Differential Diagnosis

- Cholesterol granuloma: sharply marginated without locoregional invasion.
- Epidermoid: no or scanty fatty component.
- Lipoma: high signal on both T1 and T2, suppressed on fat-sat sequence, no bony erosion.

Management Options

Symptomatic cases are usually addressed surgically.

References and Further Reading

1. Al-Muhaimeed HS, et al. Case Rep Otolaryngol. 2012. https://doi.org/10.1155/2012/548340. Accessed on 20 May 2024.
2. Behnke EE, Schindler RA. Laryngoscope. 1984. https://doi.org/10.1288/00005537-198406000-00009. Accessed on 20 May 2024.
3. Sturiale CL, et al. J Clin Neurosci. 2009. https://doi.org/10.1016/j.jocn.2009.02.010. Accessed on 20 May 2024.

Case 125

125

Clinical History

A 35-year-old woman presented with a right trigeminal neuralgia.

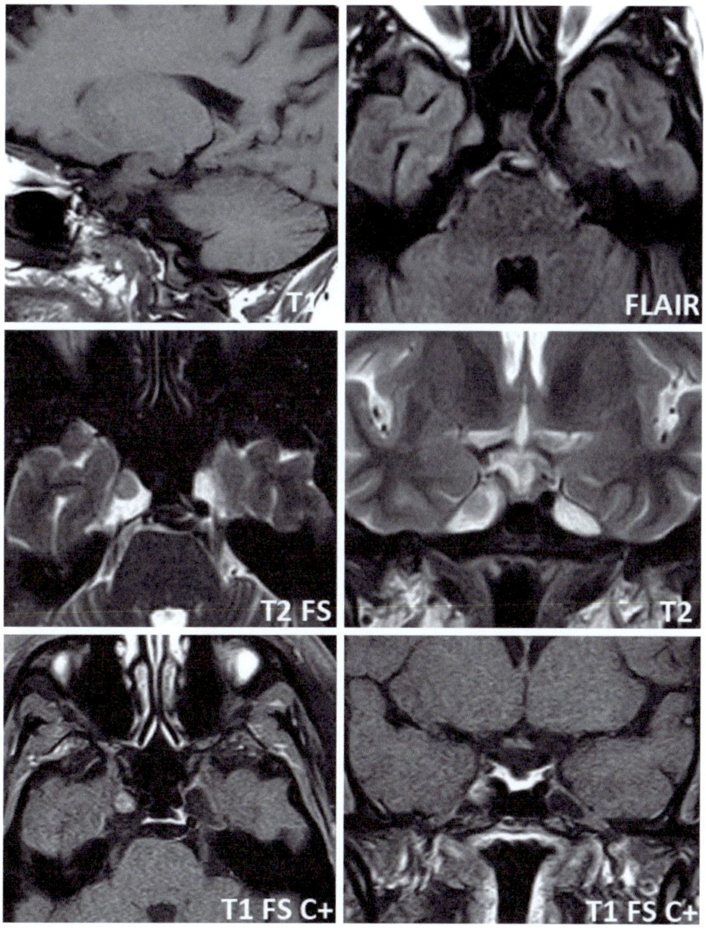

A. Haouimi et al., *Head and Neck Radiology Spot Diagnosis*,
https://doi.org/10.1007/978-3-032-14553-6_125

Findings

A tiny well-circumscribed infracentimetric nodular space-occupying lesion in the right Meckel's cave. The lesion appears isointense to the cortical grey matter on all sequences with mild to moderate homogeneous enhancement. Thickening of adjacent dura with a possible rudimentary dural tail.

Diagnosis

Meckel's cave meningioma.

Discussion

Meckel's cave or trigeminal cave is a CSF-filled dural recess in the medial aspect of the middle cranial fossa in the parasellar region. It acts as a conduit for the trigeminal nerve as it extends from the prepontine cistern to the cavernous sinus. The Meckel's cave houses the Gasserian ganglion and contains the rootlets of the trigeminal nerve; the trigeminal ganglion; and the ophthalmic (cranial nerve V_1), maxillary (cranial nerve V_2), and mandibular (cranial nerve V_3) divisions.

The incidence of Meckel's cave meningiomas is rare and represents only 1% of all intracranial meningiomas. They originate from arachnoid cells.

Smaller lesions can remain asymptomatic, and their size may remain stable. The bigger lesions create extrinsic compression on trigeminal ganglion and other neurovascular structures. The symptoms of the lesions can be trigeminal neuralgia, facial pain, and tic "douloureux."

On MRI, unlike schwannomas, the Meckel's cave meningiomas are nodular and appear isointense on all sequences. They show moderate enhancement after gadolinium.

Common Differential Diagnosis

- Schwannoma: linear, usually dumbbell shaped, T2 high-signal lesion.
- Pituitary adenoma: pituitary fossa epicenter.
- Petrous apex cephalocele: no restricted diffusion, isosignal to CSF on all sequences.
- Metastatic lesion: usually retrograde perineural spread from head and neck tumors.

Management Options

Surgical options are reserved for symptomatic and bigger lesions.

References and Further Reading

1. Haouimi A. Radiopaedia.org. 2024. https://doi.org/10.53347/rID-185804. Accessed on 03 May 2024.
2. Kontzialis, M, Kocak M. J Istanb Univ Fac Dent. 2017. https://doi.org/10.17096/jiufd.27242. Accessed on 08 June 2024.
3. Malhotra A, et al. Neuroimaging of Meckel's cave in normal and disease conditions. Insights Imaging. 2018. https://doi.org/10.1007/s13244-018-0604-7. Accessed on 15 June 2024. Epub 2018 Apr 18. PMID: 29671218; PMCID: PMC6108963.

Case 126

126

Clinical History

An 11-year-old boy presented with mild left proptosis.

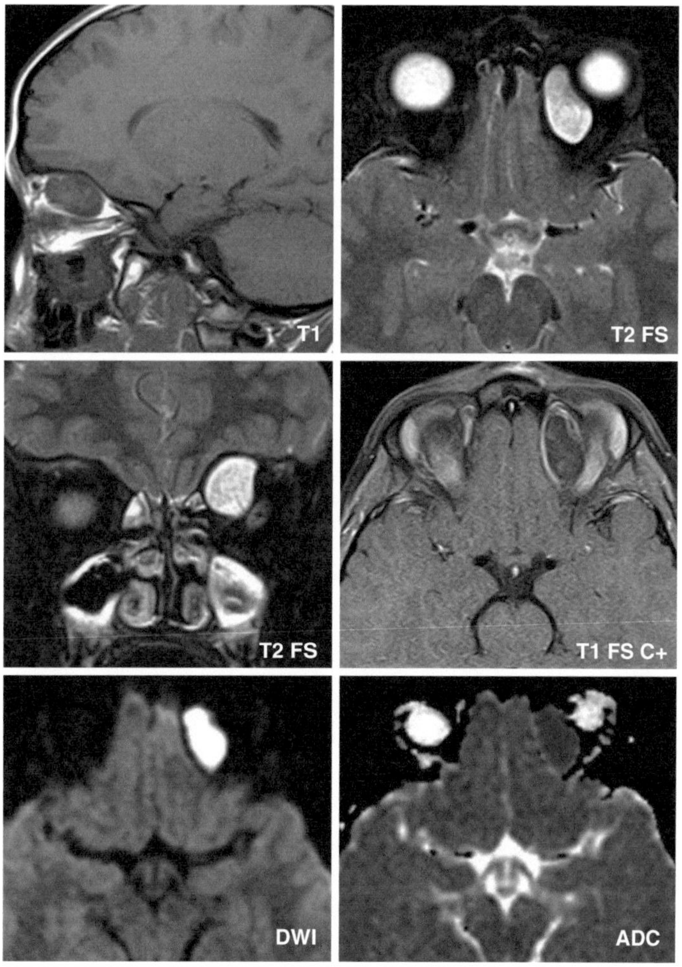

A. Haouimi et al., *Head and Neck Radiology Spot Diagnosis*,
https://doi.org/10.1007/978-3-032-14553-6_126

Findings

Well-defined extraconal left orbital cystic mass in the upper inner quadrant, displacing the superior and medial rectus muscles as well as the optic nerve and the globe laterally. It is isointense to the cortical grey matter on T1, and high signal on T2 fat sat with restricted diffusion. Thin peripheral enhancement. No calcifications or hemorrhage. Scalloping of the medial aspect of the left orbital roof, best seen on coronal T2 fat-sat image.

Diagnosis

Orbital epidermoid cyst.

Discussion

Both dermoid and epidermoid cysts are the commonest benign space-occupying lesions of the orbit. Most of the cases originate from the zygomaticofrontal suture. These cystic choristomas contain keratin, cholesterol clefts, and degenerated blood. Histologically, unlike the dermoid, the cystic wall of epidermoid cysts does not have skin appendages.

Congenital epidermoids are present since birth and may remain asymptomatic for years. Patients with orbital epidermoid may clinically present with painless subcutaneous mass that are mostly fixed to the underlying bone. Acquired lesions may arise from surgery and trauma.

On CT, the orbital lesions are hypodense, showing signs of bone remodeling (thinning, destruction with sclerotic borders), and can show punctate calcification in about 15% cases. MRI shows isosignal to vitreous on all sequences with restricted diffusion. Very thin rim enhancement may be seen on both CT and MRI.

Common Differential Diagnosis

- Idiopathic pseudotumor: acute painful proptosis, periocular edema.
- Frontal mucocele: frontal sinus epicenter, associated chronic sinusitis.
- Capillary hemangioma: infants, serpiginous flow void, compressible, lobulation, septa.

Management Options

Surgical resection in most of the cases. Anti-inflammatory drugs are indicated when ruptured.

References and Further Reading

1. Blanco G, et al. Orbital intradiploic giant epidermoid cyst. Arch Ophthalmol. 2001. https://doi.org/10.1001/archopht.119.5.771. Accessed on 16 Aug 2024.
2. Haouimi A. Orbital epidermoid cyst. Radiopaedia.org. 2024. https://doi.org/10.53347/rID-193226. Accessed on 16 Aug 2024.
3. Pushker N, et al. Orbital and periorbital dermoid/epidermoid cyst: a series of 280 cases and a brief review. Can J Ophthalmol. 2019. https://doi.org/10.1016/j.jcjo.2019.08.005. Accessed on 20 Dec 2024. Epub 2019 Nov 8. PMID: 31712044.

Case 127

127

Clinical History

A 5-year-old boy presented with a recent increase in size of a long-standing progressive right parotid swelling.

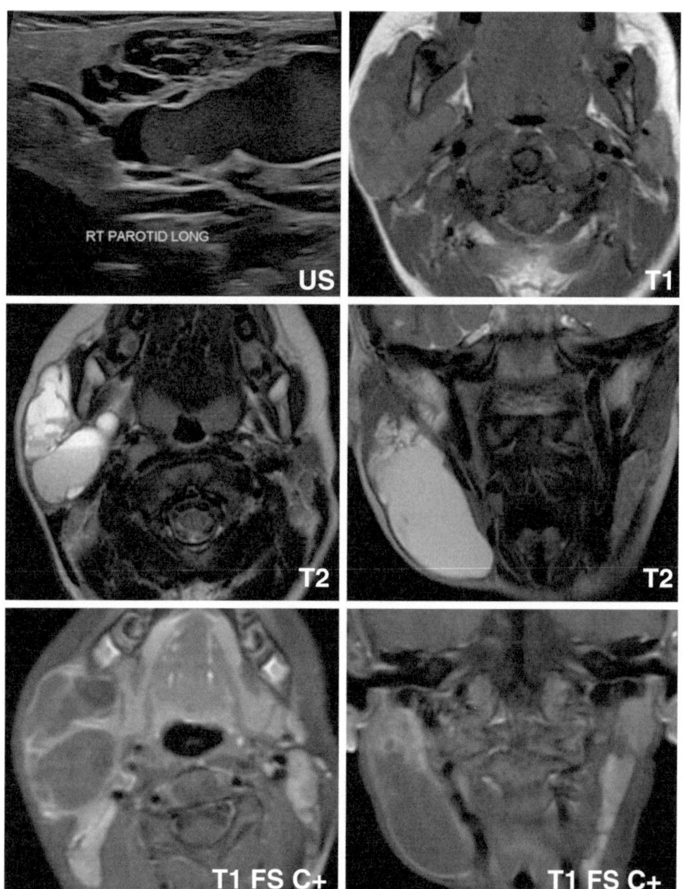

A. Haouimi et al., *Head and Neck Radiology Spot Diagnosis*,
https://doi.org/10.1007/978-3-032-14553-6_127

Findings

Multiseptated cystic lesion of the right parotid gland with thick septa seen on ultrasound. On MRI, this trans-spatial cystic lesion appears multilobulated and multiseptated, involving both parotid lobes. The lesion is iso- to low signal on T1 and heterogeneously high signal on T2 with low-signal sediments (intracystic hemorrhage). Associated septal enhancement. The lesion extends into the submandibular space, causing displacement of the submandibular gland.

Diagnosis

Cystic lymphangioma of the parotid gland.

Discussion

Cystic lymphangioma, also known as lymphatic malformation or cystic hygroma, is a slow-growing, benign congenital vascular anomaly with no potential for malignancy. These lesions consist of multiple sequestered, noncommunicating lymphatic spaces that exist alongside a normally functioning lymphatic system. They are thought to arise from abnormal development of the lymphatic sacs during embryogenesis. Cystic lymphangiomas are most commonly diagnosed in children under two years of age, predominantly affecting the head and neck region. Congenital forms are frequently associated with chromosomal abnormalities, such as Turner syndrome, whereas acquired lesions in adults are generally considered to result from trauma.

The patients present with a gradually increasing, painless, soft, doughy neck lesion.

On ultrasound, lymphangiomas are multiseptated anechoic or hypoechoic lesions with thin walls. Both CT and MRI can delineate the trans-spatial extension and appear as hypodense/hypointense on T1 and high signal on T2. Lesions may show fluid–fluid level and septal enhancement.

Common Differential Diagnosis

- Parotid abscess: acute onset, pain, fever, thick, regular ring enhancement.
- Second branchial cleft cyst: unilocular, "beak sign" or "tail sign" positive.
- Thyroglossal duct cyst: midline location.

Management Option

Treatment options are surgical for isolated unilocular lesions and sclerotherapy for trans-spatial extensive lesions with vascular component.

References and Further Reading

1. Chinnakkulam Kandhasamy S, Gunasekaran G, et al. Adult cystic lymphangioma of the parotid gland: an unwonted presentation. Cureus. 2018. https://doi.org/10.7759/cureus.2644. Accessed on 23 Aug 2024. PMID: 30034966; PMCID: PMC6051554.
2. Haouimi A. Cystic lymphangioma – parotid. Radiopaedia.org. 2021. https://doi.org/10.53347/rID-86121. Accessed on 23 Aug 2024.

Case 128

128

Clinical History

A 13-year-old boy with a history of chronic left otorrhea presented with hearing loss.

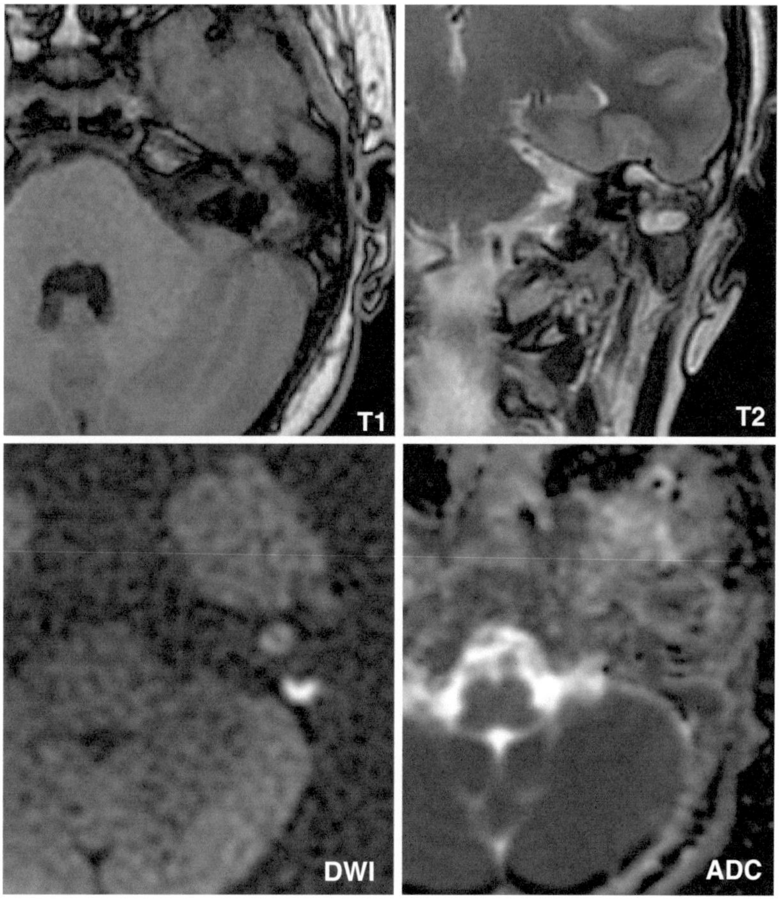

A. Haouimi et al., *Head and Neck Radiology Spot Diagnosis*,
https://doi.org/10.1007/978-3-032-14553-6_128

Findings

Soft-tissue filling the left mastoid and middle ear, showing low signal on T1 and high signal on T2 with restricted diffusion.

Diagnosis

Cholesteatoma.

Discussion

Cholesteatomas are abnormal soft-tissue growths in the middle ear, mostly resulting from repeated infection and "Eustachian tube dysfunction" with impairment of normal ventilation of the middle ear. The negative pressure ultimately causes the eardrum to retract. The collection of keratinized squamous epithelium can become trapped within the middle ear, ultimately leading to a cholesteatoma. Ninety-eight percent of cholesteatomas are acquired and only 2% are congenital.

Cholesteatomas present with painless foul-smelling otorrhea, progressive hearing loss, dizziness, and vertigo.

CT is the modality of choice and shows non-dependent soft-tissue density starting from Prussak space. It causes blunting of scutum and erosion of the bony ossicles, tegmen tympani, facial canal as well as lateral semicircular canal. The lesion extends posteriorly through aditus ad antrum to fill the mastoid air cells. The locoregional extension can lead to intracranial complications such as meningitis, brain abscess and sigmoid sinus thrombosis. MRI is helpful to assess intracranial complications.

Common Differential Diagnosis

- Cerumen: external auditory meatus.
- Cholesterol granuloma: T1 high signal, no restricted diffusion.
- Middle ear effusion: dependent collection, inflamed tonsils, nasopharyngeal carcinoma.

Management Options

Surgical excision is the mainstay of treatment.

References and Further Reading

1. Haouimi A. Cholesteatoma. Radiopaedia.org. 2021. https://doi.org/10.53347/rID-93658. Accessed on 26 Aug 2024.
2. Pachpande TG, Singh CV. Diagnosis and treatment modalities of cholesteatomas: a review. Cureus. 2022. https://doi.org/10.7759/cureus.31153. Accessed on 01 Dec 2024. PMID: 36505121; PMCID: PMC9731553.
3. Touska P, Connor SEJ. ESR Essentials: imaging of middle ear cholesteatoma-practice recommendations by the European Society of Head and Neck Radiology. Eur Radiol. https://doi.org/10.1007/s00330-024-11021-x. Accessed on 18 Sept 2025.

Case 129

129

Clinical History

A 60-year-old man (chronic smoker) with a history of progressive painless swelling of the left parotid region.

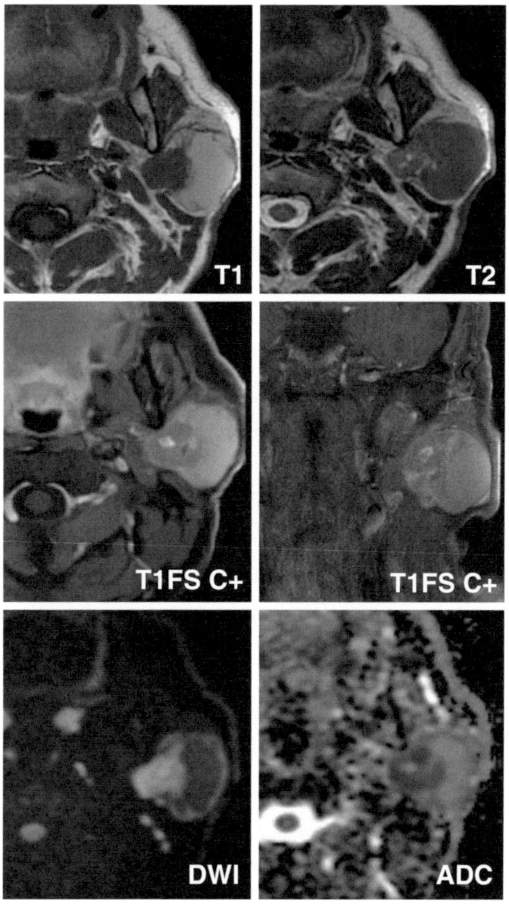

A. Haouimi et al., *Head and Neck Radiology Spot Diagnosis*,
https://doi.org/10.1007/978-3-032-14553-6_129

Findings

Well-circumscribed solid-cystic lesion of the left parotid gland. The cystic component is of high signal on T1, low signal on T2 with areas of restricted diffusion peripherally and no enhancement on postcontrast fat-sat images. The solid component shows isosignal to the muscles on T1, heterogeneous signal on T2, and early enhancement with restricted diffusion.

Diagnosis

Warthin tumor.

Discussion

Warthin tumor, also called papillary cystadenoma lymphomatosum, is a benign, slow-growing salivary gland tumor of unknown cause. Cigarette smoking is a well-known risk factor. The tumor most often develops in the tail of the parotid gland and usually affects middle-aged people, with a male predominance. It ranks as the second most common parotid gland tumor after pleomorphic adenoma.

The lesion is typically spherical or ovoid and originates from salivary duct remnants trapped within the gland tissue. Clinically, it appears as a painless mass that can be uni/bilateral, or multicentric in about 20% of cases. About one-third of these lesions contain cystic parts.

On ultrasound, these well-circumscribed inhomogeneous rounded or lobulated lesions can show both solid and cystic components. Internal cystic changes with septations are common. CT shows heterogeneous parenchyma without calcification. On MRI, the cystic component may show high signal due to cholesterol component on T1. The solid component is hypointense on T1, hyperintense on T2 with early enhancement and progressive washout within the tumor on the TIC (time–signal intensity curve). They also show a low ADC value (<30%).

Common Differential Diagnosis

- Malignant parotid lesion: ill-defined, higher washout ratio >30%, higher ADC value.
- Benign mixed tumor: lobulated, dystrophic calcifications +.
- Benign lymphoepithelial lesions: HIV seropositivity.

Management Options

Treatment option ranges from watchful waiting to surgical excision. Sclerotherapy for recurrent lesions.

References and Further Reading

1. Haouimi A. Warthin tumour – parotid gland. Radiopaedia.org. 2021. https://doi.org/10.53347/rID-94556. Accessed on 26 Aug 2024.
2. Limaiem F, Jain P. Warthin tumor. Stat Pearls Publishing. 2024. https://www.ncbi.nlm.nih.gov/books/NBK557640/. Accessed on Aug 2024.

Case 130

130

Clinical History

A 40-year-old woman presented with a foreign body sensation in the throat.

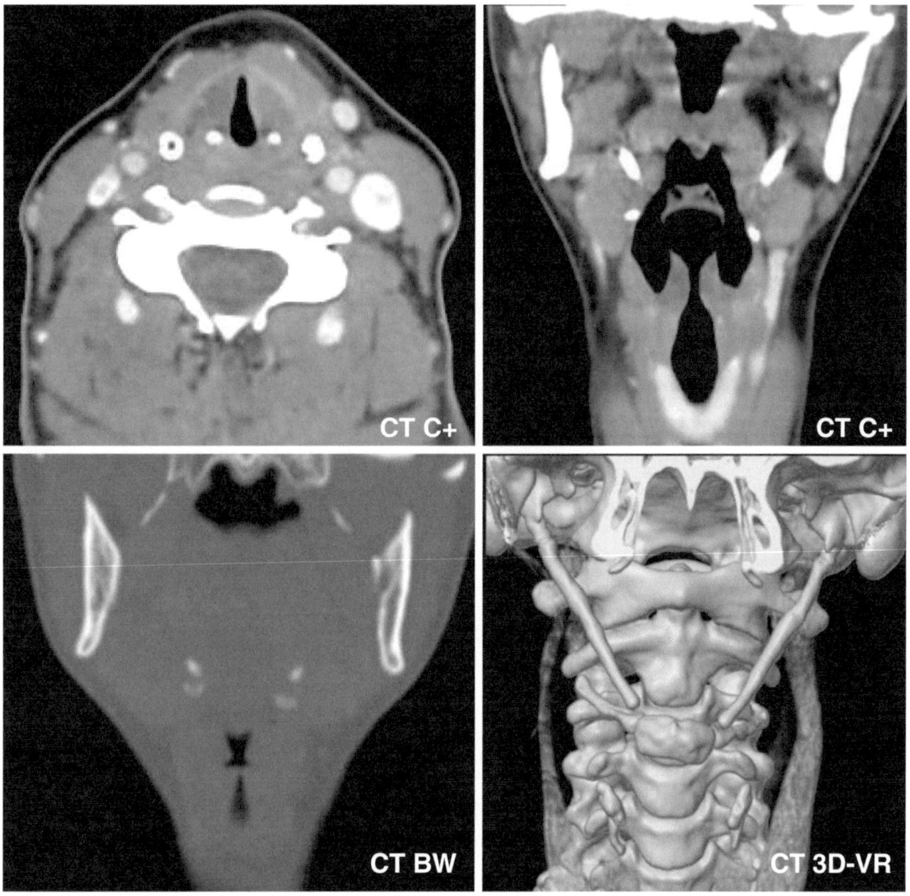

A. Haouimi et al., *Head and Neck Radiology Spot Diagnosis*,
https://doi.org/10.1007/978-3-032-14553-6_130

Findings

Bilaterally elongated and prominent styloid processes with ossification of the stylohyoid ligaments. The findings are best seen on 3D volume-rendered image.

Diagnosis

Eagle syndrome.

Discussion

Eagle syndrome is a condition when styloid process is abnormally elongated or when the ossification of stylohyoid ligament leads to a direct bony bridging between the skull base and hyoid bone. It can be both uni- or bilateral. Dr. Eagle believed that the styloid elongation is secondary to traumatic or spontaneous fracture of the styloid process. The exact etiology remains unknown.

Clinical symptoms are vague and many patients remain asymptomatic. Dysphagia is the most common symptom. Elongated styloid process may cause glossopharyngeal neuralgia. Cerebrovascular complications are extremely rare but remain a serious potential manifestation of the syndrome. Compression on the large vessels with rotational neck movement, frequently the internal carotid artery, can result in a transient ischemic attack. Occasionally, the nerve compression can even lead to vocal cord paralysis. The wide range of nonspecific symptoms makes clinical diagnosis of Eagle syndrome a challenge. CT scan is the gold standard for diagnosis.

Common Differential Diagnosis

- The diagnosis is straightforward with no differential consideration on imaging.

Management Options

Conservative treatment includes ultrasound-guided injection of steroids and NSAIDs. The most definitive treatment is surgical amputation of the elongated styloid process.

References and Further Reading

1. Haouimi A. Eagle syndrome. Radiopaedia.org. 2021. https://doi.org/10.53347/rID-88999. Accesse on 15 Mar 2024.
2. Saccomanno S, et al. Eagle's Syndrome, from clinical presentation to diagnosis and surgical treatment: a case report. Acta Otorhinolaryngol Ital. 2018. https://pubmed.ncbi.nlm.nih.gov/29967562/. Accessed on 15 Mar 2024.
3. Swanson D, et al. Eagle syndrome: pathophysiology, differential diagnosis and treatment options. Health Psychol Res. 2023. https://doi.org/10.52965/001c.67851. Accessed on 15 Mar 2024.

Case 131

131

Clinical History

A 45-year-old woman presented with a history of recurrent bilateral parotid gland swelling.

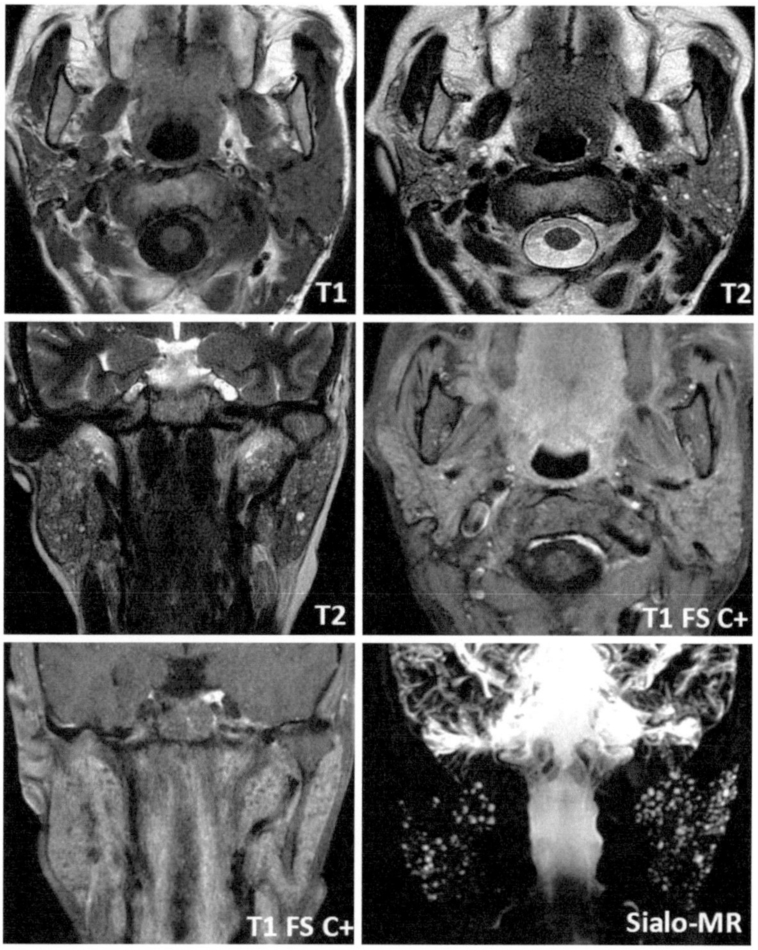

A. Haouimi et al., *Head and Neck Radiology Spot Diagnosis*,
https://doi.org/10.1007/978-3-032-14553-6_131

Findings

Moderate enlargement of both parotids. Bilateral intraglandular innumerable diffuse microcystic lesions involving both deep and superficial lobes. The microcysts appear as low signal on T1, high signal on T2 with a moderate heterogeneous enhancement. Normal submandibular glands.

Diagnosis

Chronic parotitis.

Discussion

Recurrent episodes of painful swelling of the parotids are considered as chronic recurrent parotitis. Their etiology is multifactorial but remains unclear. Genetic and hereditary factors along with immune deficiency, inflammation, recurrent infections, ductal obstruction, and allergy are considered as predisposing factors. When no definite etiology is identified, the term "chronic recurrent nonspecific parotitis" is used.

Chronic parotitis is most often seen in middle-aged patients with female predilection. Patients present with recurrent episodes of dry mouth, difficulty in swallowing, and painful mouth opening, especially while eating, in addition to pain and tenderness of parotid glands.

Ultrasound and sialography are characterized by sialectasis. Sialogram shows a typical "dots and blobs" appearance at the terminal ductules. On MRI, the enlarged glands show tiny microcystic changes, low signal on T1 and high on T2 involving both superficial and deep lobes.

Common Differential Diagnosis

- Mikulicz syndrome: lacrimal and submandibular involvement, sensitive to IgG4 titers.
- Sjögren syndrome: on ultrasound, hypoechoic foci interposed hyperechoic lines or dots.
- Sarcoidosis: systemic involvement.

Management Options

Most patients are managed conservatively with antibiotics, steroids, and analgesics. Diagnostic sialography often improves the patency of duct following cannulation and flushing during intraductal lavage.

References and Further Reading

1. Haouimi A. Chronic parotitis. Radiopaedia.org. 2019. https://doi.org/10.53347/rID-68681. Accessed on 26 Aug 2024.
2. Mahalakshmi S, et al. Chronic recurrent non-specific parotitis: a case report and review. Ethiop J Health Sci. 2017. https://doi.org/10.4314/ejhs.v27i1.13. Accessed on 26 Aug 2024. PMID: 28458496; PMCID: PMC5390234.

Case 132

132

Clinical History

A 16-year-old adolescent presented with a history of nasal obstruction and snoring.

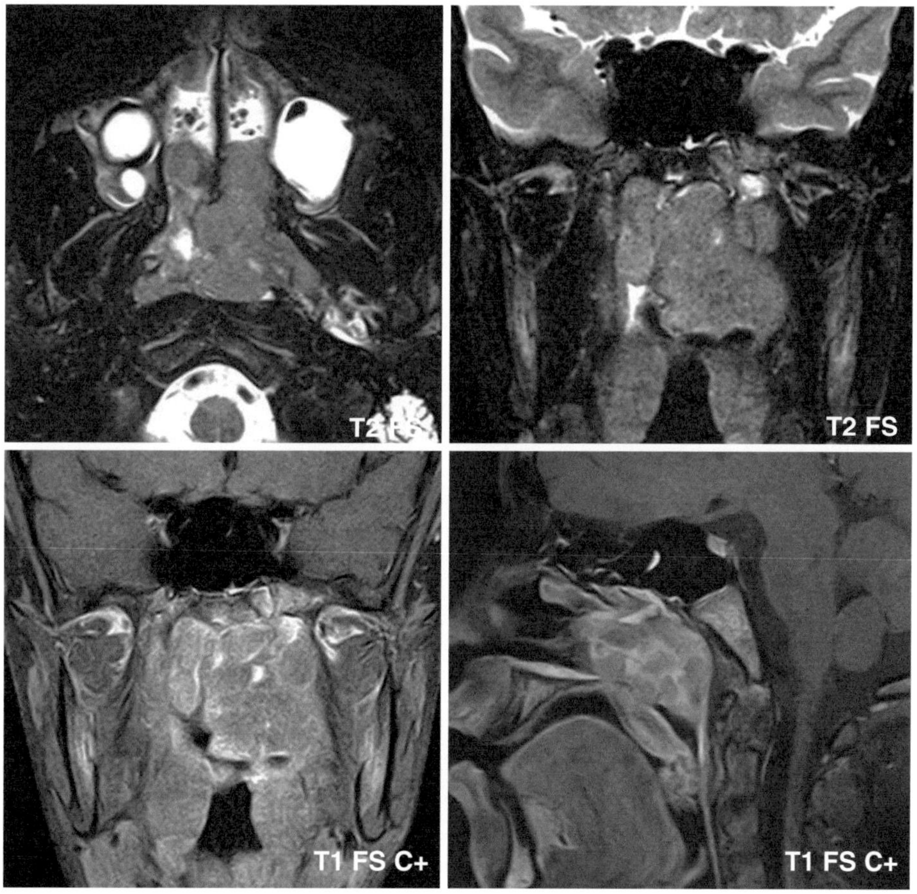

A. Haouimi et al., *Head and Neck Radiology Spot Diagnosis*,
https://doi.org/10.1007/978-3-032-14553-6_132

Findings

Large nasopharyngeal soft tissue mass obliterating the fossae of Rosenmüller and Eustachian tube openings with anterior extension obstructing the choanae. The mass appears isointense to muscles on T1, intermediate signal on T2 fat sat with moderate heterogeneous enhancement. Signs of secondary otomastoiditis and bilateral maxillary sinusitis as high signal on T2 fat sat.

Diagnosis

Burkitt lymphoma.

Discussion

Burkitt lymphoma predominantly affects children with a male predominance (4:1). The etiology of sporadic Burkitt lymphoma (American) is unknown, whereas endemic Burkitt lymphoma (African) is linked to *Plasmodium. falciparum* and Epstein-Barr virus infections. Cases have also been linked to HIV infection or immunosuppression.

Clinically, patients present with mouth breathing, dysphagia, otalgia, and occasionally with epistaxis, confusing the provisional diagnosis with juvenile nasopharyngeal angiofibroma.

Both CT and MRI are used to evaluate the extension of the lesion and staging. The lesion appears as symmetric and diffuse soft tissue mass with a propensity to spread laterally through the fat planes and along the mucosa of Waldeyer's tonsillar ring. MRI can also show the intracranial perineural extension through foramen ovale (if present).

Common Differential Diagnosis

- Nasopharyngeal carcinoma: unilateral, centered at the fossa of Rosenmüller.
- Juvenile nasopharyngeal angiofibroma: epicenter at nasopalatine foramen, male patients.
- Chordoma: spheno-occipital epicenter.

Management Options

The mainstay treatment of Burkitt lymphoma is chemotherapy with a good prognosis.

References and Further Reading

1. Haouimi A. Burkitt lymphoma. Radiopaedia.org. 2023. https://doi.org/10.53347/rID-159530. Accessed on 26 Aug 2024.
2. Hsueh CY, et al. Nasopharyngeal lymphoma. J Clin Med. 2019. https://doi.org/10.3390/jcm8101604. Accessed on 26 Aug 2024. PMID: 31623372; PMCID: PMC6833098.
3. Liu X-W, et al. Magnetic resonance imaging features of nasopharyngeal carcinoma and nasopharyngeal non-Hodgkin's lymphoma. Eur J Radiol. 2012. https://pubmed.ncbi.nlm.nih.gov/21864999/. Accessed on 26 Aug 2024.

Case 133

133

Clinical History

A 35-year-old man presented with a tongue lesion.

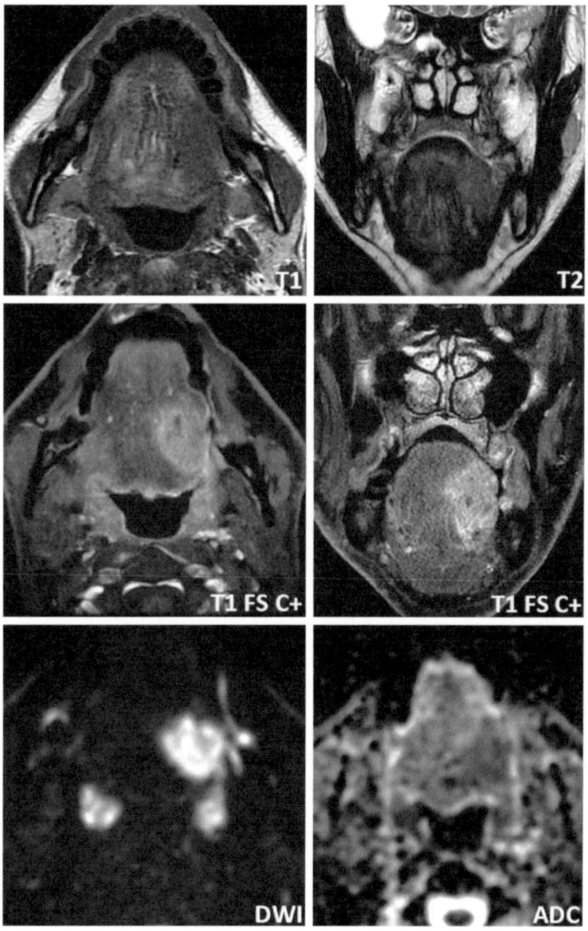

A. Haouimi et al., *Head and Neck Radiology Spot Diagnosis*,
https://doi.org/10.1007/978-3-032-14553-6_133

Findings

Left hemilingual mass involving the middle third of the tongue. It appears as a low signal on T1 and isosignal to the normal tongue tissue on T2. Intense nonhomogeneous enhancement after gadolinium. Locoregional invasion of intrinsic and extrinsic muscles, including the palatoglossus, styloglossus, and hyoglossus muscles posteriorly, as well as genioglossus medially. Intact normal lingual septum, suggesting no midline crossing.

Diagnosis

Squamous cell carcinoma of tongue.

Discussion

Cancer at anterior tongue is often diagnosed early when the tumor is small, but cancer of the base is diagnosed at a more advanced stage with locoregional invasion. Tongue base cancers may be associated with human papillomavirus. Smoking and chewing of tobacco, overindulgence to alcohol, and coal tar exposure are other major risk factors.

MR evaluation of the midline of the tongue and the contralateral neurovascular bundle is important for surgical planning, as invasion of the midline may preclude hemiglossectomy. MR allows detailed locoregional evaluation and nodal involvement.

Common Differential Diagnosis

- Lingual abscess: peripheral ring-enhancing lesion splaying genioglossus muscles.
- Epidermoid cyst: restricted diffusion, low signal on T1 and high signal on T2.
- Foregut duplication cyst: thick walled, septated, isointense on T1 and hyperintense on T2.

Management Options

Local excision or hemiglossectomy is the treatment of choice. However, combination of chemotherapy, radiotherapy, and invasive procedures is often used.

References and Further Reading

1. Haouimi A. Tongue squamous cell carcinoma. Radiopaedia.org. 2023. https://doi.org/10.53347/rID-160588. Accessed on 26 Aug 2024.
2. Okubo M, et al. Squamous cell carcinoma of the tongue dorsum: incidence and treatment considerations. Indian J Otolaryngol Head Neck Surg. 2017. https://pubmed.ncbi.nlm.nih.gov/28239570/. Accessed on 26 Aug 2024.
3. Shah S, et al. Importance and implications of neurovascular bundle involvement and other MRI findings of oral tongue squamous cell carcinoma (OTSCC) on prognosis. Oral Oncol Vol. 2021. https://doi.org/10.1016/j.oraloncology.2021.105403. Accessed on 26 Aug 2024.

Case 134

134

Clinical History

A 65-year-old woman. Incidental finding.

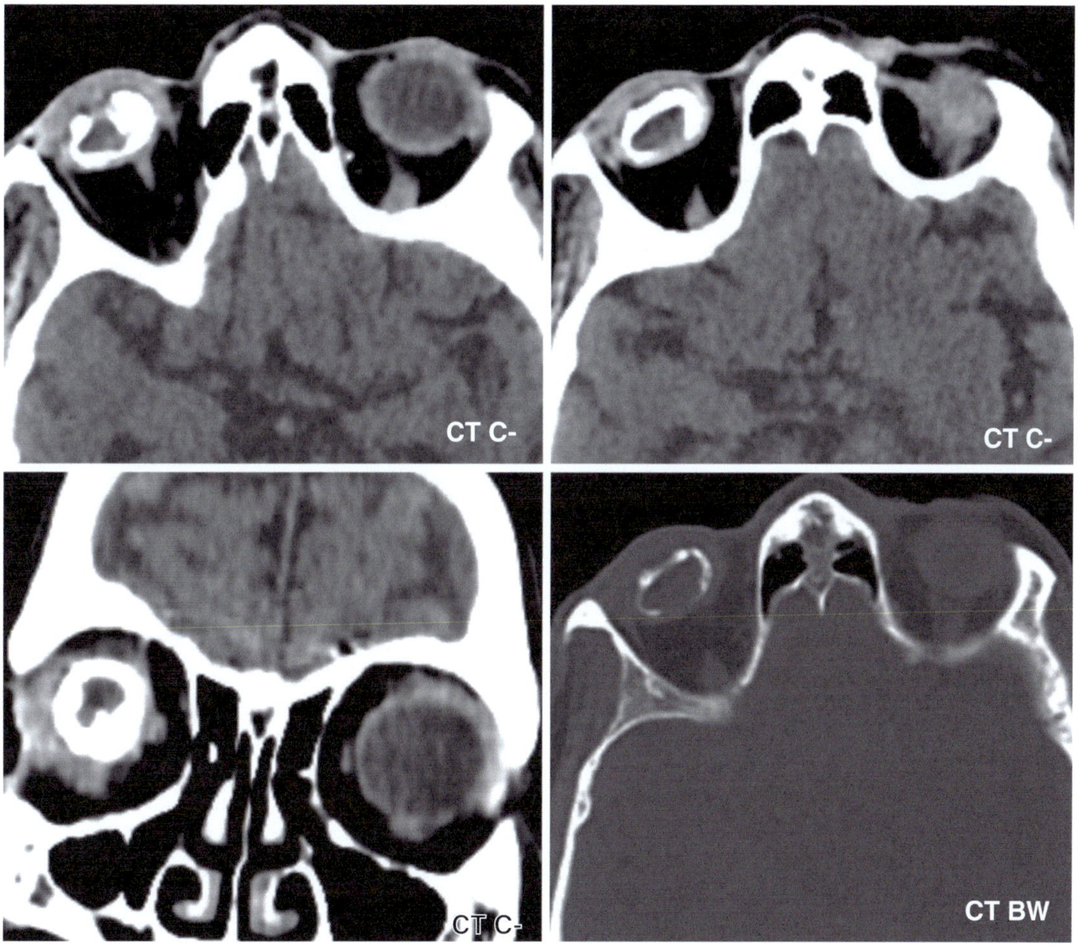

A. Haouimi et al., *Head and Neck Radiology Spot Diagnosis*,
https://doi.org/10.1007/978-3-032-14553-6_134

Findings

Small size and shrunken right globe with irregular contour and dystrophic calcification.

Diagnosis

Phthisis bulbi.

Discussion

The term phthisis bulbi is an end-stage ocular response leading to a shrunken, nonfunctional eye following severe eye disease, inflammation, neoplasm, or trauma. The condition mostly involves elderly patients. In children and adolescents, it is mostly secondary to trauma, tumor, and congenital abnormalities.

Morphologically, the globe is markedly shrunken (usually <20 mm) and deformed with a thickened/folded posterior sclera. Alterations in oxygenation and metabolism due to hypotonia, loss of plasma proteins, release of cytokines, chemotactic and angiogenic factors from the rupture of hemato-ocular barrier are believed to be involved in pathogenesis.

Patients often complain of reduced or lost vision with a small, soft, atrophic, painful eye and a positive clinical history. However, in the absence of positive history, the possibility of other causes like retinoblastoma or malignant uveal melanoma needs to be ruled out.

On CT, intraocular dystrophic calcification and occasionally, a "calcified lump" can be seen in the shrunken and deformed eye. MRI signals are heterogeneous on all sequences.

Common Differential Diagnosis

- Bourneville disease: "giant drusen," cutaneous manifestation.
- Retinoblastoma: younger children, protruding calcification in vitreous body.
- Senile calcific scleral plaques: anterior and bilateral with normal ocular size and volume.

Management Options

Once damaged and shrunken vision cannot be restored. Alleviating ocular pain and cosmetic rehabilitation after enucleation are the focus of management.

References and Further Reading

1. Gaillard F, et al. Phthisis bulbi. Radiopaedia.org. 2024. https://doi.org/10.53347/rID-1871. Accessed 25 Nov 2024.
2. Haouimi A. Phthisis bulbi. Radiopaedia.org. 2020. https://doi.org/10.53347/rID-85434. Accessed 27 Aug 2024.
3. Tripathy K, et al. Phthisis Bulbi-a clinicopathological perspective. Semin Ophthalmol. 2018. https://doi.org/10.1080/08820538.2018.1477966. Accessed 27 Aug 2024. Epub 2018 Jun 14.

Case 135

135

Clinical History

A 35-year-old woman presented with a right hemifacial pain.

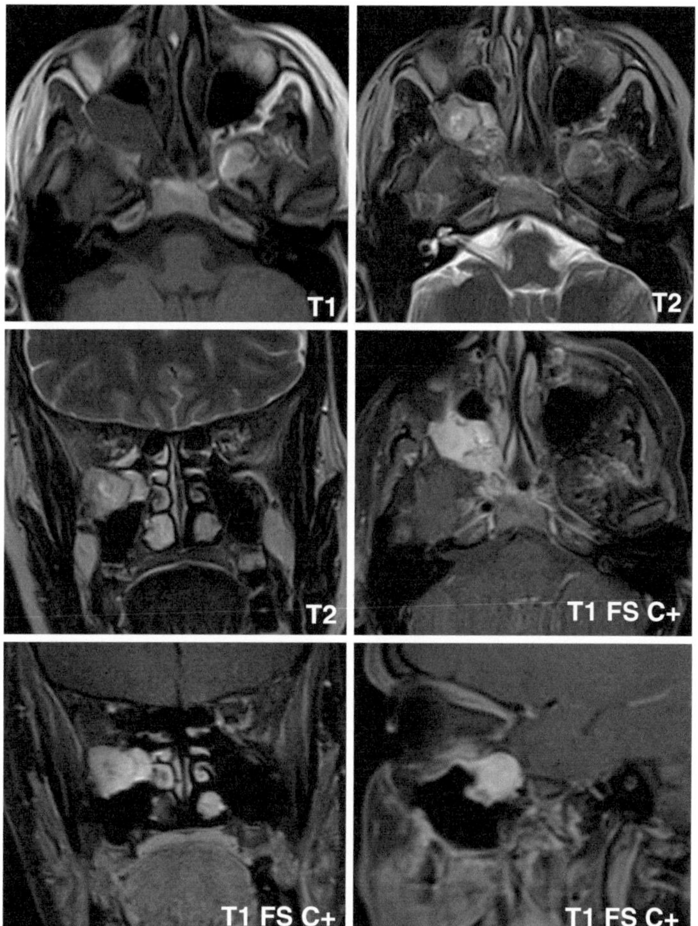

A. Haouimi et al., *Head and Neck Radiology Spot Diagnosis*,
https://doi.org/10.1007/978-3-032-14553-6_135

Findings

A lobulated soft-tissue mass of the right maxillary sinus centered on its posterosuperior wall. It is of intermediate signal on T1, high signal on T2 with a vivid enhancement. The lesion extends to the pterygomaxillary fissure posteriorly and inferomedial extraconal space superiorly with partial destruction of the orbital floor.

Diagnosis

Adenoid cystic carcinoma of the maxillary sinus.

Discussion

Maxillary sinus adenoid cystic carcinoma, previously known as cylindroma, is a rare, locally aggressive, slow-growing malignant tumor. It has a propensity for distant metastasis and a tendency to recur. The lesion originates from the mucosa of minor seromucous glands underlying the respiratory epithelium, mostly seen in the hard palate. Maxillary sinus involvement is rare. The lesions affect people between 50 and 70 years with no sex predilection.

The clinical presentation can be nonspecific. Patients present with nasal obstruction and epistaxis and may be misdiagnosed as sinusitis or allergic rhinitis. Locoregional invasion of the orbit and skull base can cause proptosis, ophthalmoplegia, otalgia, and even seizures.

CT and MRI images are highly nonspecific. 3D surface-shaded CT helps the surgeon to project the surgical approach, and MRI can show perineural invasion if present.

Common Differential Diagnosis

- Chronic sinusitis: nonaggressive, thickened sinus wall.
- Mucocele: hypodense, expansile, nonenhancing, bony thinning, and remodeling on CT.

Management Options

Curative surgery and adjuvant radiotherapy are the mainstay of treatment.

References and Further Reading

1. Dudde F, et al. Fulminant adenoid cystic carcinoma of the maxillary sinus – a rare finding: case report. In Vivo Mar. 2023. https://doi.org/10.21873/invivo.13160. Accessed 27 Aug 2024.
2. Haouimi A. Adenoid cystic carcinoma - maxillary sinus. Radiopaedia.org. 2020. https://doi.org/10.53347/rID-75261. Accessed 27 Aug 2024.
3. Lahjaouj M, et al. Advanced adenoid cystic carcinoma of maxillary sinus: rare case report and review of literature. Int J Surg Case Rep. 2021. https://doi.org/10.1016/j.ijscr.2021.02.008. Accessed 27 Aug 2024. Epub 2021 Feb 6. PMID: 33592415; PMCID.

Case 136

136

Clinical History

A 25-year-old woman presented with a history of a rapidly enlarging right orbital swelling.

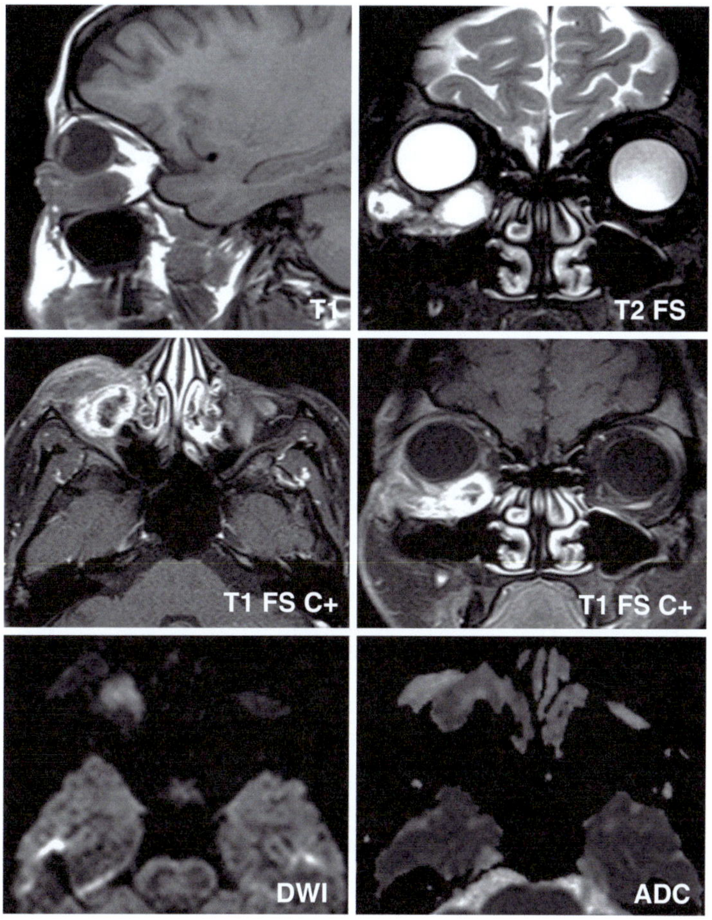

A. Haouimi et al., *Head and Neck Radiology Spot Diagnosis*,
https://doi.org/10.1007/978-3-032-14553-6_136

Findings

Right orbital extraconal mass centered on the lower inner quadrant, inseparable from the inferior rectus muscle with mass effect on the globe, which is displaced superiorly and infiltrates the lower eyelid. It shows an intermediate signal on T1, a high signal on T2 with restricted diffusion and intense heterogeneous enhancement with a central necrosis.

Diagnosis

Orbital rhabdomyosarcoma.

Discussion

Orbital rhabdomyosarcomas occur predominantly in children, most often before 16 years of age. They account for approximately 20% of all rhabdomyosarcomas arising in the head and neck region. These tumors originate from primitive mesenchymal cells having the potential to differentiate into striated muscle fibers. The embryonal subtype commonly involves the superior orbit, whereas the alveolar subtype more frequently affects the inferior orbital region.

Clinically, the patients present with rapidly developing proptosis over weeks, ptosis, globe displacement, blepharoptosis, and ocular pain.

On imaging, the lesions are mostly extraconal but inseparable from the extraocular muscles without enlarging the muscle belly. Smaller lesions are well-circumscribed, homogeneous, isodense/isointense soft-tissue masses. Bigger lesions are heterogeneous on both CT and MRI due to hemorrhagic and necrotic components. On T2, the lesions are usually hyperintense and show restricted diffusion. Distortion and displacement of the globe can occur in bigger lesions as well as bony erosion. Moderate to marked enhancement is seen after gadolinium.

Common Differential Diagnosis

- Orbital lymphoma: separable from extraocular muscles.
- Orbital pseudotumor: enlargement of the muscle belly and involvement of tendons.
- Orbital capillary hemangioma: serpiginous, flow voids, homogeneous enhancement, lobulated appearance with thin septa.

Management Option

A combination of radio- and chemotherapy remains the mainstay of treatment.

References and Further Reading

1. Gaillard F, et al. Rhabdomyosarcoma (orbit). Radiopaedia.org. 2024. https://doi.org/10.53347/rID-8338. Accessed 29 Dec 2024.
2. Haouimi A. Orbital rhabdomyosarcoma - embryonal subtype. Radiopaedia.org. 2020. https://doi.org/10.53347/rID-73163. Accessed 27 Aug 2024.
3. Jurdy L, et al. 2013. Orbital rhabdomyosarcomas: a review Saudi J Ophthalmol. https://doi.org/10.1016/j.sjopt.2013.06.004. Accessed 27 Aug 2024.

Case 137

137

Clinical History

A 35-year-old woman presented with a painless submental swelling.

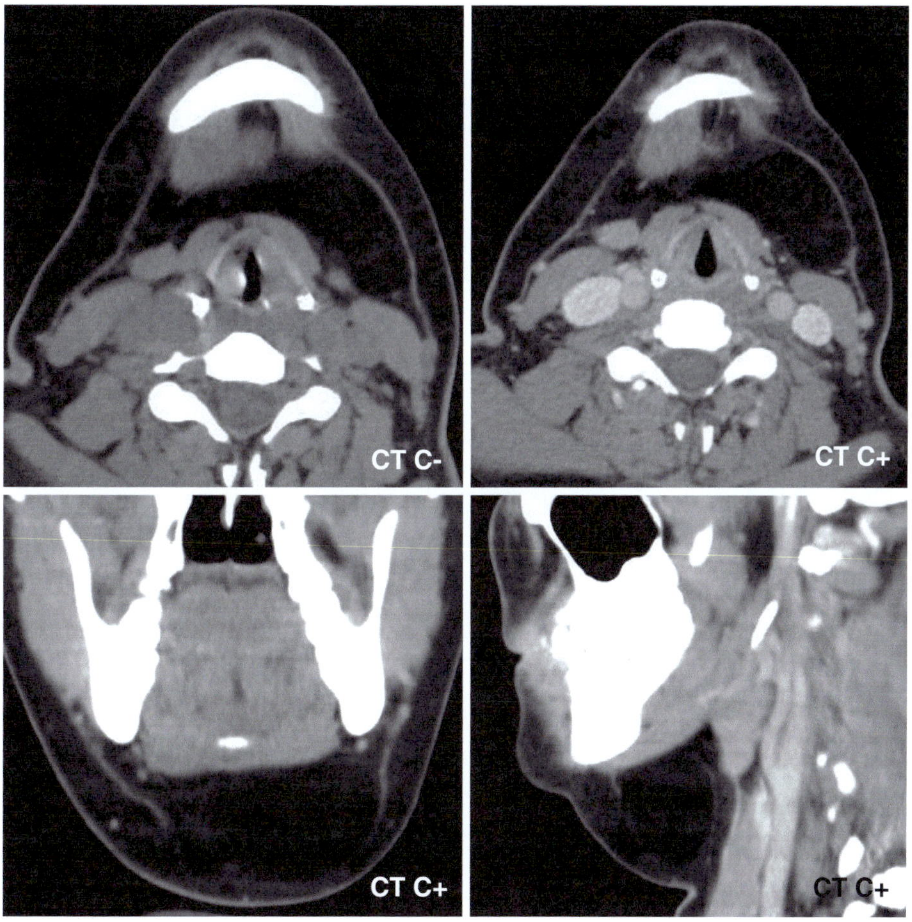

A. Haouimi et al., *Head and Neck Radiology Spot Diagnosis*,
https://doi.org/10.1007/978-3-032-14553-6_137

Findings

A large subcutaneous well-encapsulated fatty lesion in the submental region showing isodensity to subcutaneous fat. No calcification, no thick septation or contrast enhancement.

Diagnosis

Submental lipoma.

Discussion

Lipomas are well-defined, nonepithelial, capsulated benign lesions usually seen subcutaneously. They are infrequent in the head and neck region. They are the most common neoplasms of mesenchymal origin and are typically seen between the fifth and sixth decades. Males are 10 times more prone to develop lipomas. Malignant degeneration to liposarcoma is extremely rare.

Submental lipomas present as a slow-developing facial contour deformity that can give rise to cosmetic concerns.

On ultrasound, the lesions are well-defined iso- or hypoechoic solid masses without acoustic shadow. Lesions are homogeneously hypodense on CT, showing no enhancement. MRI is the modality of choice for tissue characterization. The lesions appear as well-defined high signal on T1 and relatively less high signal on T2. The fat-suppression sequences allow complete suppression of signal and help to reach a near histologic diagnosis.

Common Differential Diagnosis

- Liposarcoma: infiltrative, nonadipose tissue +, thick nodular septa, enhancement ++.
- Angiolipoma: nonhomogeneous, low signal on T1 and high signal on T2 for vascular components and intense enhancement.
- Ludwig's angina: clinical history, clouding of fat plane, abscess +/−.

Management Options

Surgical excision is the definitive treatment. Liposuction and steroid injections are alternative, less popular options.

References and Further Reading

1. Cree M, et al. Lipomas, Lipoma variants, and well-differentiated liposarcomas. AJR. 2012. https://www.ajronline.org/doi/10.2214/ajr.182.3.1820733. Accessed 25 Sept 2024.
2. Haouimi A. Submental lipoma. Radiopaedia.org. 2024. https://radiopaedia.org/cases/194855. Accessed 25 Sept 2024.
3. Medina CR, et al. Giant submental lipoma: case report and review of the literature. Can J Plast Surg. 2007. https://doi.org/10.1177/229255030701500405. Accessed 25 Sept 2024. PMID: 19554181; PMCID: PMC2696007.

Case 138

138

Clinical History

A 5-year-old girl with a history of a recurrent left peripheral facial palsy.

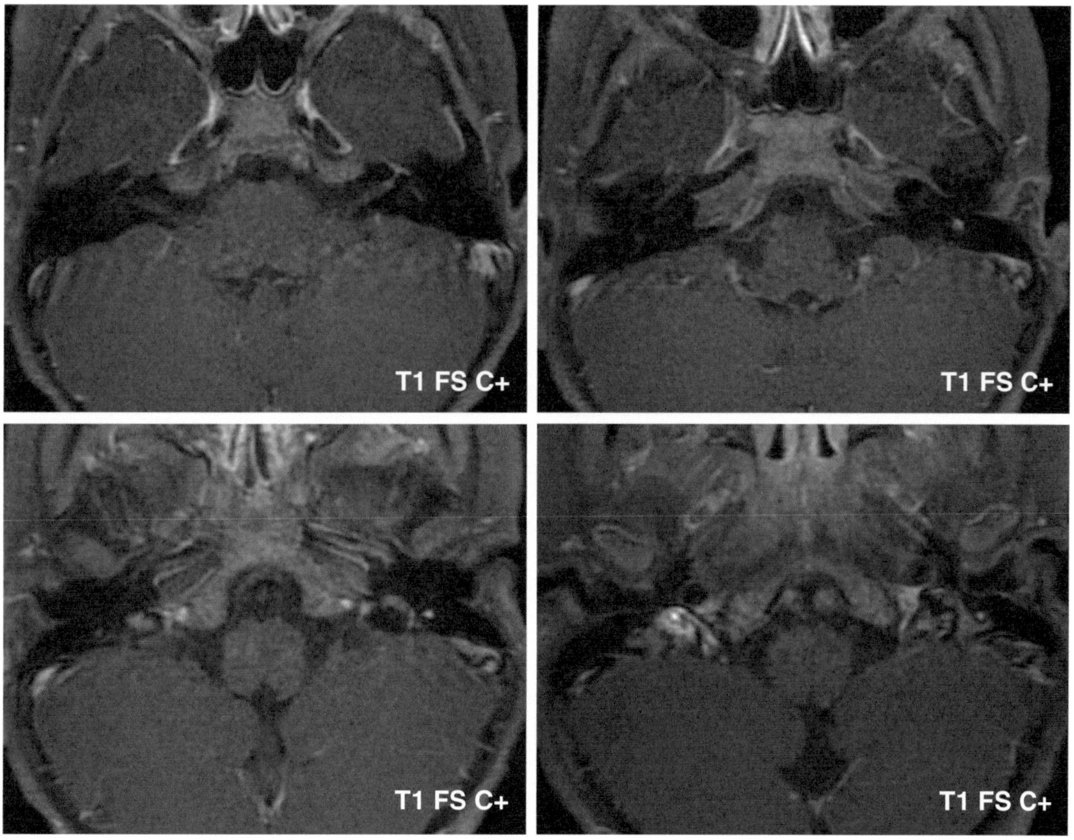

A. Haouimi et al., *Head and Neck Radiology Spot Diagnosis*,
https://doi.org/10.1007/978-3-032-14553-6_138

Findings

Non nodular thickening and enhancement of the left facial nerve extending along the entire length from the meatal segment and geniculate ganglion to the level of stylomastoid foramen.

Diagnosis

Facial neuritis.

Discussion

Facial neuritis, also known as "Bell's palsy," is one of the most common causes of lower motor neuron facial paralysis. It causes temporary inability to control the facial muscles and spontaneous resolution occurs within 6–8 weeks without any identifiable etiology.

Clinically, the patients present with acute and rapidly progressing (over a couple of hours) unilateral facial paralysis reaching its peak usually at 72 h. The peak age of presentation is between 15 and 50 years. There is no gender predilection.

Clinically, retro-auricular pain precedes complete or partial paralysis of facial nerve. Unilateral facial numbness, lack of facial expression, drooping of the eyelid, inability to wrinkle the forehead, or inability to close the eye are the major complaints.

The diagnosis is clinical by exclusion of other causes. MRI shows intratemporal, long-segment linear, nonnodular enhancement of the facial nerve, more intense than the contralateral normal facial nerve. The enhancement may persist for up to 1 year beyond clinical improvement, but the size gradually regresses.

Common Differential Diagnosis

- Facial neuroma: insidious onset, focal nodular enhancement, steroid resistant.
- Ramsay Hunt syndrome: clinical history, following activation of varicella-zoster virus.
- Lyme disease: clinical history of tick bite, mostly bilateral.
- Perineural spread of tumor: history of cancer in the vicinity.

Management Options

The mainstay of treatment is with oral corticosteroids. Oral glucocorticoids will reduce the severity, improve the nerve function, and shorten the recovery time.

References and Further Reading

1. Gaillard F, et al. Bell palsy. Radiopaedia.org. 2025. https://doi.org/10.53347/rID-973. Accessed 27 Nov 2024.
2. Gupta S, et al. Imaging the facial nerve: a contemporary review. Radiol Res Pract. 2013. https://doi.org/10.1155/2013/248039. Accessed 27 Nov 2024.
3. Haouimi A. Facial neuritis. Radiopaedia.org. 2024. https://radiopaedia.org/cases/194862. Accessed 14 Nov 2024.

Case 139

139

Clinical History

A 40-year-old woman with a history of painless swelling of the right submandibular region.

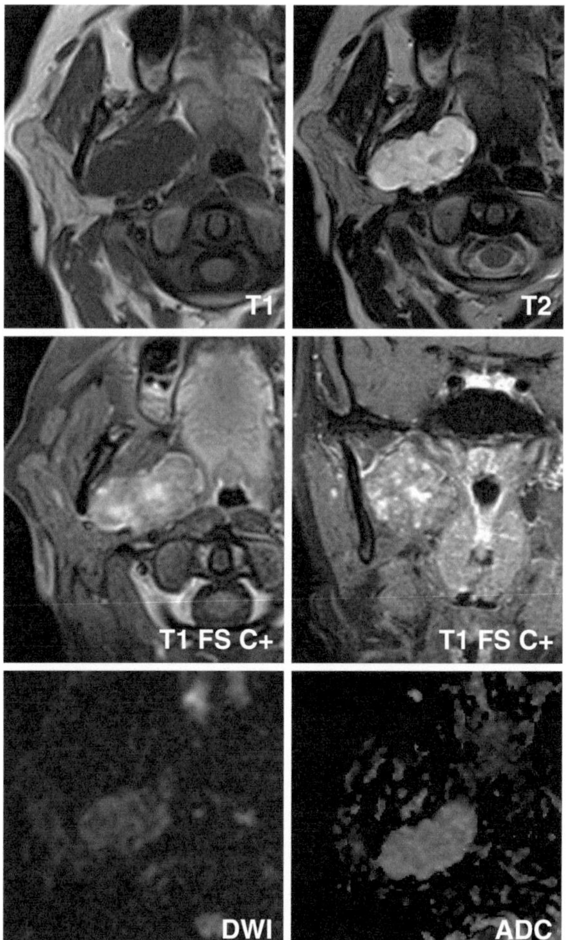

A. Haouimi et al., *Head and Neck Radiology Spot Diagnosis*,
https://doi.org/10.1007/978-3-032-14553-6_139

Findings

Well-circumscribed right prestyloid parapharyngeal space (PPS) enhancing mass in contact with the deep parotid lobe. The mass displaces the adjacent pharyngeal tonsil anteromedially and the internal carotid artery and the internal jugular vein posteriorly. It shows low signal on T1 and high signal on T2 with no restricted diffusion.

Diagnosis

Parapharyngeal pleomorphic adenoma.

Discussion

Pleomorphic tumors are the most common tumors of the PPS, originating mostly from the deep parotid lobe. The distensible medial wall of the space allows the lesions to reach a large size without giving rise to a visible neck mass. The tumor reaches the PPS, herniating through the stylomandibular tunnel. Pleomorphic tumors are situated in the anterior (prestyloid) portion of the PPS.

On CT and MRI, pleomorphic adenomas of PPS can appear entirely extraparotid without visible fat plane and widened stylomandibular tunnel. Lesions are of low signal on T1 and high signal on T2 with homo/heterogeneous enhancement. Peripheral T2-low signal represents the fibrous capsule. CT scan can show areas of calcification. Normal surrounding fat planes.

Common Differential Diagnosis

- Schwannoma: positive neurologic signs
- Parapharyngeal abscess: acute onset, fever, phlegmon, ring enhancement, clouding of fat
- Cystic hygroma: no enhancement

Management Options

Surgical excision is the best option.

References and Further Reading

1. Akın I, et al. Pleomorphic adenomas of the parapharyngeal space. Case Rep Otolaryngol. 2014. https://doi.org/10.1155/2014/168401. Accessed 28 Aug 2024. Epub 2014 Jul 22. PMID: 25140265; PMCID: PMC4129673.
2. Haouimi A. Parapharyngeal pleomorphic adenoma. Radiopaedia.org. 2019. https://doi.org/10.53347/rID-68833. Accessed 28 Aug 2024.
3. Malhotra V, et al. Largest De Novo parapharyngeal pleomorphic adenoma: a rare case removed via minimal access approach. Ann Maxillofac Surg. 2017. https://doi.org/10.4103/2231-0746.208640. Accessed 28 Aug 2024. PMID: 28713752; PMCID: PMC5502501.

Case 140

140

Clinical History

A 30-year-old HIV positive man presented with a painless swelling of the right parotid region.

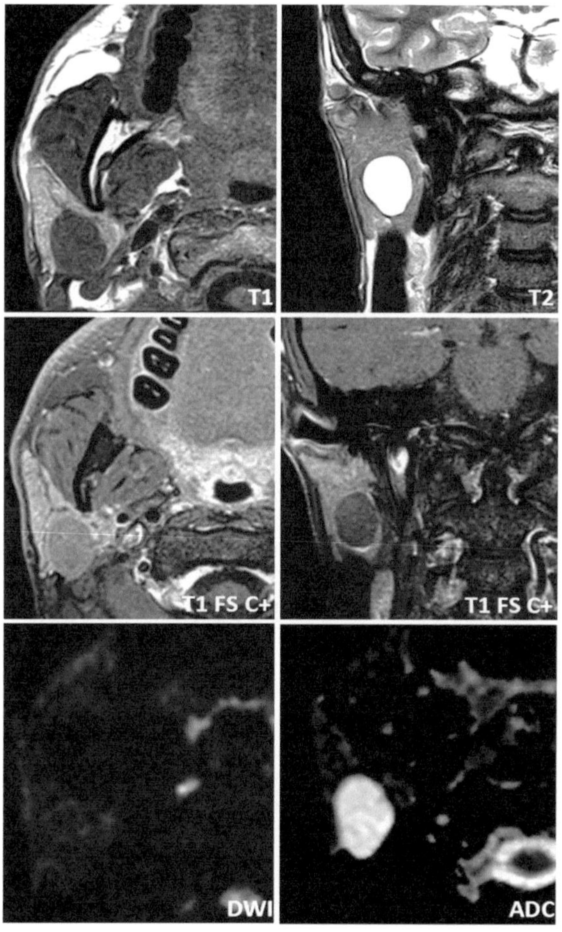

A. Haouimi et al., *Head and Neck Radiology Spot Diagnosis*,
https://doi.org/10.1007/978-3-032-14553-6_140

Findings

Well-marginated unilocular cystic lesion of the right parotid, showing low signal on T1 and high signal on T2 with no restricted diffusion. Thin, smooth, and regular peripheral rim enhancement after gadolinium. Normal left parotid gland without cervical lymphadenopathy.

Diagnosis

Parotid lymphoepithelial cyst.

Discussion

Lymphoepithelial parotid cysts represent lymphocytic infiltration of the major salivary glands and are frequently associated with Sjogren's syndrome or HIV infection. Up to 5% of HIV patients may develop lymphoepithelial parotid cysts. HIV associated lymphoepithelial cysts arise due to hyperplasia of intraparenchymal lymph nodes and associated ductal obstruction. The cysts may also result sporadically from intraparenchymal ductal dilation of the parotid gland, periparotid lymph node, or branchial cleft remnants. Associated nasopharyngeal adenoid hyperplasia may be seen in up to 35% of HIV positive patients. Uni- or bilateral painless cystic salivary gland mass in HIV patients, with or without cervical lymphadenopathy, should always raise the suspicion of the diagnosis.

Common Differential Diagnosis

- Sjögren syndrome: clinical history, multiple microcysts, solid lesions +/–.
- Pleomorphic tumor: complex lobulated solid-cystic components, dystrophic calcification.
- Parotid abscess: clinical history, restricted diffusion.

Management Options

HIV-associated cases are treated conservatively with antiretroviral therapy. Aspiration, drainage, and sclerotherapy are other options. Surgery is not performed unless there is a cosmetic compromise.

References and Further Reading

1. Gaillard F, et al. Benign lymphoepithelial lesions. Radiopaedia.org. 2023. https://doi.org/10.53347/rID-977. Accessed 23 Nov 2024.
2. Haouimi A. Parotid lymphoepithelial cyst. Radiopaedia.org. 2022. https://doi.org/10.53347/rID-149218. Accessed 28 Aug 2024.
3. Sujatha D, et al. Parotid lymphoepithelial cysts in human immunodeficiency virus: a review. J Laryngol Otol. 2013. https://doi.org/10.1017/S0022215113002417. Accessed 28 Aug 2024. Epub 2013 Oct 29.

Case 141

141

Clinical History

A 55-year-old man presented with a history of painless swelling in the superolateral aspect of the right orbit.

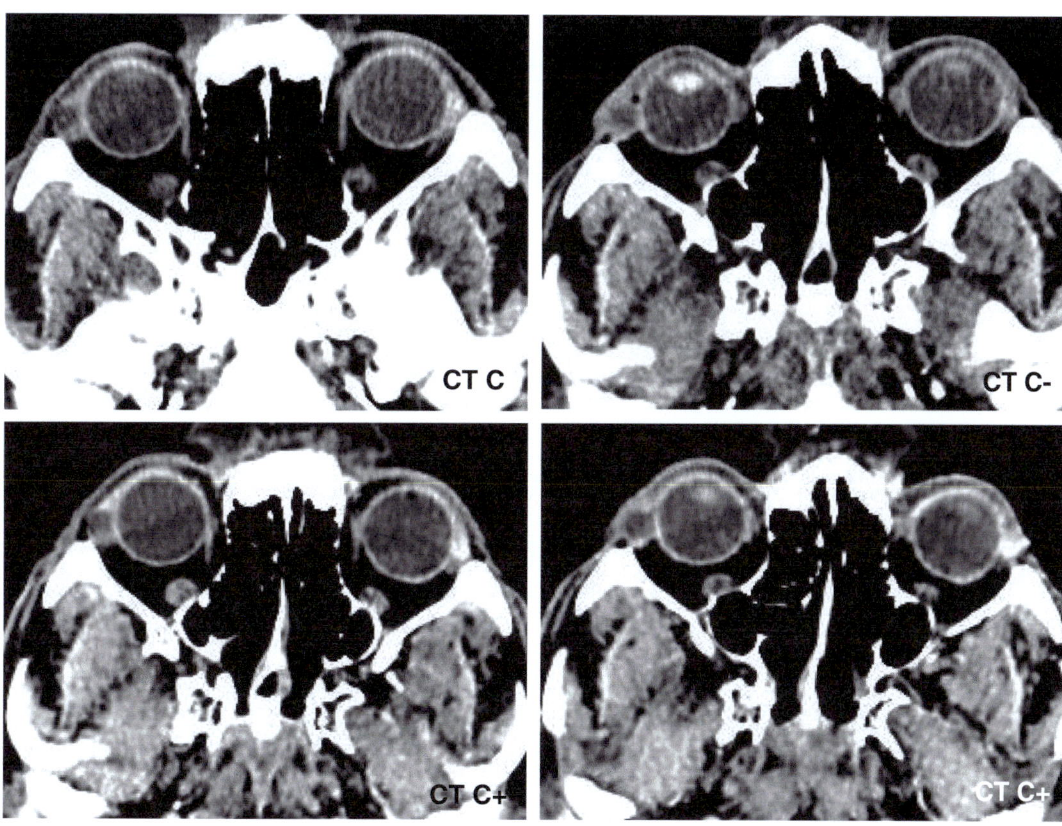

A. Haouimi et al., *Head and Neck Radiology Spot Diagnosis*,
https://doi.org/10.1007/978-3-032-14553-6_141

Findings

A well-defined cystic lesion of the right lacrimal gland showing a homogeneous fluid content with no calcification, solid component, or enhancement. No associated bony erosion or destruction. Normal left lacrimal gland as well as the ocular globes.

Diagnosis

Dacryops, also known as lacrimal gland duct cyst.

Discussion

Dacryops or lacrimal gland cyst is a benign condition. Clinically, the patient presents with a slowly progressive painless swelling at the superolateral aspect of the orbit. On examination, the lesions appear as a bluish-gray rubbery mobile nodule. The diagnosis is made on clinical grounds. On transillumination testing, the cysts have a bluish hue. Imaging is indicated if there is suspicion of a cancerous growth. Most cases are unilateral. Bilateral cases raise suspicion of systemic disease like sarcoidosis, Sjögren syndrome, Mikulicz syndrome, and other lymphoproliferative disorders. Though the lesion is largely considered benign, transformation into squamous cell carcinoma has been reported. Cysts may get infected and fistulize at superotemporal fornix. In that case, an air-fluid level may be evidenced on imaging.

Common Differential Diagnosis

- Dermoid cyst: punctate calcification +/−, fatty component shows T1 high signal.
- Dacryocystocele: bony remodeling.
- Adenoid cystic carcinoma: infiltrative, bony destruction, enhancement.

Management Options

Excision or marsupialization is reserved for patients with symptoms and cosmetic reasons. Incomplete excision may result in recurrence. Argon laser photocoagulation has also been described.

References and Further Reading

1. Haouimi A. Dacryops. Radiopaedia.org. 2022. https://doi.org/10.53347/rID-156627. Accessed 28 Aug 2024.
2. Tanaboonyawat S, et al. Dacryops - a review. Orbit. 2020. https://doi.org/10.1080/01676830.2019.1608564. Accessed 25 Sept 2024. Epub 2019 Sep 12. PMID: 31512543.
3. Tejasvi S, et al. Dacryops. Radiopaedia.org. 2024. https://doi.org/10.53347/rID-84181. Accessed 25 Sept 2024.

Case 142

142

Clinical History

A 75-year-old man with a history of painless swelling of the left parotid gland.

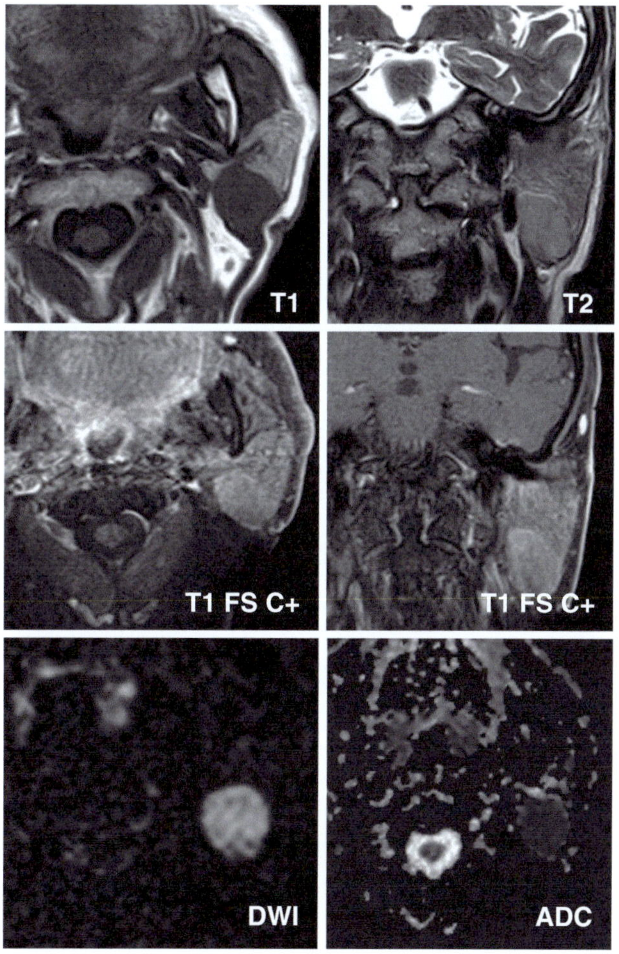

A. Haouimi et al., *Head and Neck Radiology Spot Diagnosis*,
https://doi.org/10.1007/978-3-032-14553-6_142

Findings

A well-defined lobulated ovoid mass at the superficial lobe of the left parotid gland showing low signal on T1 and mildly elevated signal on T2 with a peripheral hypointense capsule. There is restricted diffusion and a low ADC value. The TIC (not shown) reveals an early enhancement and low wash-out within the tumor. The right parotid gland appears normal.

Diagnosis

Non-Hodgkin lymphoma (non-MALT) of the parotid gland.

Discussion

Primary parotid gland NHL is rare and represents only 2% of all parotid tumors. They often occur in association with autoimmune diseases such as Sjögren syndrome. There are two histological subtypes based on the association of mucosa: MALT and non-MALT. The subtypes vary in their prognosis and treatment.

Patients usually present with nonspecific symptoms such as a progressively enlarging painless parotid swelling that is largely indistinguishable from conditions like mixed parotid tumor or Warthin tumor. However, a positive clinical history of autoimmune disease with clinically appreciable lymphadenopathy should raise the index of suspicion.

CT may show an ill-defined, homogeneous, isodense, or solid-cystic mass. Homogeneous low signal on T1 and low-to-high signal intensity on T2 with variable enhancement is seen on MRI. MALT lymphoma often demonstrates a solid-cystic texture, whereas non-MALT lymphoma is usually solid.

Common Differential Diagnosis

- Warthin tumor: adult, smoker, no history of Sjögren syndrome.
- Metastatic necrotic lymph nodes: clinical history.
- Pleomorphic adenoma: lobulated, dystrophic calcification.

Management Options

Treatment depends on the stage, age and the subtype. Parotidectomy, can be used to remove the lesion and to make a diagnosis. Other options are chemotherapy and radiation therapy.

References and Further Reading

1. Haouimi A. Non-Hodgkin lymphoma - parotid gland. Radiopaedia.org. 2019. https://doi.org/10.53347/rID-71531. Accessed 28 Aug 2024.
2. Zhu L, et al. Non-Hodgkin lymphoma involving the parotid gland: CT and MR imaging findings. Dentomaxillofac Radiol. 2013. https://doi.org/10.1259/dmfr.20130046. Accessed 28 Aug 2024. Epub 2013 Aug 23. PMID: 23975113; PMCID.

143 Case 143

Clinical History

A 6-year-old boy presented with a painless, superficial mobile swelling of the left neck.

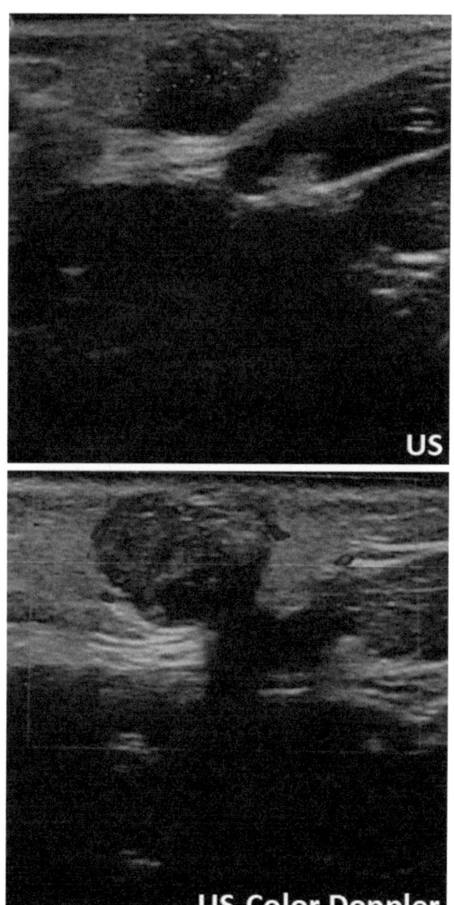

A. Haouimi et al., *Head and Neck Radiology Spot Diagnosis*,
https://doi.org/10.1007/978-3-032-14553-6_143

Findings

A small, well-defined ovoid subcutaneous heterogeneously hypoechoic mass, containing microcalcifications, with posterior acoustic shadows. Slightly increased echogenicity of the surrounding subcutaneous fat. On color Doppler, the flow was mainly peripheral.

Diagnosis

Pilomatricoma.

Discussion

Pilomatricoma, also known as calcifying epithelioma of Malherbe, is a benign tumor arising from cutaneous adnexa with remote malignant potential. About 50% of pilomatricoma occur in the head and neck region, which is more common in Caucasian children. This condition was first described by Malherbe and Chenantias in 1880. After epidermoid cyst, pilomatricomas are the second most frequently excised pediatric skin lesions.

The diagnosis is clinical and histological. The lesions appear as slow-growing, bluish-red, hard, mobile superficial nodules. The lesions can be isolated or be a syndromic component in Gardner syndrome and Turner syndrome.

On ultrasound, it is seen as an ovoid complex hypoechoic mass containing microcalcifications with focal thinning of the overlying dermis. The lesions may show a hypoechoic capsule. CT shows well-defined, subcutaneous lesions with microcalcifications. The nodules are iso- to hypointense on T1. T2 signal and enhancement pattern are variable.

Common Differential Diagnosis

- Gardner syndrome: associated with multiple colonic polyps.
- Epidermal cysts: normal colored overlying skin, low signal on T1 and high signal on T2.
- Ossifying hematoma: clinical history.

Management Options

The treatment is surgical excision.

References and Further Reading

1. Garioni E, Danesino GM, Madonia L. Pilomatricoma: sonographic features. J Ultrasound. 2008. https://doi.org/10.1016/j.jus.2008.03.001. Accessed 28 Aug 2024. Epub 2008 Apr 25. PMID: 23396664; PMCID: PMC3553250.
2. Haouimi A. Pilomatricoma. Radiopaedia.org. 2018. https://doi.org/10.53347/rID-61482. Accessed 28 Aug 2024.
3. Holland M, et al. Pilomatricoma. Radiopaedia.org. 2024. https://doi.org/10.53347/rID-19245. Accessed 28 Nov 2024.

Case 144

144

Clinical History

A 50-year-old man presented with a tingling sensation of the upper limbs.

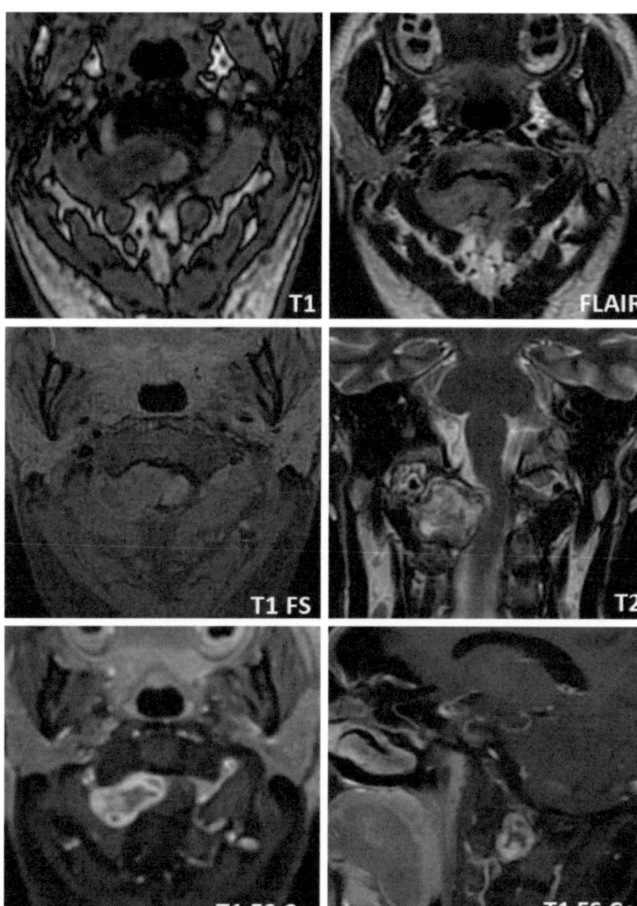

A. Haouimi et al., *Head and Neck Radiology Spot Diagnosis*,
https://doi.org/10.1007/978-3-032-14553-6_144

Findings

A well-demarcated transforaminal intradural extramedullary dumbbell-shaped soft-tissue lesion with both intra- and extracanalar components at right C1-C2 level. It shows low signal on T1, isosignal on FLAIR, and nonhomogeneous high signal on T2 with intense heterogeneous enhancement. Widening of the neural foramen with slight scalloping of the C2 vertebral body. Posterior and left lateral displacement of spinal cord without sign of myelopathy.

Diagnosis

Cervical schwannoma.

Discussion

Schwannomas are the most common benign, slow-growing intradural extramedullary tumor of the spine. They arise mostly from Schwann cells at the spinal nerve sensory roots and may occur spontaneously or in conjunction with clinical syndromes such as schwannomatosis and Carney complex. Most lesions are solitary and sporadic. Multiple lesions can be seen as a component of neurofibromatosis type 2.

Patients may experience pain, limb weakness, and other signs of myelopathy.

On imaging, the lesions show bony remodeling and widening of the neural foramina. Most lesions have well-circumscribed dumbbell configuration appearing iso- or hypointense on T1 and heterogeneously hyperintense on T2. Moderate to severe heterogeneous enhancement seen after contrast. On CT, the lesions are isodense. Neurofibromas and schwannomas may look identical on imaging. However, schwannomas, unlike neurofibromas, are frequently associated with hemorrhage, thrombosis, and cyst formation.

Common Differential Diagnosis

- Meningioma: broad dural base, no extracanalar extension.
- Neurofibroma: homogeneous, no cystic or hemorrhagic component.
- Perineural root sleeve cyst: low signal T1 and high signal T2, no enhancement.

Management Options

Wait-and-see approach for smaller and asymptomatic patients. Surgical resection is usually curative for patients with sporadic cases.

References and Further Reading

1. Airlangga P, et al. Schwannoma of the upper cervical spine–a case report. Chin J Traumatol. 2019. https://doi.org/10.1016/j.cjtee.2019.07.005. Accessed 9 Aug 2025. https://www.ncbi.nlm.nih.gov/pubmed/31653502.
2. Haouimi A. Schwannoma-cervical. Radiopaedia.org. 2022. https://doi.org/10.53347/rID-155265. Accessed 8 Dec 2024.

Case 145

145

Clinical History

A 64-year-old woman with a history of pyogenic meningitis, complicated by hearing loss, presented for cochlear implant assessment.

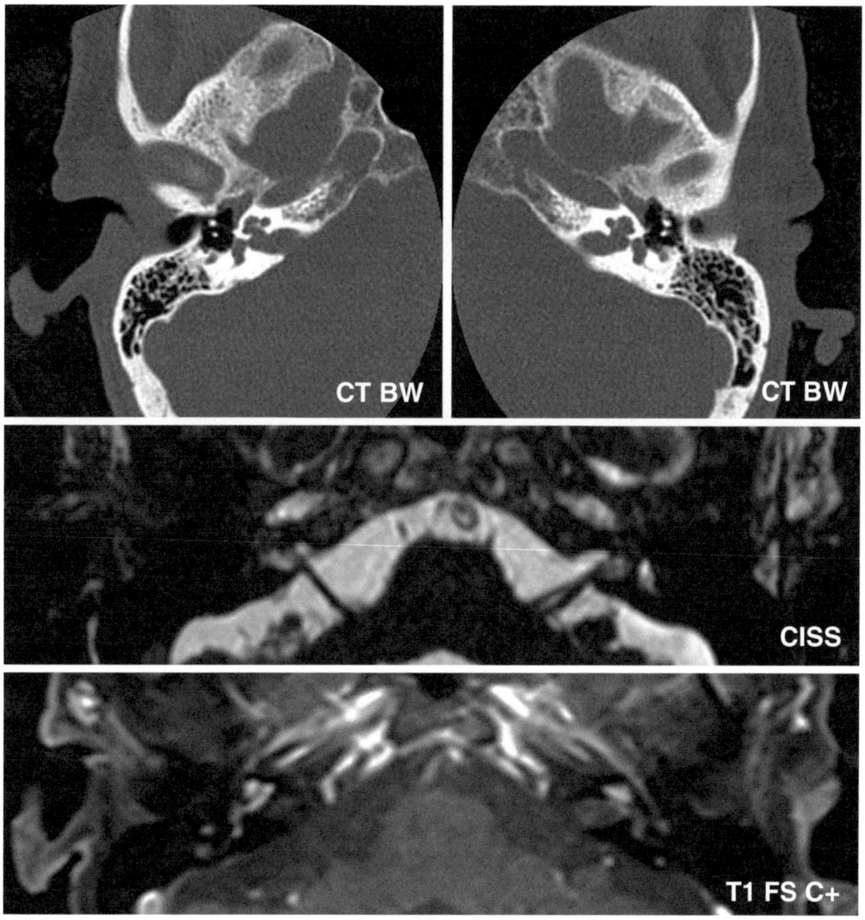

A. Haouimi et al., *Head and Neck Radiology Spot Diagnosis*,
https://doi.org/10.1007/978-3-032-14553-6_145

Findings

The unenhanced CT scan shows preserved shape and density of the inner ear structures. The axial CISS MRI demonstrates high T2-signal intensity of bilateral cochleae and right vestibule. Enhancement of the affected sites is seen on the postcontrast axial T1 FS image.

Diagnosis

Acute labyrinthitis.

Discussion

Acute labyrinthitis refers to sudden inflammation of the membranous labyrinth. Though most of the patients achieve complete recovery, some may be left with residual balance or hearing deficits. In most cases, the etiology is due to viral infection or following an episode of flu. Other less common causes include bacterial infections, trauma, autoimmune disorders, and hemorrhage. Organisms can extend to the inner structures through the meninges (via the vestibular or cochlear aqueduct) or the middle ear (via the oval or round windows). Irreversible injury to the labyrinthine structures can lead to ossification and sclerosis.

Patients can present with sudden intense spinning sensation worsening with head movement, dizziness, headache, and vomiting and can later progress to hearing loss.

CT appearance of the inner ear structures is usually normal in acute labyrinthitis. MRI will show postcontrast enhancement, restricted diffusion, and high T2 signal of the labyrinthine structures due to edema.

Common Differential Diagnosis

- Vestibular neuronitis: no hearing loss.
- Ménière disease: recurrent episodes, fluctuating hearing, no enhancement.
- Schwannoma: cochlear involvement extremely uncommon.

Management Options

Treatment is tailored to the etiology and symptom control. Steroids can help in recovering from hearing loss if started early. Cochlear implants are the treatment of choice for hearing loss, and imaging is critical to determine the stage and onset of sclerosis and ossification.

References and Further Reading

1. Taxak P, Chithra R. Labyrinthitis and Labyrinthitis Ossificans - a case report and review of the literature. J Radiol. 2020. https://doi.org/10.3941/jrcr.v14i5.3706. Accessed 16 Nov 2024.
2. Barkwill D, Arora R. Labyrinthitis. Stat Pearls Publishing; 2023. https://www.ncbi.nlm.nih.gov/books/NBK560506/. Accessed 16 Nov 2024.

Case 146

146

Clinical History

A 6-month-old infant presented with bilateral leukocoria.

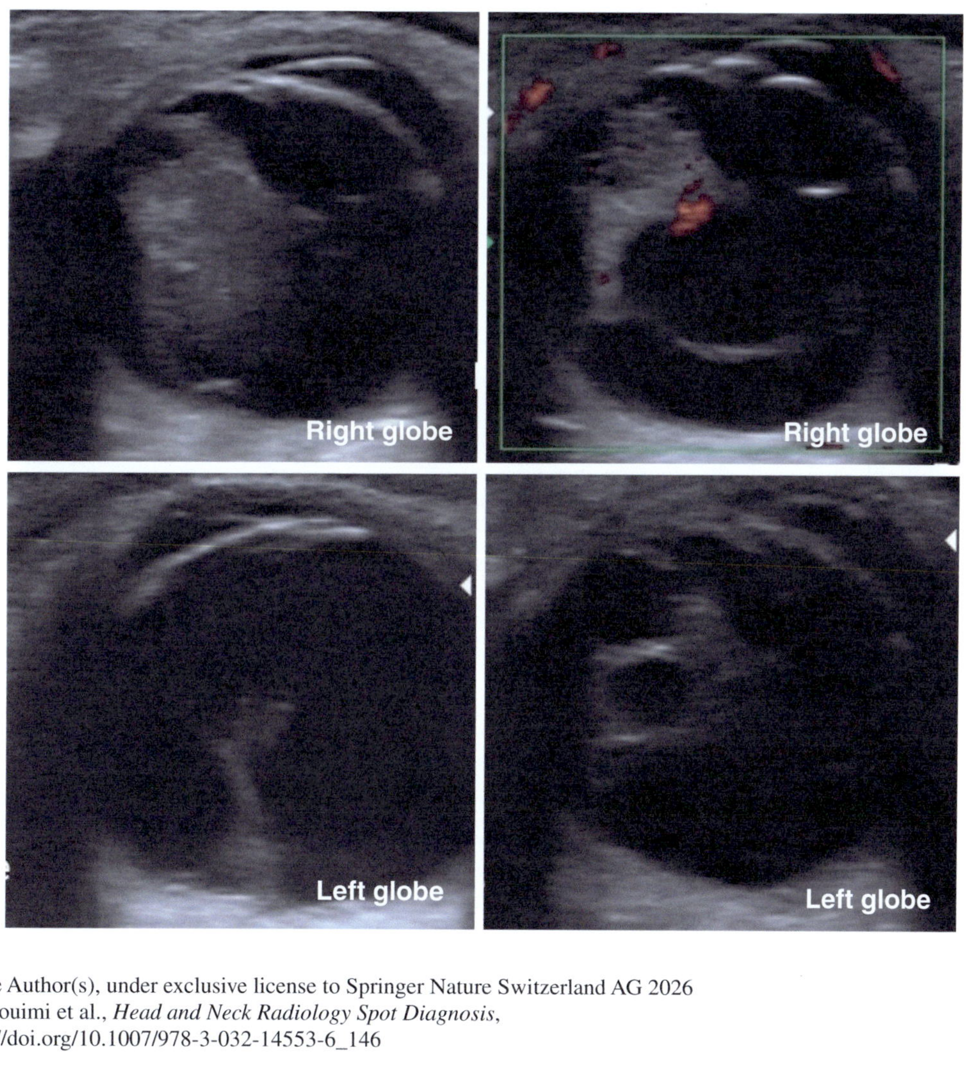

A. Haouimi et al., *Head and Neck Radiology Spot Diagnosis*,
https://doi.org/10.1007/978-3-032-14553-6_146

Findings

Heterogeneous mass within the anterior segment of the vitreous of the right globe. An echogenic band extending posteriorly to the optic disc, revealing arterial blood flow within on color Doppler. Left globe shows an echogenic band in the posterior segment of the vitreous body in contact with the optic disc.

Diagnosis

Persistent hyperplastic primary vitreous.

Discussion

Persistent hyperplastic primary vitreous, also known as persistent fetal vasculature (PFV), is a benign congenital retinoblastoma mimic. The fetal hyaloid artery typically regresses completely by 29 weeks of gestation. PFVs are intraocular anatomical remnants due to the failure of regression of these fetal vessels. The lesions are mostly unilateral and 10% bilateral. Both genetic and hereditary factors have been postulated as the etiology. *ATOH7* and *NDP* genes are probably playing a major role during the pathogenesis.

Patients may present with the classical clinical triad of leukocoria, microphthalmia, and cataract at birth. As the baby continues to grow, strabismus and amblyopia gradually develop due to a traction effect. Conditions such as Norrie syndrome and Walker–Warburg syndrome can be associated with PFV.

An echogenic band along the course of Cloquet's canal can be seen on ultrasound with possible arterial blood on Doppler. On MRI, the retrolental triangular soft tissue shows low signal on T1 and high signal on T2, resembling a "martini glass" appearance.

Common Differential Diagnosis

- Retinoblastoma: microphthalmia, calcification.
- Congenital cataract: no intraocular anatomical remnant. No retinal traction.
- Retinopathy of prematurity: usually bilateral, premature babies.

Management Options

The goal of management is to clear the opacity to allow visual development and to prevent the potential complications from PFV.

References and Further Reading

1. Haouimi A. Persistent hyperplastic primary vitreous. Radiopaedia.org. 2019. https://doi.org/10.53347/rID-71013. Accessed 28 Aug 2024.
2. Weerakkody Y, et al. Persistent hyperplastic primary vitreous. Radiopaedia.org. 2024. https://doi.org/10.53347/rID-19170. Accessed 28 Nov 2024.

Case 147

147

Clinical History

A 55-year-old man with a history of painless hard swelling of the left mandibular region.

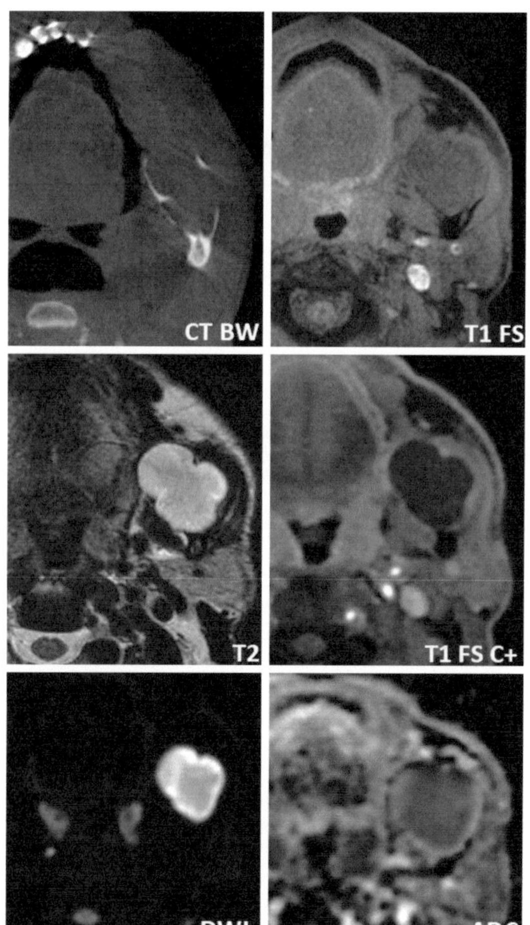

A. Haouimi et al., *Head and Neck Radiology Spot Diagnosis*,
https://doi.org/10.1007/978-3-032-14553-6_147

Findings

An expansile "dumbbell-shaped" lytic lesion centered on the ramus of the left mandible with cortical thinning and areas of cortical breach on CT scan. On MRI, this lytic lesion demonstrates low signal on T1 fat sat, high signal on T2 with restricted diffusion, and thin rim of peripheral enhancement.

Diagnosis

Epidermoid cyst of the mandible.

Discussion

Epidermoid cysts are benign developmental lesions derived from ectoderm, containing cheesy keratin-filled cysts and lined by squamous epithelium. Traumatic and inflammatory conditions have been hypothesized as the mechanism in acquired form. Mandibular epidermoid cysts are rare, slow-growing lesions. They are believed to develop from dental lamina.

The lesions remain asymptomatic and are discovered incidentally. The lesion can be painful when infected.

On panoramic X-ray and CT scan, the epidermoid appears as a well-marginated unilocular radiolucent lesion. There can be associated bony expansion with cortical thinning and breaching. The lesions show low signal on T1 and moderate-to-high signal on T2 with restricted diffusion.

Common Differential Diagnosis

- Odontogenic keratocyst: unilocular, osteolytic, minimal buccolingual expansion.
- Ameloblastoma: multilocular, septal enhancement, mural nodule.
- Dentigerous cyst: unilocular osteolytic around crown of impacted tooth.

Management Options

Surgical excision is recommended for symptomatic cases.

References and Further Reading

1. Borghesi A, et al. Odontogenic keratocyst: imaging features of a benign lesion with an aggressive behaviour. Insights Imaging. 2018. https://doi.org/10.1007/s13244-018-0644-z. Accessed 28 Nov 2024. Epub 2018 Jul 31. PMID: 30066143; PMCID.
2. Haouimi A. Epidermoid cyst - mandible. Radiopaedia.org. 2024. https://radiopaedia.org/cases/194988. Accessed 28 Nov 2024.
3. Loxha MP, et al. Epidermoid cyst of mandible ramus: case report. Med Arch. 2016. https://doi.org/10.5455/medarh.2016.70.238-240. Accessed 28 Nov 2024. Epub 2016 May 31. PMID: 27594757; PMCID: PMC5010063.

Case 148

148

Clinical History

A 55-year-old man presented with a painful swelling in the left parotid region with fever and elevated inflammatory markers. History of resection of a cyst at the same place.

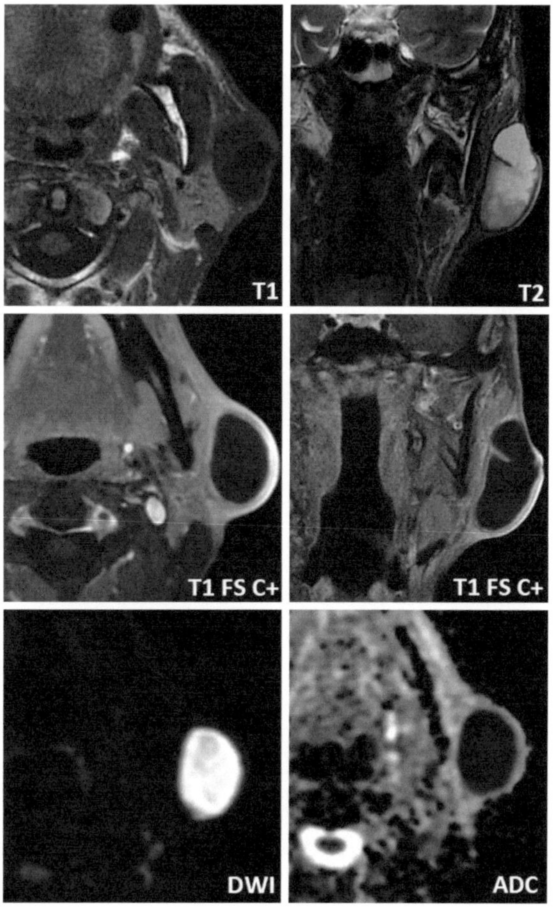

A. Haouimi et al., *Head and Neck Radiology Spot Diagnosis*,
https://doi.org/10.1007/978-3-032-14553-6_148

Findings

A well-defined septated cystic mass around the left pinna, superficial to the left parotid gland. It displays a low signal on T1, inhomogeneously high signal on T2 with thick enhanced wall. Restricted diffusion on DWI/ADC. Normal ipsilateral parotid gland parenchyma.

Diagnosis

Infected first branchial cleft cyst.

Discussion

First branchial cleft cysts are congenital lesions secondary to incomplete fusion of the cleft between the first and second branchial arches. Type 1 (periauricular) is extremely rare and histologically is purely ectodermal. They are seen posteromedially to the pinna and postero-inferiorly to the external auditory canal. Type 2 (periparotid) lesions contain both ectodermal and mesodermal components and are seen near the angle of mandible, mostly deep to the facial nerve.

Clinically, patients present with a compressible, painless cystic lesion neighboring the pinna or concha. The diagnosis can be difficult in newborns. Otorrhea in the absence of chronic otitis, along with the presence of a fistula or sinus tract, can help with the diagnosis. The sinus tract associated with type 1 is above the jawline, whereas the sinus tract with type 2 is below the jawline. A wide tract inferior to the auditory canal is considered as a diagnostic sign for type 1 first branchial cleft cyst.

Ultrasound reveals the cystic nature of the lesion without any vascular component in the parotid space superficial to the parotid gland. Connection to the parotid gland (if present) is a distinctive feature. Ultrasound may not adequately evaluate the extent and depth of the lesion. MRI confirms the cystic nature as low and high signal on T1 and T2, respectively. Infected lesions can show nonhomogeneous contents with thick peripheral enhancement and restricted diffusion.

Common Differential Diagnosis

- Lymphangioma: multilocular, insinuating, rarely seen at parotid space.
- Suppurative parotid lymph node: fever, intraparotid, thick peripheral enhancement.
- Benign lymphoepithelial cyst of HIV: bilateral, multiple, associated parotid cysts.

Management Options

Complete surgical resection is always preferable to avoid the development of fistulous tract.

References and Further Reading

1. Finn DG, et al. First branchial cleft cysts: clinical update. Laryngoscope. 1987. https://doi.org/10.1288/00005537-198702000-00003. Accessed 28 Nov 2024.
2. Haouimi A. Infected first branchial cleft cyst. Radiopaedia.org. 2024. https://radiopaedia.org/cases/197016. Accessed 28 Nov 2024.

Case 149

149

Clinical History

A 50-year-old woman presented with a neglected right hemiparesis.

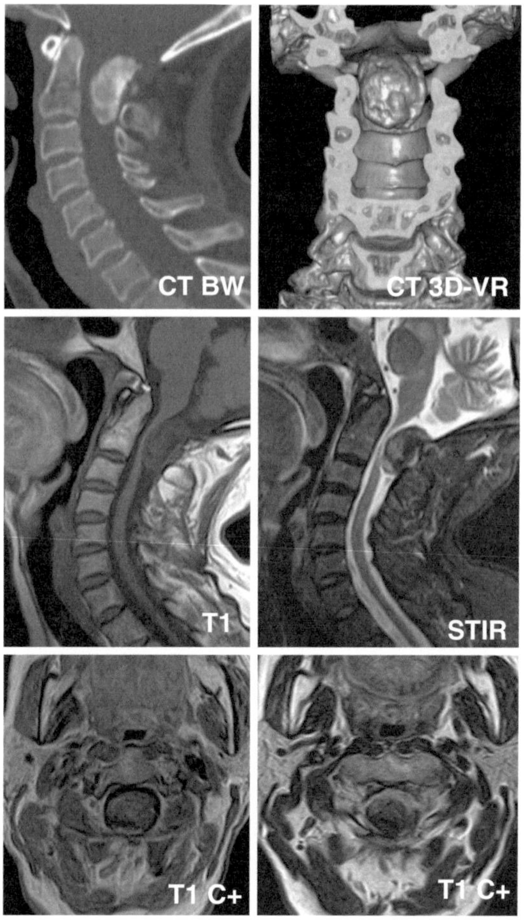

A. Haouimi et al., *Head and Neck Radiology Spot Diagnosis*,
https://doi.org/10.1007/978-3-032-14553-6_149

Findings

A broad-based intradural extramedullary iso- to hypointense lesion seen on all MRI sequences posterior to the spinal cord below the foramen magnum. It shows moderate nonhomogeneous enhancement, causing extrinsic medullary compression and displacement of spinal cord anteriorly. Focal T2 intramedullary high signal consistent with compressive myelopathy. On CT, the lesion appears to be calcified.

Diagnosis

Calcified meningioma of cervical spine.

Discussion

Spinal meningiomas are benign, slow-growing, non-life-threatening WHO grade 1 tumor. Malignant transformation is extremely rare. Spinal meningiomas represent only a minority of all meningiomas with a peak incidence in the sixth to eighth decades and with female predominance. Childhood ionizing radiation and trauma are risk factors. Spinal meningiomas can also be seen as a component of neurofibromatosis.

As the lesions grow, they can cause extrinsic medullary compression leading to myelopathy. Cervical meningiomas can also cause cervicalgia and radiating arm pain due to compression on adjacent nerve roots as well as sensory deficits.

MRI findings demonstrate well-demarcated isointense broad-based dural lesions on all sequences with moderate to intense enhancement. "Dural tail sign" and "Ginko leaf sign" can be positive. CT can show calcification when present.

Common Differential Diagnosis

- Schwannoma: extracanalicular extension, may be hemorrhagic, widened neural foramina.
- Neurofibroma: often multiple, low-intensity central region on T2 and T1 C+ images.
- Metastasis: clinical history, no dural base.

Management Options

Depending on its size, location, and symptoms, the meningioma may simply be observed or surgically removed. Surgical removal is not always mandatory. Less than 10% may experience recurrence.

References and Further Reading

1. Gaillard F, et al. Spinal meningioma. Radiopaedia.org. 2024. https://doi.org/10.53347/rID-19063. Accessed 4 Jan 2025.
2. Haouimi A. Calcified meningioma - cervical canal. Radiopaedia.org. 2022. https://doi.org/10.53347/rID-70136. Accessed 8 Dec 2024.
3. Lee JW, et al. CT and MRI findings of calcified spinal meningiomas: correlation with pathological findings. Skeletal Radiol. 2010. https://doi.org/10.1007/s00256-009-0771-1. Accessed 4 Jan 2025.

Case 150

150

Clinical History

A 75-year-old woman presented with a painless left-sided cheek swelling.

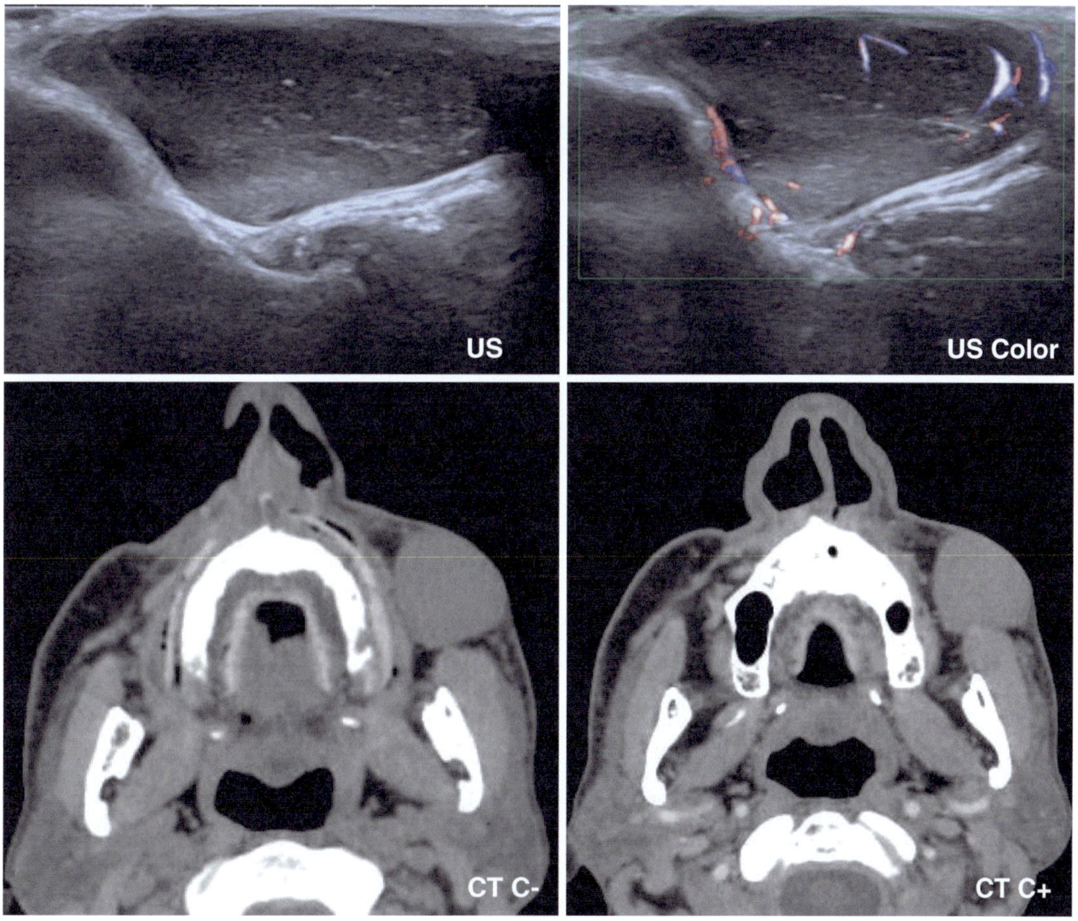

A. Haouimi et al., *Head and Neck Radiology Spot Diagnosis*,
https://doi.org/10.1007/978-3-032-14553-6_150

Findings

A well-defined homogeneous hypoechoic mass of the left cheek with internal vascularity on Doppler. On CT, the subcutaneous mass is iso- to hypodense, showing moderate homogeneous enhancement. No fatty interface between the mass and skin.

Diagnosis

Dermatofibrosarcoma protuberans (DFSP).

Discussion

Dermatofibrosarcoma protuberans (DFSP) is an uncommon, low-grade cutaneous sarcoma originating within the dermis and extending into adjacent tissues through characteristic tentacle-like projections. Most cases are associated with a specific chromosomal translocation involving chromosomes 17 and 22. Ultraviolet radiation exposure and previous trauma are also thought to play contributory roles in its development. DFSP most often affects individuals between 30 and 50 years of age. The lesions may enlarge more rapidly during pregnancy, and additional nodules can occasionally develop over time.

Clinically, the tumor usually begins as a firm, slowly enlarging plaque that may appear pink or violaceous.

On ultrasound, DFSP presents as a well-circumscribed, hypoechoic subcutaneous nodule with moderate internal vascularity, more prominent at the periphery on Doppler imaging. CT typically demonstrates an isodense, noncalcified nodule with mild, homogeneous enhancement. High-resolution MRI shows low signal intensity on T1-weighted images, high signal on T2 (slightly greater than subcutaneous fat), and moderate enhancement with tentacle-like infiltration into adjacent fat, best appreciated on fat-suppressed sequences.

Common Differential Diagnosis

- Benign peripheral nerve sheath tumor (BPNST): no external skin color change.
- Nodular fasciitis: T2 isointense, needs biopsy.
- Keloid: T1 hyperintensity, history, may need biopsy.

Management Options

Treatment options are Mohs surgery, radiation, and targeted therapy with drugs like imatinib.

References and Further Reading

1. Haouimi A. Dermatofibrosarcoma protuberans (DFSP) - cheek. Radiopaedia.org. 2024. https://radiopaedia.org/cases/196387. Accessed 25 Sept 2024.
2. Menon G, et al. Dermatofibrosarcoma protuberans. Stat Pearls Publishing; 2024. https://www.ncbi.nlm.nih.gov/books/NBK513305/. Accessed 25 Sept 2024.
3. Torreggiani WC, et al. Dermatofibrosarcoma protuberans: MR imaging features. AJR Am J Roentgenol. 2002. https://doi.org/10.2214/ajr.178.4.1780989. Accessed 25 Sept 2024.

Case 151

151

Clinical History

A 63-year-old woman presented with a long-standing headache and cervicalgia.

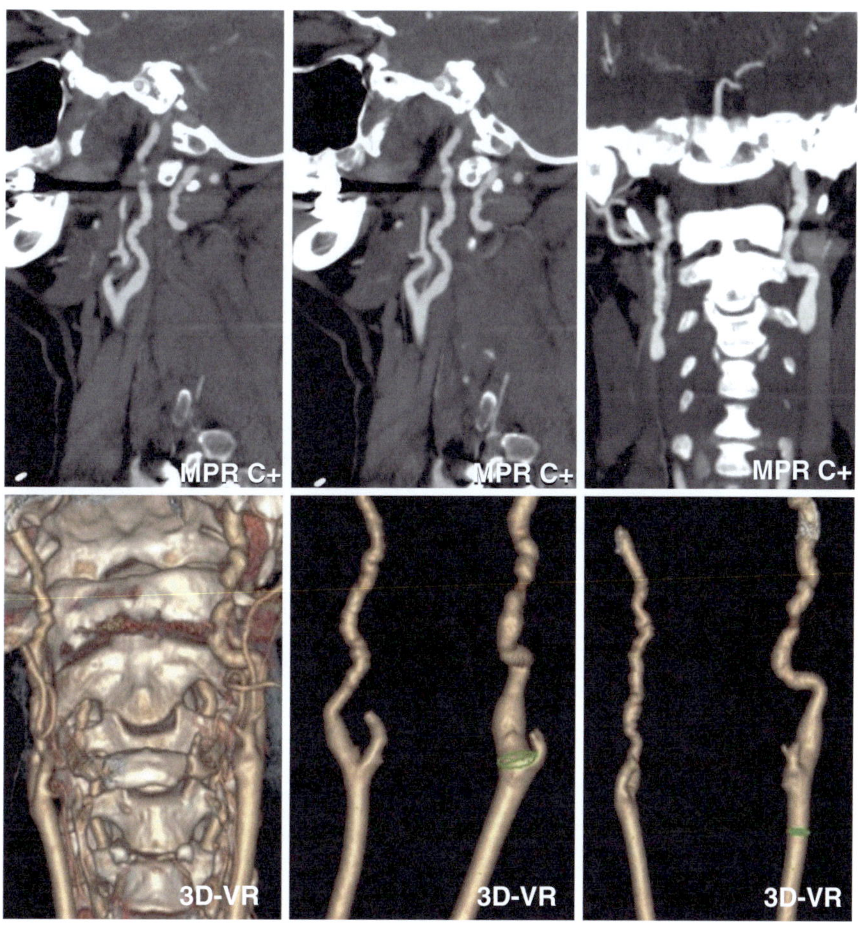

A. Haouimi et al., *Head and Neck Radiology Spot Diagnosis*,
https://doi.org/10.1007/978-3-032-14553-6_151

Findings

Tortuous and ectatic extracranial internal carotid arteries showing a "string of beads" appearance. Slight fusiform dilatation of the left proximal internal carotid immediately beyond the carotid bifurcation.

Diagnosis

Bilateral carotid artery fibromuscular dysplasia (FMD).

Discussion

FMD is a rare, benign, idiopathic, nonatherosclerotic, noninflammatory condition of the vascular wall involving the small and medium-sized arteries. The etiology remains unknown. However, environmental and genetic factors have been reported. Conditions such as Marfan syndrome, Ehler–Danlos syndrome, Bourneville disease, and von Recklinghausen disease have also been found in association with FMD. The exact prevalence is not known due to underdiagnosis. FMD usually involves the midsegment of the arteries with a female predominance between their 40s and 70s.

Many patients remain asymptomatic. Headache, cervicalgia, pulsatile tinnitus, dizziness, and vertigo are the major clinical presentations in symptomatic carotid FMD patients. Occasionally, the condition can lead to TIA or even stroke. Renal artery FMD can cause hypertension.

Both CT and catheter angiography show a classical "string of beads" appearance.

Common Differential Diagnosis

- Atherosclerosis: short segment, usually involves the origin of the artery, calcification +/−.
- Vasculitides: elevated sedimentation rate, fever +/−.
- Vasospasm: diffuse narrowing, clinical history.
- Carotid dissection: trauma +/−, outpouching from pseudoaneurysm +/−, irregular stenosis.

Management Options

No known cure for FMD. Treatment focuses on relieving associated symptoms. Transluminal angioplasty without stenting is the primary modality of choice for revascularization.

References and Further Reading

1. Baradhi KMP. Fibromuscular dysplasia. Stat Pearls Publishing; 2023. https://www.ncbi.nlm.nih.gov/books/NBK493204/. Accessed 5 Jan 2025.
2. Sharma R, et al. Fibromuscular dysplasia. Radiopaedia.org. 2025. https://doi.org/10.53347/rID-3842. Accessed 3 Dec 2025.

Case 152

152

Clinical History

A 50-year-old woman presented with signs of left oculomotor palsy.

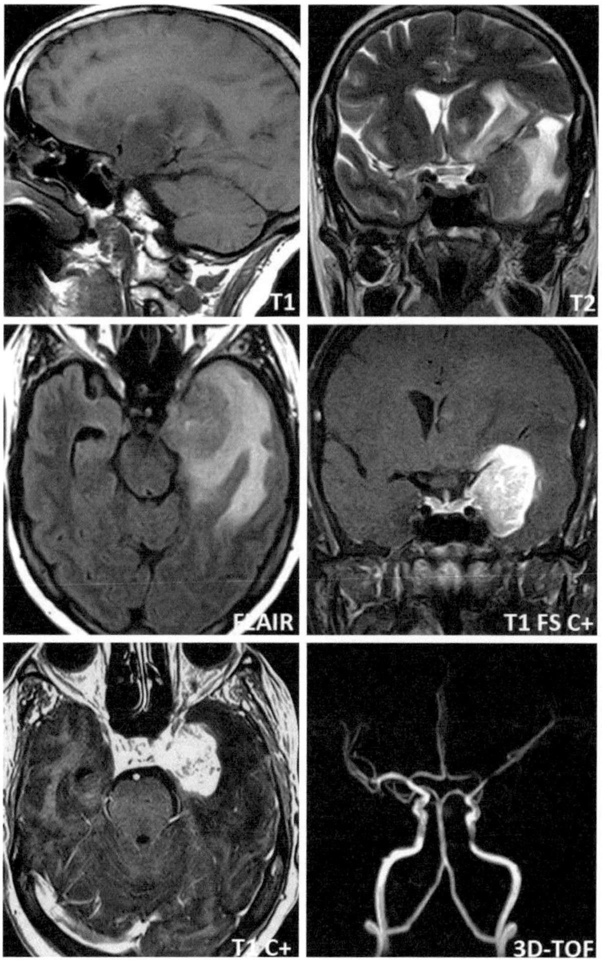

A. Haouimi et al., *Head and Neck Radiology Spot Diagnosis*,
https://doi.org/10.1007/978-3-032-14553-6_152

Findings

An extraaxial lesion of left cavernous sinus epicenter showing isosignal on all sequences encasing the terminal ICA and the proximal MCA with luminal narrowing. Intense homogeneous enhancement. 3D TOF images better show the narrowed vascular lumen. Extrinsic compression causing indentation on the adjacent temporal lobe and vasogenic edema.

Diagnosis

Cavernous sinus meningioma.

Discussion

Tumors of the cavernous sinus are rare. Anatomically, the cavernous sinus extends from the supraorbital fissure anterosuperiorly to Meckel's cave posteroinferiorly. Meningiomas typically arise from the lateral wall. Several cranial nerves, including III, IV, V1, and the ophthalmic and maxillary branches of CN V, traverse the cavernous sinus, accounting for the cranial nerve deficits observed with lesions in this region.

Clinically, these tumors exhibit unpredictable behavior with slow progression. Small lesions may remain clinically silent due to their indolent growth and can go undetected for extended periods. Manifestations such as ophthalmoplegia, diplopia, ptosis, and anisocoria reflect involvement of CN III, CN IV, and CN VI. Hemifacial numbness or pain, along with trigeminal dysfunction, results from the involvement of CN V branches. Lesions in proximity to CN II or the pituitary gland may cause visual field disturbances or endocrine abnormalities due to compressive effects. Vascular compression of the internal carotid artery (ICA) can lead to ischemic complications. On MRI, these tumors typically demonstrate isointense signals across sequences with marked, homogeneous contrast enhancement.

Common Differential Diagnosis

- Pituitary adenoma: midline epicenter, englobement but no narrowing of carotid artery.
- Perineural extension of head-neck tumors: enlarged foramen oval, caudocranial extension.
- Chordoma: midline spheno-occipital epicenter, T2 bright signal.

Management Options

The challenge in treating this lesion is the functional outcomes and needs "do not harm" approach. Management options are observation, microsurgical resection, and radiosurgery.

References and Further Reading

1. Amelot A, et al. Natural history of cavernous sinus meningiomas. J Neurosurg. 2018. https://doi.org/10.3171/2017.7.JNS17662. Accessed 21 Dec 2024.
2. Haouimi A. Meningioma - cavernous sinus. Radiopaedia.org. 2022. https://doi.org/10.53347/rID-99835. Accessed 21 Dec 2024.

Case 153

153

Clinical History

A 65-year-old woman presented with a right parietal painless swelling. No history of cancer or endocrinopathy.

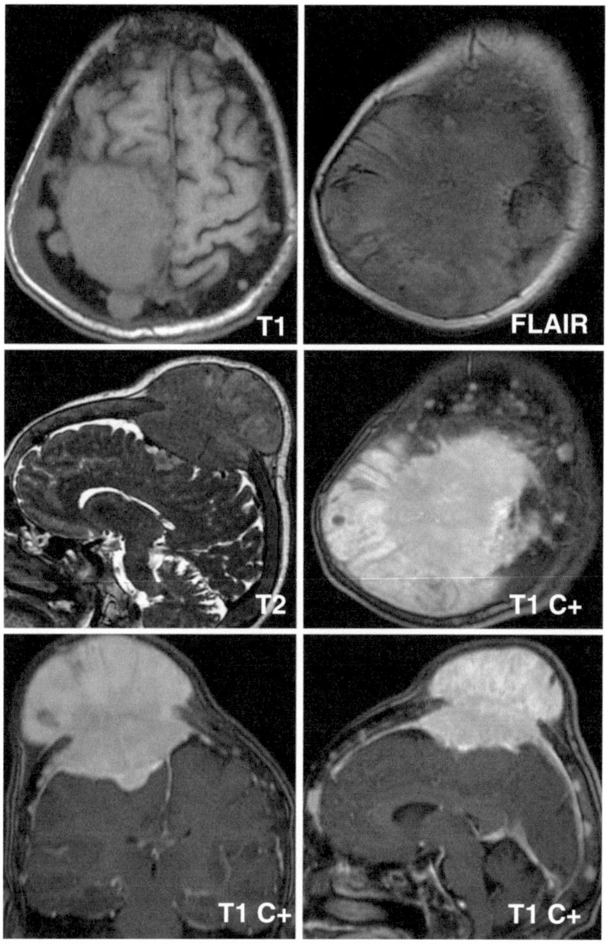

A. Haouimi et al., *Head and Neck Radiology Spot Diagnosis*,
https://doi.org/10.1007/978-3-032-14553-6_153

Findings

"Raindrop skull" with one well-defined humongous lesion epicentered on the right parietal bone showing both intra and extracranial extension. The mass causes indentation on brain parenchyma. The mass shows intermediate signal on T1 and FLAIR series. On T2, the lesions are isointense to white matter and there is intense homogeneous enhancement. Invasion of adjacent superior sagittal sinus.

Diagnosis

Multiple myeloma with a large skull plasmacytoma.

Discussion

Multiple myeloma accounts for roughly about 10% of all hematologic cancers. It is a clonal plasma cell neoplasm that replaces bone marrow and is characterized by excessive production of monoclonal immunoglobulins. Grossly, these tumors appear as brownish, gelatinous masses and are commonly linked with trabecular bone rarefaction. Microscopically, they demonstrate sheets of plasma cells with eccentric nuclei and basophilic cytoplasm. The underlying mechanism involves a disruption of the normal balance between osteoblastic bone formation and osteoclastic resorption. The median age at presentation is around 70 years, with a slight male predominance. Therapy though can control the disease but is generally not curative.

On imaging, multiple myeloma typically presents with lytic bone lesions. At times, distinguishing these from metastatic deposits can be challenging, and whole-body scintigraphy is recommended for comprehensive evaluation.

Common Differential Diagnosis

- Solitary plasmacytoma: unique lesion, normal bone marrow
- Skull metastasis: history of cancer, poorly defined multiple lesions
- Pepper pot skull: hyperparathyroidism, mottling of skull vault

Management Options

Medical treatment with melphalan, prednisolone, thalidomide, and bortezomib. Autologous stem cell therapy remains another therapeutic option.

References and Further Reading

1. Albagoush SA, Shumway C, Azevedo AM. Multiple myeloma. Stat Pearls Publishing; 2023. https://www.ncbi.nlm.nih.gov/books/NBK534764/. Accessed 24 Oct 2024.
2. Haouimi A. Multiple myeloma with a large skull plasmacytoma. Radiopaedia.org. 2020. https://doi.org/10.53347/rID-80944. Accessed 24 Oct 2024.
3. Moore C, et al. Multiple myeloma. Radiopaedia.org. 2025. https://doi.org/10.53347/rID-9555. Accessed 2 Jan 2025.

Case 154

154

Clinical History

A 60-year-old woman presented with headache and slowly deteriorating visual impairment.

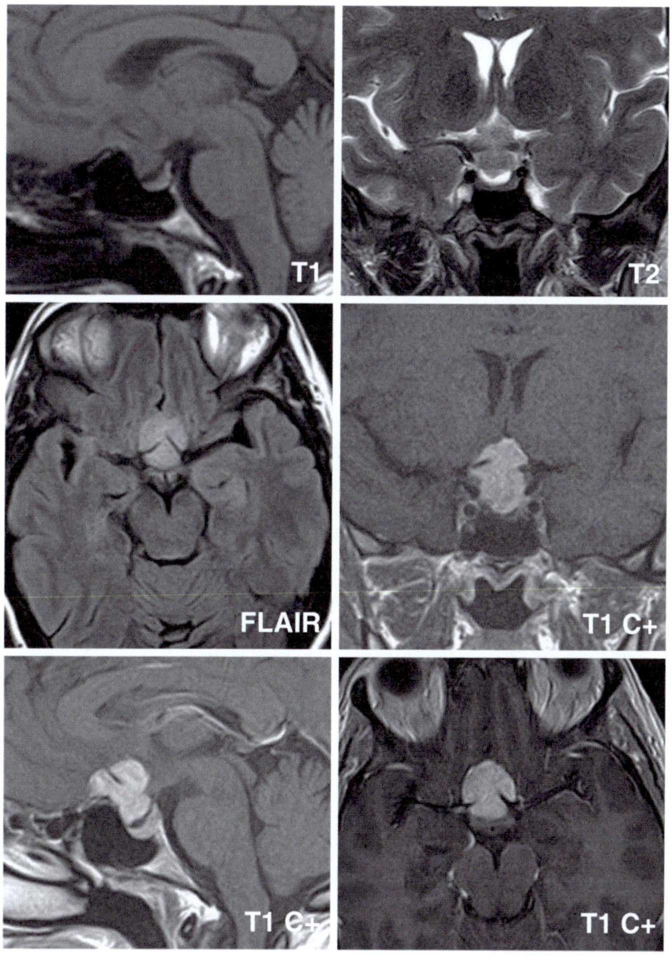

A. Haouimi et al., *Head and Neck Radiology Spot Diagnosis*,
https://doi.org/10.1007/978-3-032-14553-6_154

Findings

An extraaxial well-defined lobulated suprasellar mass epicentered on the tuberculum sellae. It is isointense to the cortical grey matter on both T1 and T2 and hyperintense on FLAIR with a homogeneous enhancement. The "beak of kiwi sign" is better appreciated on sagittal postcontrast images anteriorly. The lesion causes chiasmatic compression and encases mainly the proximal anterior cerebral arteries. Normal pituitary gland seen at the pituitary fossa.

Diagnosis

Tuberculum sellae meningioma.

Discussion

Tuberculum sellae meningioma can arise from the dura of (a) tuberculum sellae, (b) anterior clinoid process, (c) diaphragma sellae, and (d) planum sphenoidale. They account for up to 10% of all intracranial meningiomas. These slow-growing (yearly growth is about 2–4 mm) tumors are close to eloquent brain structures, pituitary gland, optic nerve, ICA, and ACA. Clinically, tuberculum sellae meningiomas cause progressive visual impairment and hemianopsia due to chiasmatic and optic nerve compression as well as hydrocephalus.

MRI shows isosignal on both T1 and T2 with avid enhancement. MRI may show a tapered anterior extension giving rise to the "beak of kiwi sign."

Common Differential Diagnosis

- Pituitary macroadenoma: upward convexity of diaphragma sellae, "figure of eight sign"
- Rathke cleft cyst: low signal on T1 and high signal on T2, no enhancement, "claw sign"
- Saccular aneurysm: partially thrombosed (T1 high signal), residual lumen: phase artifact

Management Options

Most symptomatic cases are managed surgically depending on a case-by-case basis.

References and Further Reading

1. Haouimi A. Tuberculum sellae meningioma. Radiopaedia.org. 2024. https://radiopaedia.org/cases/200063. Accessed 7 Dec 2024.
2. Taylor SL, et al. Magnetic resonance imaging of tuberculum sellae meningiomas: preventing preoperative misdiagnosis as pituitary macroadenoma. Neurosurgery. 1992. https://doi.org/10.1227/00006123-199210000-00002. PMID: 1407446. Accessed 7 Dec 2024.
3. Zhang Q, et al. A case of tuberculum sellae meningioma with beak of Kiwi bird enhancement on MRI: surgical resection and nursing care. Transl Cancer Res. 2016. https://doi.org/10.21037/tcr.2016.03.06. Accessed 7 Dec 2024.

Case 155

155

Clinical History

An 80-year-old man presented with a longstanding dysphagia.

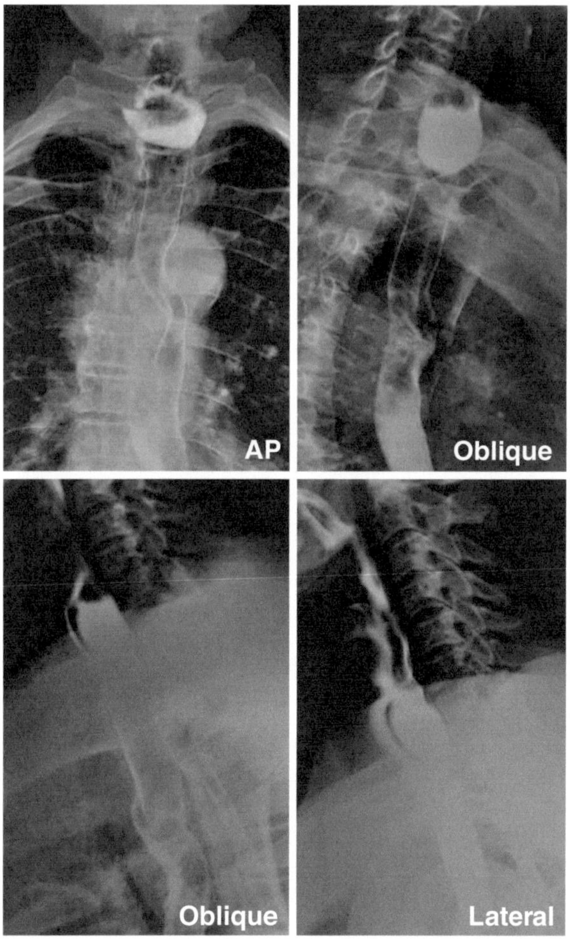

A. Haouimi et al., *Head and Neck Radiology Spot Diagnosis*,
https://doi.org/10.1007/978-3-032-14553-6_155

Findings

Posterior pharyngeal midline outpouching of contrast from the pharynx at C6 level.

Diagnosis

Zenker diverticulum.

Discussion

Zenker diverticulum is a mucosal and submucosal herniation of the hypopharynx through the Killian dehiscence. This area of muscular weakness is always seen at the posterior aspect of the distal pharynx, superior to the cricopharyngeus muscle. It is rare in young adults but not uncommon in the elderly between 60 and 80 years.

Pathologically, Zenker diverticulum is a pulsion pseudodiverticulum (forming a sac) through the Killian triangle between the fibers of the esophageal wall muscles. The etiology is not clear, but most hypotheses revolve around the abnormal structure and physiology. Overtightening of the cricopharyngeus causes the distal pharynx to outpouch. Food particles as well as liquid can be trapped in this sac when the neck of the sac is anatomically narrow. The distension of the dilated sac from trapped food can cause extrinsic esophageal compression. Most of the cases are associated with hiatal hernia and/or gastroesophageal reflux. Fluoroscopic cine deglutition is the most appropriate radiologic modality to document these abnormalities.

Clinically, patients with Zenker diverticulum complain of halitosis, regurgitation, dysphagia, hoarse voice, persistent cough, and feel like something is stuck in their throat.

On barium swallow with video fluoroscopy, Zenker's diverticulum shows a posterior midline outpouching "image d'addition" of contrast from the distal pharynx at the C5 and C6 level.

Common Differential Diagnosis

- Laimer diverticulum: inferior to cricopharyngeus muscle
- Killian-Jamieson diverticulum: from the left side of the proximal esophagus at C5-C6 level

Management Options

Zenker diverticulum carries an increased risk for aspiration. Larger cases are treated surgically.

References and Further Reading

1. Haouimi A. Zenker diverticulum. Radiopaedia.org. 2020. https://doi.org/10.53347/rID-73954. Accessed 10 Dec 2024.
2. Mous A, et al. Zenker diverticulum. Radiopaedia.org. 2024. https://doi.org/10.53347/rID-2297. Accessed 10 Dec 2024.
3. Nesheiwat Z, Antunes C. Zenker diverticulum. Stat Pearls Publishing; 2023. https://www.ncbi.nlm.nih.gov/books/NBK499996/. Accessed 10 Dec 2024.

Case 156

156

Clinical History

A 50-year-old hypertensive man presented with a gradual increase of left facial numbness.

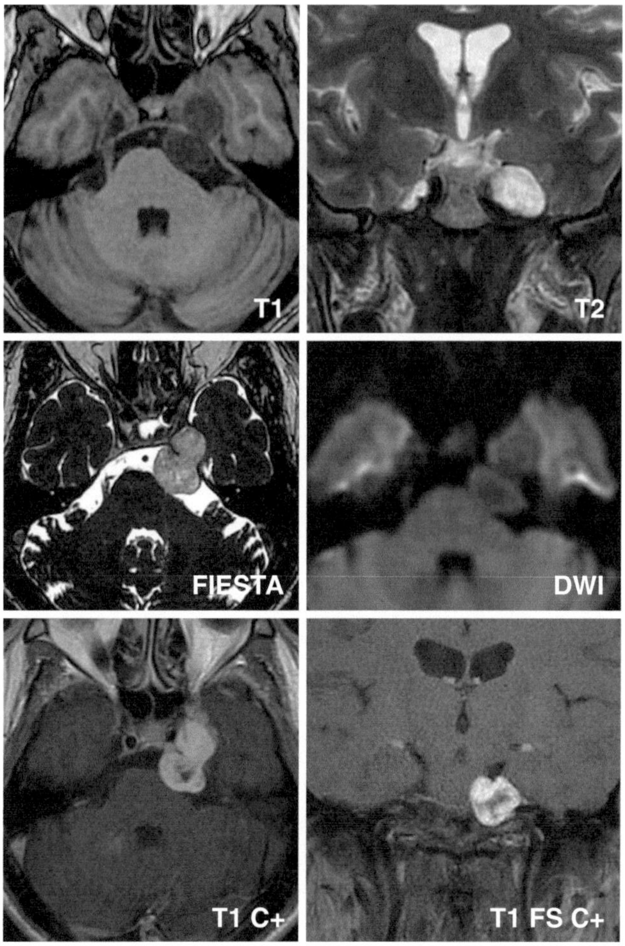

A. Haouimi et al., *Head and Neck Radiology Spot Diagnosis*,
https://doi.org/10.1007/978-3-032-14553-6_156

Findings

A dumbbell-shaped extraaxial mass, extending from the left trigeminal nerve "root entry zone" to the left cavernous sinus. It shows a low signal on T1 and a high signal on T2 and FLAIR. No restricted diffusion, no calcification, and no hemorrhage. Thick regular neural enhancement and minimal indentation on adjacent pons and left temporal lobe.

Diagnosis

Trigeminal schwannoma.

Discussion

Schwannomas are slow-growing benign tumors arising from Schwann cells in the nerve sheath. They are often seen in individuals in their fourth and fifth decades, with a slight female predominance. Any segment: cisternal, ganglionic, or postganglionic may be affected, either as isolated or multisegmental lesions.

Clinical presentations are facial numbness, neurasthenia, and masticator muscle weakness.

MRI serves as the gold standard for assessing trigeminal schwannomas. The solid portions of the tumor usually appear isointense on T1-weighted images and hyperintense on T2-weighted images, following the path of the trigeminal nerve, with vivid contrast enhancement. When both cisternal and cavernous segments are affected, the mass often demonstrates a "figure-of-eight" appearance, with the constricted portion corresponding to the porus trigeminus. Cystic degeneration may result in heterogeneous signals, with the cystic regions showing low intensity on T1. Computed tomography (CT) can depict bone remodeling, particularly when the tumor extends beyond the cranial cavity through skull base foramina.

Common Differential Diagnosis

- Vestibular schwannoma: extension to internal auditory canal, "ice cream cone sign"
- Petrous apex meningioma: "dural tail sign," calcification +
- Sympathetic plexus schwannoma: situated medial to the carotid artery, carotid canal widening on CT

Management Options

Schwannomas are typically treated by surgery. Other options are observation or radiosurgery.

References and Further Reading

1. Agrawal A, et al. Trigeminal schwannoma. Natl J Maxillofac Surg. 2017. https://doi.org/10.4103/njms.NJMS_82_14. Accessed 27 Dec 2024. PMID: 29386819; PMCID: PMC5773990.
2. Haouimi A. Trigeminal schwannoma. Radiopaedia.org. 2023. https://doi.org/10.53347/rID-173898. Accessed 7 Dec 2024.

Case 157

157

Clinical History

A 70-year-old woman with a known history of breast cancer on follow-up. Recent complaints of headache and left orbital swelling.

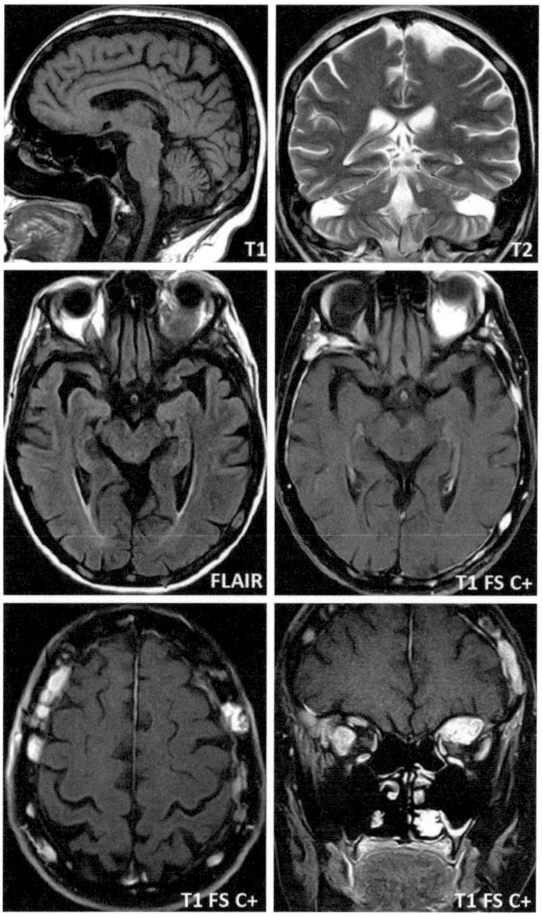

A. Haouimi et al., *Head and Neck Radiology Spot Diagnosis*,
https://doi.org/10.1007/978-3-032-14553-6_157

Findings

Extensive bilateral dural thickening with enhancement. Multiple enhancing lesions involving the calvarium. Bilateral orbital enhancing masses, the larger on the left, surrounding the superior rectus muscle. No intraaxial cerebellar or cerebral lesion.

Diagnosis

Metastatic breast cancer (pachymeningeal, orbital, and skull).

Discussion

Breast cancer is the most common malignancy in women. When the initial breast cancer is diagnosed with metastasis, it is often called "de novo metastatic breast cancer." Metastatic breast cancers are considered as stage 4. Invasive ductal carcinomas often metastasize to the brain, bones as well as lungs and liver. In general, metastatic breast cancer has a poor prognosis. About one-third of the patients diagnosed with early-stage breast cancer develop metastatic breast cancer at some point. The 5-year survival rate after diagnosis of metastatic breast cancer is about 30%. Some of the patients can live longer, up to 10 years or even more.

PET scans, whole body scintigraphy, CT, and MRI are all available to detect secondary metastasis.

Common Differential Diagnosis

- In an appropriate clinical context, no other reasonable differential diagnosis.

Management Options

No cure for stage 4 breast cancer. The focus of management is symptomatic treatment and continuous monitoring. Treatment options are chemotherapy, hormonal therapy, immunotherapy, and targeted therapy.

References and Further Reading

1. Haouimi A. Pachymeningeal, skull and orbital metastases from breast carcinoma. Radiopaedia.org. 2023. https://doi.org/10.53347/rID-170386. Accessed 20 July 2024.
2. Park M, et al. Breast cancer metastasis: mechanisms and therapeutic implications. Int J Mol Sci. 2022. https://doi.org/10.3390/ijms23126806. Accessed 20 July 2024. PMID: 35743249; PMCID: PMC9224686.
3. Pesapane F, et al. Imaging diagnosis of metastatic breast cancer. Insights Imaging. 2020. https://doi.org/10.1186/s13244-020-00885-4. Accessed 20 July 2024. PMID: 32548731; PMCID: PMC7297923.

Case 158

158

Clinical History

A 75-year-old man presented with a gradual, painless swelling at the right side of the floor of the mouth.

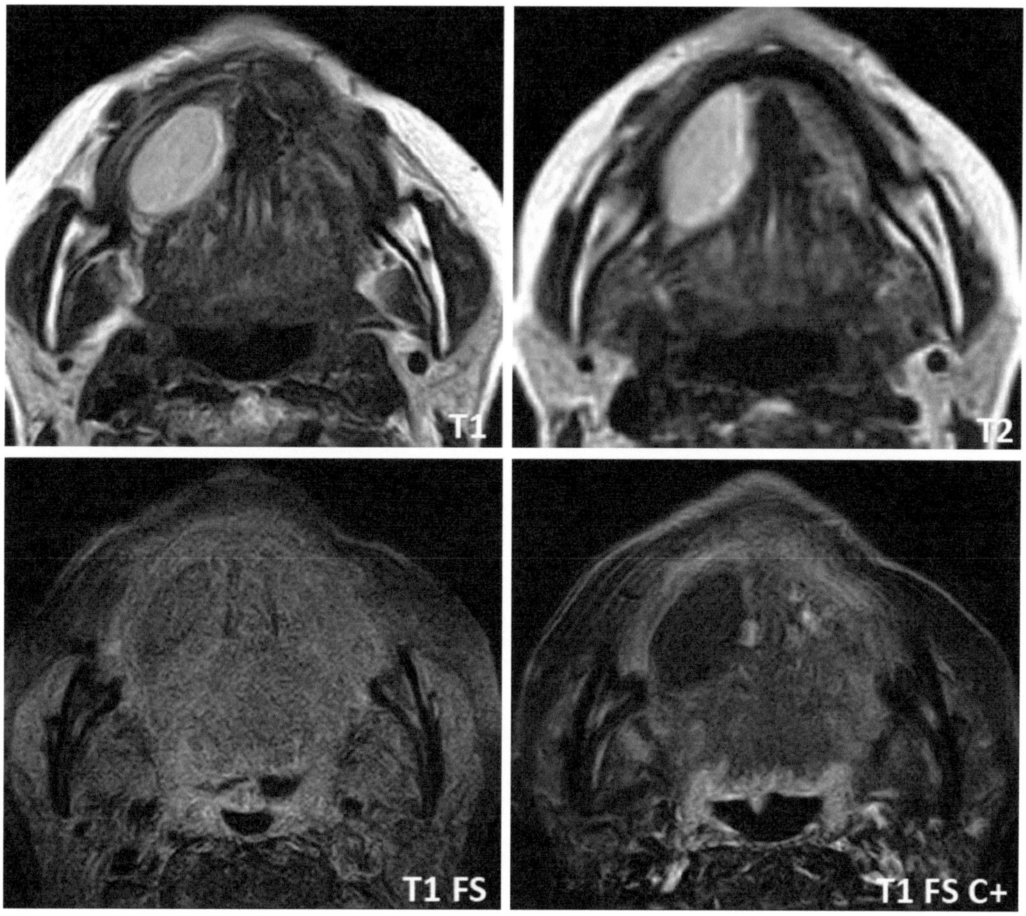

A. Haouimi et al., *Head and Neck Radiology Spot Diagnosis*,
https://doi.org/10.1007/978-3-032-14553-6_158

Findings

An ovoid lesion at the floor of the mouth on the right side, interposed between mylohyoid and geniohyoid muscles. It appears homogeneously high signal on both T1 and T2 with no contrast enhancement. Complete suppression of high signal on fat-suppression sequence.

Diagnosis

Lipoma of the floor of the mouth.

Discussion

Lipomas are benign fatty tissue lesions representing the most common mesenchymal neoplasms. Incidence in the oral cavity is rare and less than 5% of all cases. It is mostly found in ages between 50 and 60 and very uncommon in children.

Floor-of-mouth lipomas are mostly asymptomatic. However, patients may complain of a painless, sessile, or pedunculated nodule of soft consistency. Larger lesions may compress surrounding structures, causing mechanical dysfunction.

All oral cavity sublingual masses need a comprehensive workup due to intricate anatomy. While reporting MRI, it is very important to mention the size and location. Special attention is needed to look for signs of liposarcoma. Larger size, deeper intramuscular extension, lack of homogeneity, intralesional thickened septations, nonadipose nodularity, and enhancement are all suggestive of malignant liposarcoma.

Common Differential Diagnosis

- Ranula: cystic lesion, low T1 signal intensity, may be trans-spatial
- Squamous cell carcinoma: locoregional invasion, bony destruction
- Oral cavity abscess: clinical history, uni- or multilocular, smooth, thick, enhancing wall

Management Options

Oral cavity asymptomatic lipomas are "do not touch" lesions. Conservative local excision for those lesions causing issues. The recurrence is extremely rare.

References and Further Reading

1. Gibson K, et al. Large lipoma of the mouth floor. Cureus. 2021. https://doi.org/10.7759/cureus.18420. Accessed 25 July 2024.
2. Haouimi A. Lipoma - mouth floor. Radiopaedia.org. 2023. https://doi.org/10.53347/rID-159370. Accessed 25 July 2024.
3. Raj AA, et al. Lipoma of the floor of the mouth: report of an unusually large lesion. J Maxillofac Oral Surg. 2014. https://doi.org/10.1007/s12663-011-0204-2. Accessed 25 July 2024. Epub 2011 Apr 7. PMID: 25018608; PMCID: PMC4082549.

Case 159

159

Clinical History

A 60-year-old man presented with headache, gradual onset of visual disturbances, and papilledema.

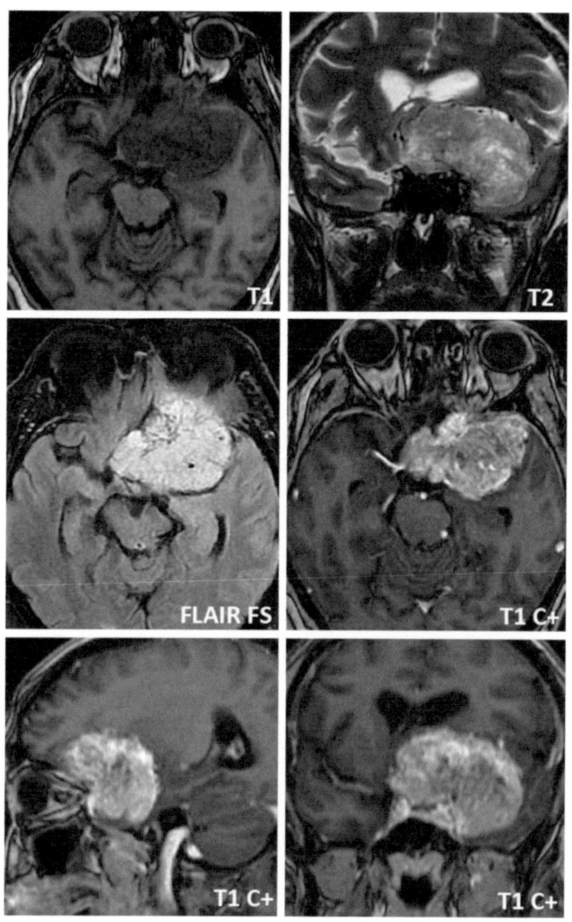

A. Haouimi et al., *Head and Neck Radiology Spot Diagnosis*,
https://doi.org/10.1007/978-3-032-14553-6_159

Findings

A well-circumscribed left middle cranial fossa lesion with sphenoid wing epicenter having a broad dural base with peripheral CSF clefts and signal voids. Midline shift toward the right. Indentation upon adjacent brain parenchyma, causing buckling of the white-gray matter interface. Scanty perilesional edema. The lesion is heterogeneously isointense on T1 and slightly hyperintense on T2 and FLAIR. Intense nonhomogeneous enhancement with "dural tail sign." "Sunburst" appearance of intralesional vasculatures in a radiating pattern may be seen. This mass extends into the suprasellar cistern, causing chiasmatic involvement and invasion of the adjacent cavernous sinus, leading to encasement and narrowing of the left ICA.

Diagnosis

Sphenoid wing meningioma.

Discussion

Sphenoid wing meningiomas account for approximately 20% of all meningiomas and are frequently asymptomatic. When symptoms do occur, they typically include headache, gradually progressive painless proptosis, visual disturbance, and oculomotor weakness.

On CT, these lesions are enhancing isodense extraaxial masses, often exhibiting a wide dural attachment and associated hyperostosis of adjacent bone. MRI findings usually demonstrate isointensity on T1-weighted images and iso- to mildly hyperintense signals on T2-weighted sequences, accompanied by strong and homogeneous postcontrast enhancement.

Common Differential Diagnosis

- Calvarial hemangioma: marked T2 hyperintensity, centripetal filling on dynamic scan
- Fibrous dysplasia: ground glass appearance on CT
- Secondary metastasis: often in the context of a known primary

Management Options

The management options for sphenoid wing meningioma include observation, surgery, and radiotherapy.

References and Further Reading

1. Haouimi A. Meningioma - sphenoid wing. Radiopaedia.org. https://doi.org/10.53347/rID-183522. Accessed 14 June 2024.
2. Hussaini SM, et al. Intraosseous meningioma of the sphenoid bone. Radiol Case Rep. 2015. https://doi.org/10.2484/rcr.v5i1.357. Accessed 14 June 2024. PMID: 27307848; PMCID: PMC4898218.
3. Watts J, et al. Magnetic resonance imaging of meningiomas: a pictorial review. Insights Imaging. 2014. https://doi.org/10.1007/s13244-013-0302-4. Accessed 14 June 2024. Epub 2014 Jan 8. PMID: 24399610; PMCID: PMC3948902.

Case 160

160

Clinical History

A 59-year-old man presented with right otalgia, hemifacial pain, dysphagia, and headache.

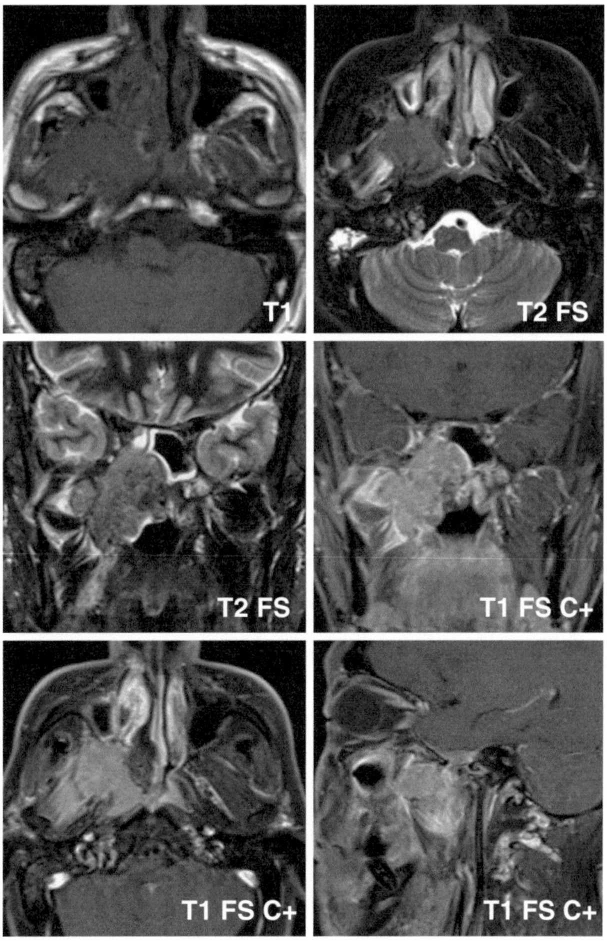

A. Haouimi et al., *Head and Neck Radiology Spot Diagnosis*,
https://doi.org/10.1007/978-3-032-14553-6_160

Findings

An invasive lesion involving the nasopharyngeal mucosal space, epicentered at the fossa of Rosenmüller, causing obstruction of the Eustachian tube and secondary otomastoiditis. There is a narrowing of the nasopharyngeal lumen. This lesion is isointense on T1 and slightly hyperintense on T2 with intense enhancement after gadolinium. There is a locoregional extension to posterior nasal cavity, cavernous sinus, and infiltration of the masticator space. Incidental right chronic maxillary sinusitis.

Diagnosis

Nasopharyngeal carcinoma (NPC).

Discussion

NPC is a rare malignancy, but the incidence is considerably higher in Southeast Asia, North Africa, and Southern China. It arises from a multifactorial etiology involving genetic susceptibility, environmental influences, and viral infection. A strong link has been seen with Epstein–Barr virus, and specific HLA polymorphisms have been identified as important genetic risk factors for the undifferentiated form of NPC.

Clinically, patients present with the classic triad of unilateral serous otitis media, conductive hearing loss, epistaxis or blood-stained nasal discharge, and cervical nodal enlargement. As the tumor grows, nasal obstruction and multiple cranial nerve palsies may appear, reflecting perineural invasion and potential spread to the cavernous sinus.

Enhanced MRI with fat suppression is the modality of choice for diagnosing the primary lesion, evaluating extension, and staging. CT imaging is more effective in demonstrating bony erosion, while PET scanning plays a crucial role in detecting distant metastatic involvement.

Common Differential Diagnosis

- Antro-choanal polyp: maxillary antrum is full, noninvasive
- Juvenile nasopharyngeal angiofibroma: wide pterygopalatine fossa, male patients
- Esthesioneuroblastoma: intracranial component, "figure of eight" configuration

Management Options

Radiotherapy is the mainstay of treatment. Combined radio and chemotherapy is another option.

References and Further Reading

1. Gaillard F, et al. Nasopharyngeal carcinoma. Radiopaedia.org. 2025. https://doi.org/10.53347/rID-9544. Accessed 10 Dec 2024.
2. Shah AB, Nagalli S. Nasopharyngeal carcinoma. Stat Pearls Publishing; 2024. https://www.ncbi.nlm.nih.gov/books/NBK554588/. Accessed 12 Apr 2024.
3. King AD, Bhatia KS. Magnetic resonance imaging staging of nasopharyngeal carcinoma in the head and neck. World J Radiol. 2010. https://doi.org/10.4329/wjr.v2.i5.159. Accessed 10 Dec 2024. PMID: 21161030; PMCID: PMC2999022.

Case 161

161

Clinical History

A 15-year-old boy presented with a recurrent episode of epistaxis and nasopharyngeal mass.

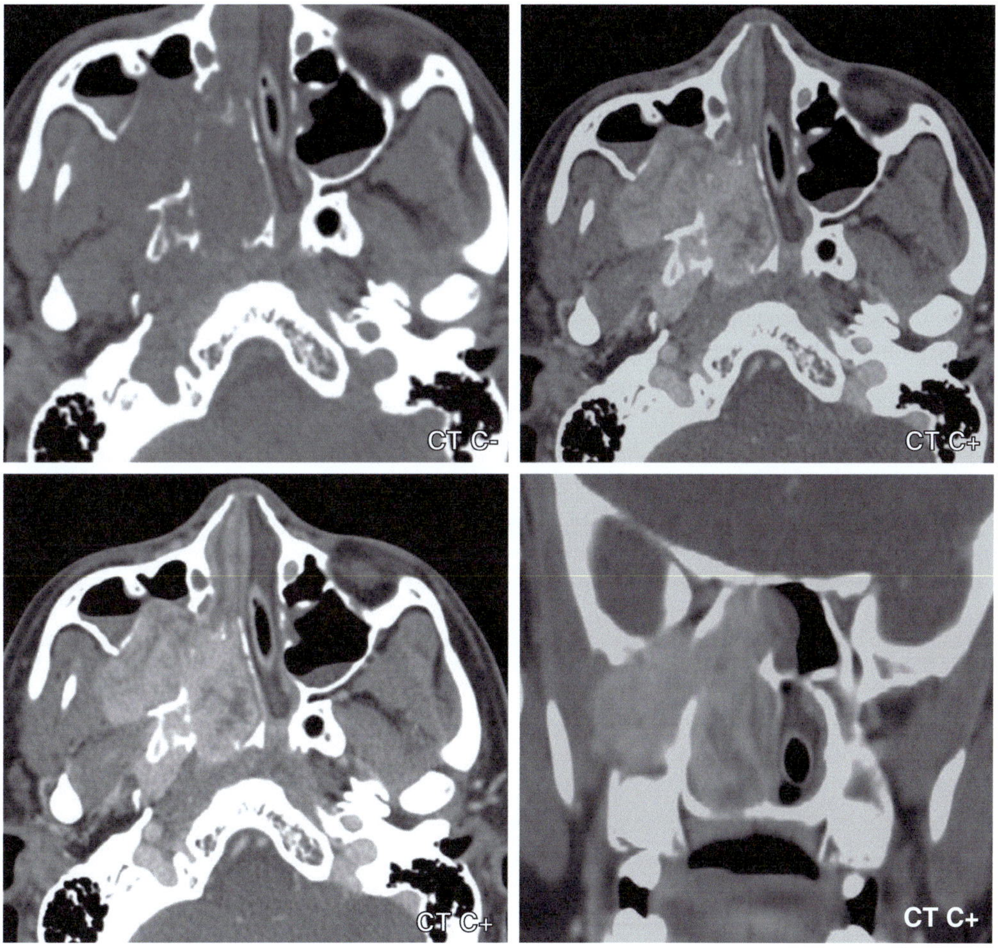

A. Haouimi et al., *Head and Neck Radiology Spot Diagnosis*,
https://doi.org/10.1007/978-3-032-14553-6_161

Findings

A large lobulated isodense expansile lesion epicentered at the right sphenopalatine foramen, causing widening of the pterygopalatine fossa. The lesion extends to the nasopharynx through the right nasal cavity and right sphenoid sinus. Locoregional expansion causing erosion and bowing of posterior wall of maxillary antrum, erosion of lateral wall of sphenoid sinus, and lateral nasal wall as well as partial resorption and destruction of the pterygoid process. Intense enhancement with slight heterogeneity in the nasal component of the lesion.

Diagnosis

Juvenile nasopharyngeal angiofibroma.

Discussion

Juvenile nasopharyngeal angiofibromas are benign, nonencapsulated, locally aggressive, highly vascular lesions of primitive mesenchymal origin. Macroscopically, they are reddish-purple nodular masses exclusively affecting males. The lesion originates near the sphenopalatine foramen and can extend into the nasal cavity, nasopharynx, and pterygopalatine fossa. The tumor is believed to be influenced by androgens, genetic, and vascular factors such as abnormal angiogenesis, as well as environmental factors.

Clinically, the adolescent males present with recurrent epistaxis and unilateral nasal obstruction.

On CT, the lesions are isodense and show intense enhancement. MRI postcontrast fat-sat sequences are best to evaluate the locoregional extension.

Common Differential Diagnosis

- Antrochoanal polyp: maxillary antrum is full, no enhancement
- Nasopharyngeal carcinoma: nasopharyngeal epicenter, normal pterygopalatine fossa
- Esthesioneuroblastoma: intracranial component, "figure of eight" configuration

Management Options

Spontaneous regression is rare. Surgical treatment is curative. Radiation is an option. Estrogen therapy is controversial.

References and Further Reading

1. Alimli AG, et al. Juvenile nasopharyngeal angiofibroma: magnetic resonance imaging findings. J Belg Soc Radiol. 2016. https://doi.org/10.5334/jbr-btr.1090. Accessed 10 Dec 2024. PMID: 30038985; PMCID: PMC5854277.
2. Gaillard F, et al. Juvenile nasopharyngeal angiofibroma. Radiopaedia.org. 2025. https://doi.org/10.53347/rID-1541. Accessed 10 July 2025.

Case 162

162

Clinical History

A 41-year-old man presented with dysphagia, stridor, and neck swelling following extubation for 1 week (intubated for chest infection). Known ESRD and heart failure.

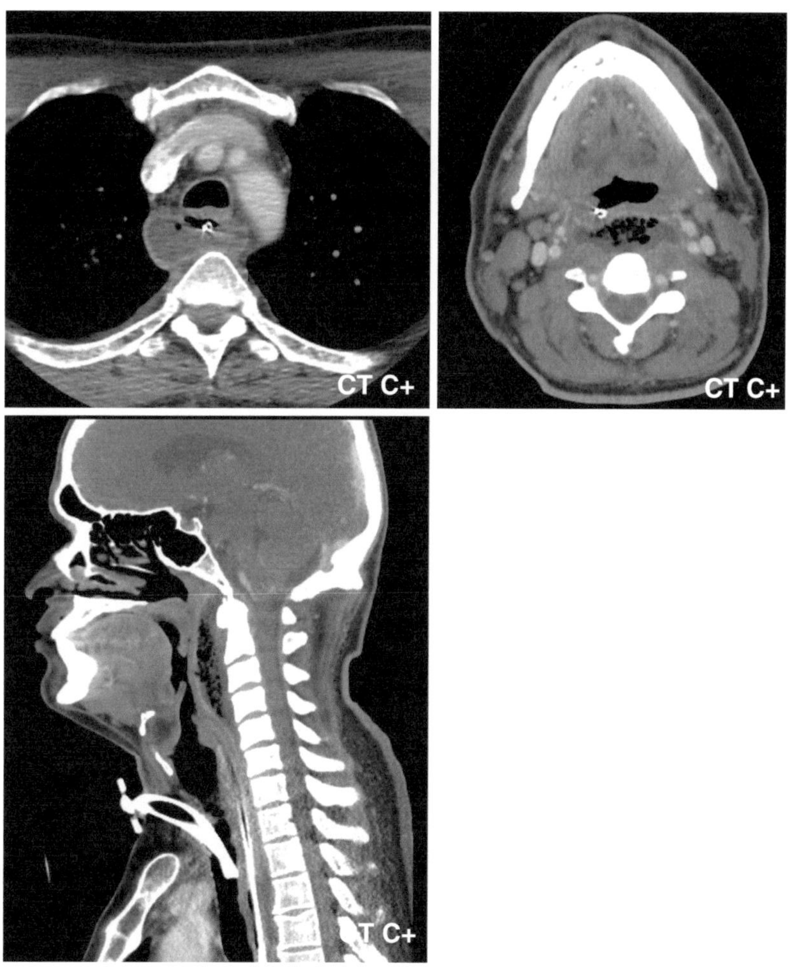

A. Haouimi et al., *Head and Neck Radiology Spot Diagnosis*,
https://doi.org/10.1007/978-3-032-14553-6_162

Findings

Enhanced CT scan of the neck shows a large, peripheral rim-enhancing, retropharyngeal collection containing air bubbles extending from the skull base to the upper mediastinum. Mass effect on the oropharynx with luminal narrowing. Normal cervical spine without any sign of discitis or osteomyelitis. The airway is secured with a tracheostomy.

Diagnosis

Retropharyngeal abscess.

Discussion

The retropharyngeal space extends behind the posterior pharyngeal wall from the clivus to the upper thoracic level. It is separated from the danger space by the deep layer of the cervical fascia, and both spaces are indistinguishable on imaging. Infections can easily spread from the true retropharyngeal space to the danger space, which can act as a conduit for the spread of infection into the mediastinum.

Retropharyngeal abscesses are commonly seen in children and are caused by the rupture of a suppurative lymph node or the spread of infection from adjacent structures (middle ear or oropharynx). Other less common causes include penetrating injury to the posterior pharyngeal wall by trauma, foreign body, or surgery.

Lateral neck radiographs can be done for initial evaluation of retropharyngeal abscesses, but CT remains the gold standard for diagnosis and detection of complications.

Common Differential Diagnosis

- Prevertebral abscess: associated discitis or osteomyelitis, epidural extension
- Boerhaave syndrome: esophageal tear, contrast spillage, associated pneumomediastinum
- Necrotic or suppurative retropharyngeal node: often bilateral

Management Options

IV antibiotic targeting anaerobic bacteria is the main management. Immediate ENT consultation to secure the airway. Surgical intervention is considered in cases of airway compromise or those cases not responding to medical treatment within 24–48 h.

References and Further Reading

1. Guelfguat M, et al. Clinical guidelines for imaging and reporting ingested foreign bodies. Am J Roentgenol. 2014. https://doi.org/10.2214/AJR.13.12185. Accessed 10 Dec 2024.
2. Hoang JK, et al. Multiplanar CT and MRI of collections in the retropharyngeal space: is it an abscess? Am J Roentgenol. 2011. https://doi.org/10.2214/AJR.10.5116. Accessed 10 Dec 2024.
3. Jain H, et al. Retropharyngeal Abscess. Stat Pearls Publishing; 2025. http://www.ncbi.nlm.nih.gov/books/NBK441873/. Accessed 10 July 2024.

Case 163

163

Clinical History

A 50-year-old woman presented with a right-sided hearing loss. There is a past history of breast cancer for 5 years, treated by surgery and chemotherapy.

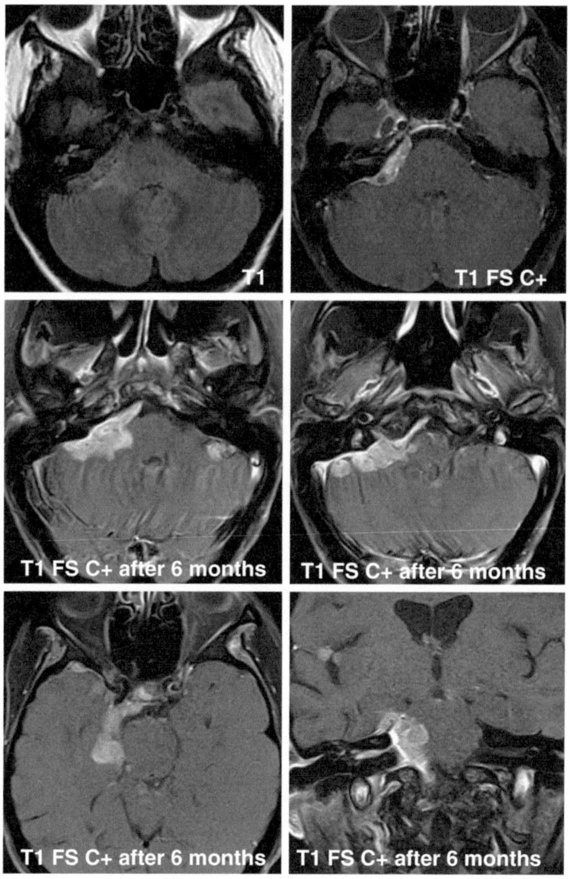

A. Haouimi et al., *Head and Neck Radiology Spot Diagnosis*,
https://doi.org/10.1007/978-3-032-14553-6_163

Findings

A broad dural-based right cerebellopontine angle (CPA) enhancing lesion seen on initial examination. On subsequent 6-month follow-up, the lesion has increased in size and extended further craniocaudally. Appearance of new, enhancing additional lesions elsewhere, including left CPA, right Sylvian fissure, and right cerebellum.

Diagnosis

Cerebellopontine angle (CPA) metastases.

Discussion

This case was initially diagnosed as meningioma. But considering the clinical history, the appearance of additional lesions and rapid growth on subsequent follow-up, the case was diagnosed as metastatic disease.

CPA metastasis is rare and, when present, is usually seen in breast and lung cancers. CSF dissemination and/or leptomeningeal extension are possible pathways of metastatic spread.

In the absence of history of cancer, the isolated CPA metastasis is a diagnostic challenge. Rapidly progressive acute symptoms in patients with history of treated breast and lung cancer carry a high index of suspicion for CPA metastasis. In the absence of systemic metastases, histopathological diagnosis may be required to confirm this rare condition.

Common Differential Diagnosis

- Vestibular schwannoma: "ice-cream cone" lesion, intracanalar extension +, enlarged IAC
- Meningioma: broad dural base, slow growth
- Epidermoid cyst: isointense to CSF, very bright on diffusion MRI, thin peripheral enhancement

Management Options

The treatment of metastatic CPA lesion varies. Often, a combination of surgery and/or radiation therapy is needed. The role of chemotherapy is questionable.

References and Further Reading

1. Chiong Y, et al. Isolated metastasis to the cerebellopontine angle secondary to breast cancer. Can J Surg. 2009. https://pubmed.ncbi.nlm.nih.gov/19865565/. Accessed 25 Nov 2024. PMID: 19865565; PMCID: PMC2769124.
2. Haouimi A. Cerebellopontine angle metastasis. Radiopaedia.org. https://doi.org/10.53347/rID-97861. Accessed 25 Nov 2024.
3. Mingshan Z, et al. Metastases in cerebellopontine angle from the tumors of central nerve system. J Clin Neurosci. 2017. https://doi.org/10.1016/j.jocn.2017.04.011. Accessed 25 Nov 2024.

Case 164

164

Clinical History

A 56-year-old woman referred with severe bilateral sensorineural hearing loss for cochlear implant assessment.

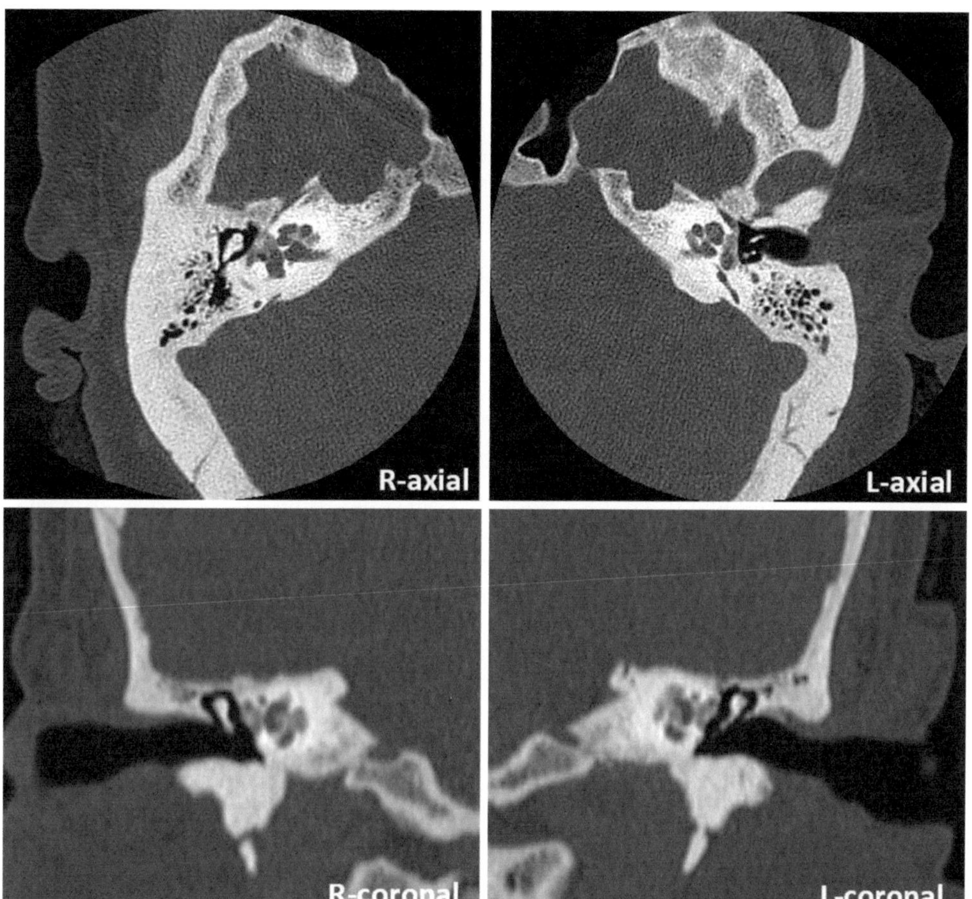

A. Haouimi et al., *Head and Neck Radiology Spot Diagnosis*,
https://doi.org/10.1007/978-3-032-14553-6_164

Findings

Bilateral otic capsule lucencies at oval windows, the cochlear promontory, fissula ante fenestram, as well as lucency around the cochlear aperture and basal turn of the cochlea.

Diagnosis

Otosclerosis (fenestral and retro-fenestral).

Discussion

Otosclerosis is an autosomal dominant disorder of the otic capsule characterized by replacement of normal endochondral bone with spongy, vascularized bone. Approximately 80–85% of cases are bilateral, with a female-to-male ratio of 2:1. The condition most commonly presents between the second and fourth decades of life and is more frequent in Caucasian populations. Depending on the site of involvement, otosclerosis can be classified as fenestral (stapedial), retro-fenestral (cochlear), or bipolar, affecting both stapedial and cochlear regions.

The hallmark symptom is progressive hearing loss, often accompanied by tinnitus and vertigo. Otoscopic and audiometric findings are generally nonspecific, whereas noncontrast CT of the temporal bone remains the diagnostic gold standard. Commonly affected areas include the region of the embryonic fissula ante fenestram, the promontory, the round window niche, and the tympanic segment of the facial nerve canal. The disease may extend to the stapes footplate and eventually involve the cochlea.

Common Differential Diagnosis

- Osteogenesis imperfecta: generalized, Wormian bone +
- Paget disease: multifocal, "cotton wool" pattern
- Fibrous dysplasia: "ground glass" matrix, bony expansion

Management Options

Stapes surgery is the earliest intervention used in cases of conductive hearing loss. Hearing aids are an alternative for patients who are not surgical candidates or those needing correction of sensorineural hearing loss.

References and Further Reading

1. Batson L, et al. Otosclerosis: an update on diagnosis and treatment. JAAPA. 2017. https://doi.org/10.1097/01.JAA.0000511784.21936.1b. Accessed 25 Nov 2024.
2. Gredilla M, et al. Update on the imaging diagnosis of otosclerosis. Radiología (English Edition). 2016. https://doi.org/10.1016/j.rxeng.2016.07.005. Accessed 25 Nov 2024.
3. Manning PM, et al. Role of radiologic imaging in otosclerosis. Curr Otorhinol Rep. 2022. https://doi.org/10.1007/s40136-021-00377-z. Accessed 25 Nov 2024.

Case 165

165

Clinical History

A 45-year-old woman presented with a progressive painless left parietal swelling. History of breast cancer.

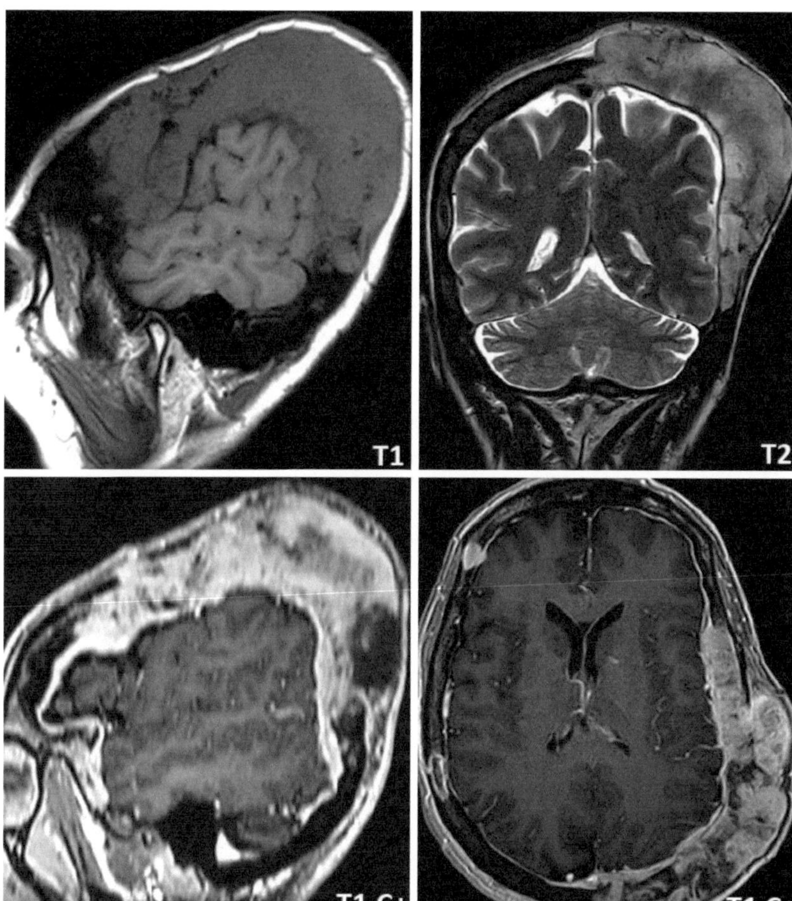

A. Haouimi et al., *Head and Neck Radiology Spot Diagnosis*,
https://doi.org/10.1007/978-3-032-14553-6_165

Findings

A large soft-tissue mass of the thickened cranial vault centered at left parietal region, hypointense on T1 and heterogeneously hyperintense on T2. Heterogeneous enhancement along with bilateral thickened patchy meningeal infiltrations. A few tiny enhancing intradiploic lesions in right frontoparietal region. Invasion of adjacent segment of superior sagittal sinus.

Diagnosis

Skull and meningeal metastases.

Discussion

The most frequent sites of breast cancer metastasis are the bones and lungs, whereas involvement of the meninges is comparatively uncommon. In women presenting with pachymeningeal or skull metastases, breast cancer is often suspected as the primary malignancy. Generally, smaller primary breast tumors are associated with a lower likelihood of metastatic spread. A considerable proportion of patients with meningeal or skull metastases may remain asymptomatic, making clinical suspicion difficult. In many cases, the primary breast tumor is only identified at the time metastases are discovered.

Approximately half of patients experience nonspecific headaches as a presenting symptom. While around 25% of patients with metastatic breast cancer may survive up to 5 years, the mean survival is closer to 3 years. Imaging modalities such as bone scintigraphy and PET scans are frequently more sensitive and can detect smaller metastatic lesions. On MRI, fat-suppression sequences are useful to differentiate true enhancement from normal hyperintense marrow and scalp fat.

Common Differential Diagnosis

- Plasmacytoma: clinical history, characteristic laboratory findings.
- Intraosseous hemangioma: well-defined sunburst lesions, no meningeal infiltration.
- Osteomyelitis: periosteal reaction and reactive sclerosis, may show abscess.

Management Options

Systemic treatment includes a combination of chemo, hormone therapy, and immunotherapy. Targeted intrathecal chemo and radiation are recommended in palliative cases to slow the progression.

References and Further Reading

1. Haouimi A. Large skull metastasis from breast cancer. Radiopaedia.org. 2021. https://doi.org/10.53347/rID-90535. Accessed 25 Nov 2024.
2. Mitsuya K, et al. Metastatic skull tumors: MRI features and a new conventional classification. J Neurooncol. 2011. https://doi.org/10.1007/s11060-010-0465-5. Accessed 25 Nov 2024.

Case 166

166

Clinical History

An 8-year-old girl presented with visual disturbances.

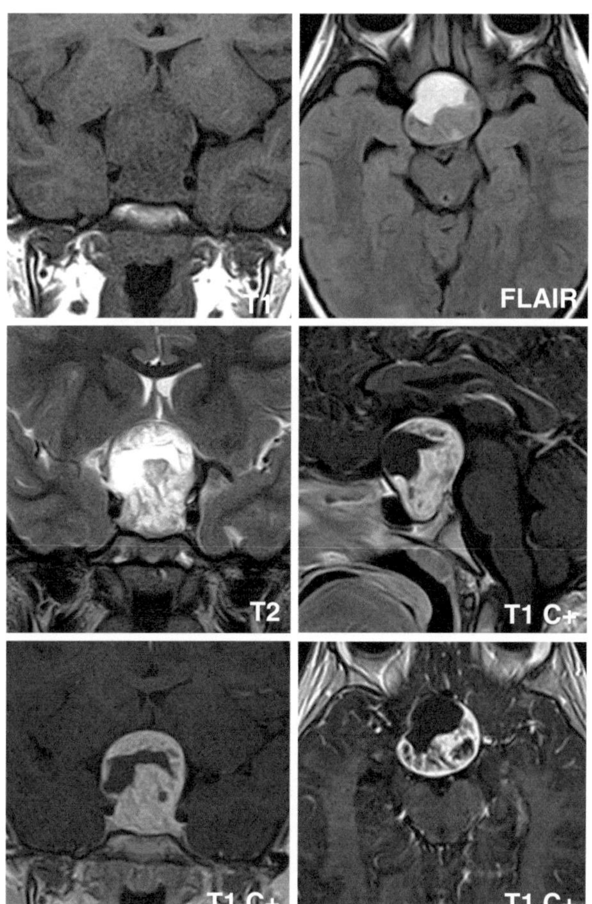

A. Haouimi et al., *Head and Neck Radiology Spot Diagnosis*,
https://doi.org/10.1007/978-3-032-14553-6_166

Findings

A well-defined solid-cystic suprasellar lesion with intrasellar extension. The solid component shows low signal on T1, high signal on FLAIR and T2 with heterogeneous enhancement. The cystic component is isosignal to central gray matter on T1 and high signal on FLAIR and T2. Chiasmatic elevation and compression on the third ventricular floor without hydrocephalus.

Diagnosis

Adamantinomatous craniopharyngioma.

Discussion

Craniopharyngiomas are rare benign neoplastic lesions primarily affecting children and young adults. They are believed to derive from Rathke's cleft. The lesions have a bimodal age distribution and are seen in the sellar/suprasellar region. The first peak is between 5 and 15 years, consisting almost exclusively of the adamantinomatous subtype.

Though the lesions are benign, the location can cause diverse clinical issues. As they continue to grow slowly, at some point they can cause extrinsic compression on the adjacent optic pathway, pituitary gland, and hypothalamic structures. Apart from signs of increased intracranial pressure, the clinical symptoms can include visual changes, signs of endocrinopathy, and hypothalamic syndrome, depending on the size of the lesion.

The lesions are usually lobulated having solid, cystic, and calcified components. The calcified component is difficult to appreciate on MRI and CT will be very important in that regard. There is always an enhancement of the solid component.

Common Differential Diagnosis

- Rathke cleft cyst: no enhancement, no calcification, "claw sign."
- Pituitary adenoma: mostly sellar with suprasellar extension, occasionally bleeds.
- Thrombosed giant aneurysm: contains blood product and SWI is recommended.

Management Options

The goal of treatment is to reduce the size to preserve visual, hormonal, and hypothalamic functional balance and prevent hydrocephalus. The treatment is surgical. Stereotactic aspiration can be an option.

References and Further Reading

1. Hald J, Eldevik O, Skalpe I. Acta Radiol. 1995. https://www.ncbi.nlm.nih.gov/pubmed/7710792. Accessed 18 Mar 2022.
2. Haouimi A. Adamantinomatous craniopharyngioma. Radiopaedia.org. 2020. https://doi.org/10.53347/rID-85427. Accessed 25 Nov 2024.

Case 167

167

Clinical History

A 6-year-old boy presented with a painless worsening of right eye vision.

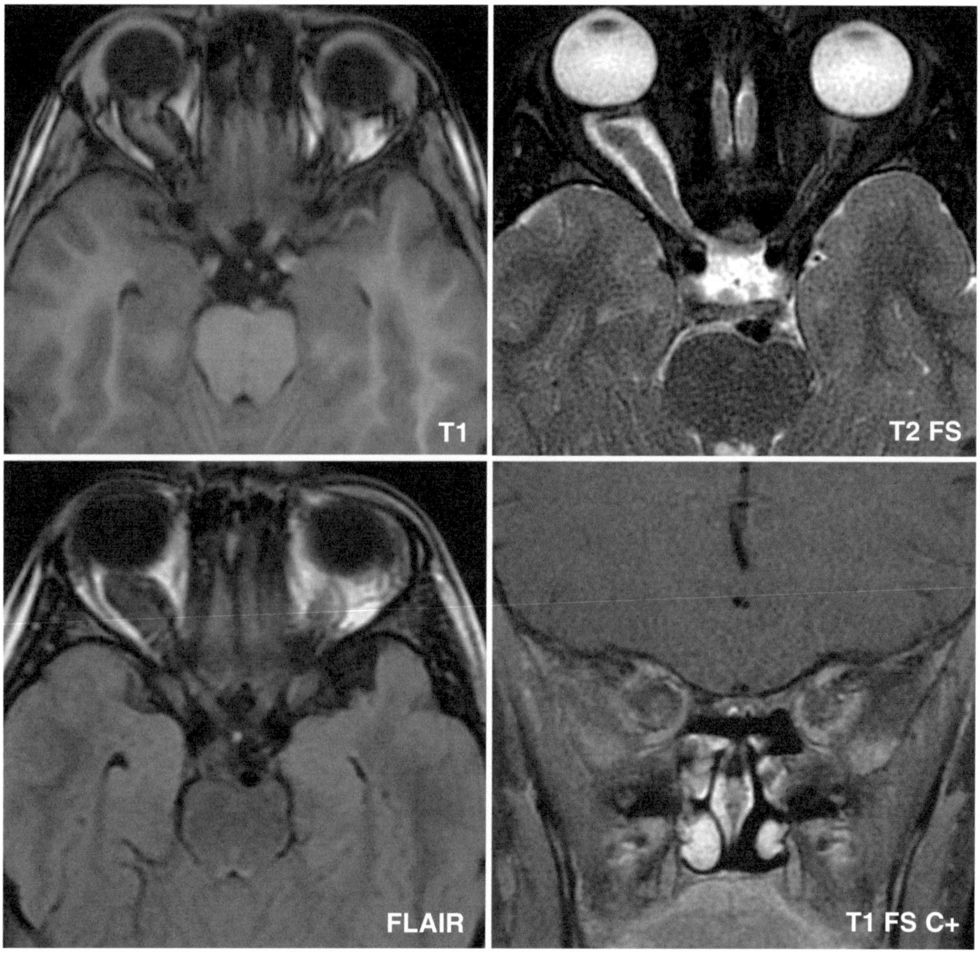

A. Haouimi et al., *Head and Neck Radiology Spot Diagnosis*,
https://doi.org/10.1007/978-3-032-14553-6_167

Findings

Mild right ocular proptosis. Kinking with fusiform enlargement of right intraorbital and intracanalicular optic nerve, showing isosignal on T1, T2, and FLAIR with mild heterogeneous enhancement. Enlarged perineural CSF space of right intraorbital optic nerve.

Diagnosis

Optic nerve glioma.

Discussion

Optic nerve gliomas are the most common type of brain tumor in children under the age of 10 and represent about 5% of all childhood brain tumors. The lesions can be either sporadic or syndromic, associated with von Recklinghausen's disease and adult-onset type. The lesions may stop growing and disappear in some cases associated with von Recklinghausen's disease.

Pathologically, the optic nerve gliomas are WHO grade 1 pilocytic astrocytomas with varying degrees of cystic changes. The tumors may be lobulated, eccentric, or fusiform.

MRI is the investigation of choice, showing isosignal on T1 and iso to slightly high signal on T2. There may be kinking and buckling of the thickened optic nerve. CT can reveal the enlarged optic canal. Calcification is absent and is an important finding to differentiate between optic nerve sheath meningioma.

Common Differential Diagnosis

- Optic neuritis: acute painful ophthalmoplegia, mild enhancement.
- von Recklinghausen disease (NF1): cutaneous involvement, "café au lait" skin lesions.
- Optic nerve sheath meningioma: marked enhancement. "Tram track" calcification on CT.

Management Options

Treatment is initiated following disease progression with either reduction in visual acuity or growth pattern on follow-up neuroimaging. Management options include chemotherapy and radiotherapy in selected cases. The surgical option is controversial.

References and Further Reading

1. Fu L, et al. Lagophthalmos. Pearls Publishing; 2023. https://www.ncbi.nlm.nih.gov/books/NBK560661/figure/article-24008.image.f2/. Accessed 2 Jan 2025.
2. Gaillard F, et al. Optic pathway glioma. Radiopaedia.org. 2025. https://doi.org/10.53347/rID-6665. Accessed 2 Jan 2025.
3. Haouimi A. Optic nerve glioma. Radiopaedia.org. 2020. https://doi.org/10.53347/rID-83006. Accessed 24 Oct 2024.

Case 168

168

Clinical History

A 55-year-old woman presented with a right-sided gradual hearing loss.

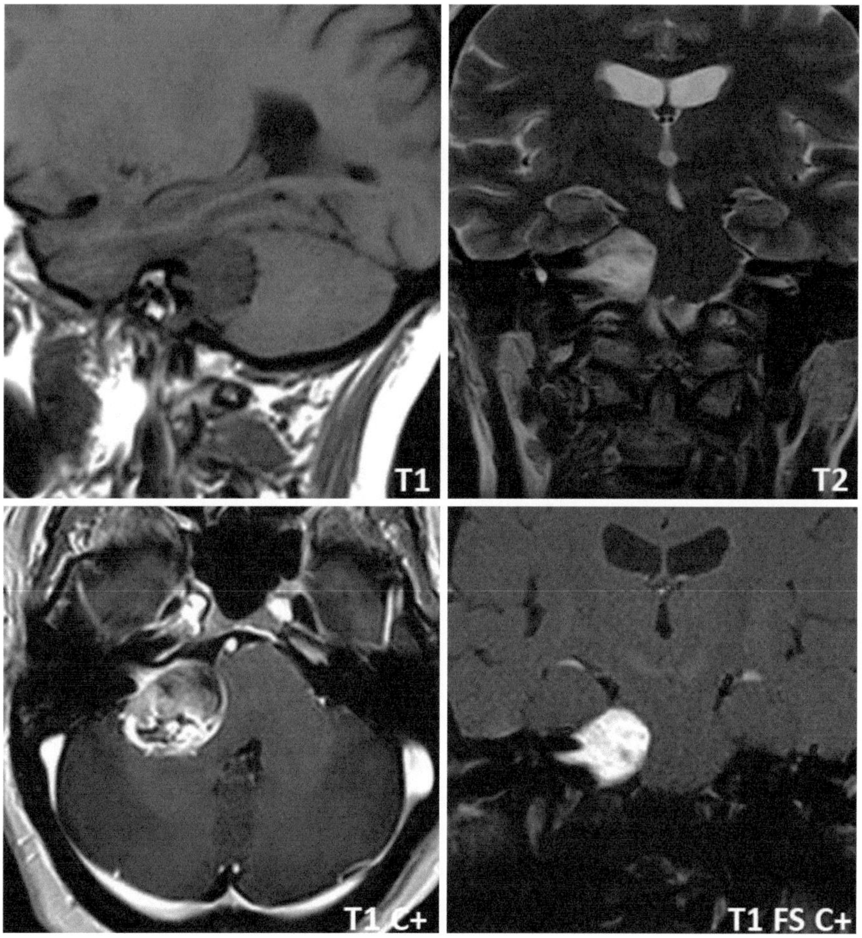

A. Haouimi et al., *Head and Neck Radiology Spot Diagnosis*,
https://doi.org/10.1007/978-3-032-14553-6_168

Findings

An extraaxial well-defined right cerebellopontine angle (CPA) "ice-cream cone" lesion with intracanalicular extension. It displays a low signal on T1 and a nonhomogeneous high signal on T2 with intense heterogeneous enhancement. Mass effect on the right middle cerebellar peduncle with displaced fourth ventricle toward the left. No hydrocephalus.

Diagnosis

Vestibular schwannoma.

Discussion

Ninety percent of the lesions involving the CPA are vestibular schwannomas, also known as acoustic neuromas. These benign encapsulated slow-growing lesions (growth rate less than 1 mm per year) arise from glial-Schwann cells, typically from the vestibular portion of vestibulocochlear nerve. They are a grade 1 type of WHO lesion.

The common symptoms are unilateral sensorineural hearing loss, tinnitus, vertigo, and facial numbness. On rare occasions, the lesion can grow rapidly to compress the brainstem and may interfere with vital functions. The lesions are often sporadic but when bilateral, one should consider the diagnosis of neurofibromatosis type 2.

Any unilateral enhancing lesion along the presumed trajectory of the vestibulocochlear bundle can be considered as a vestibular neuroma until proven otherwise. MRI is the investigation of choice. CT scan is less sensitive. A CT feature may include widening of internal acoustic meatus with or without erosion, on bone window.

Common Differential Diagnosis

- Meningioma: "dural tail sign" +/−, may calcify, usually no intracanalar extension.
- Epidermoid cyst: isointense to CSF on T1 and T2 with restricted diffusion.
- Arachnoid cyst: isointense to CSF on T1 and T2, no restricted diffusion or enhancement.
- Endolymphatic sac tumor: posteroinferior to the IAC, often bone erosion.

Management Options

Multidisciplinary approach including surgery, radiosurgery, and conservative management. Resection only prevents further hearing loss but does not restore the hearing already lost.

References and Further Reading

1. Haouimi A. Acoustic neuroma with intracanalicular extension. Radiopaedia.org. https://radiopaedia.org/cases/195149. Accessed 7 Dec 2024.
2. Kabashi S, et al. The role of magnetic resonance imaging (MRI) in diagnostics of acoustic schwannoma. Acta Inform Med. 2020. https://doi.org/10.5455/aim.2020.28.287-291. Accessed 7 Dec 2024.

Case 169

169

Clinical History

A 40-year-old woman presented with a right trigeminal neuralgia.

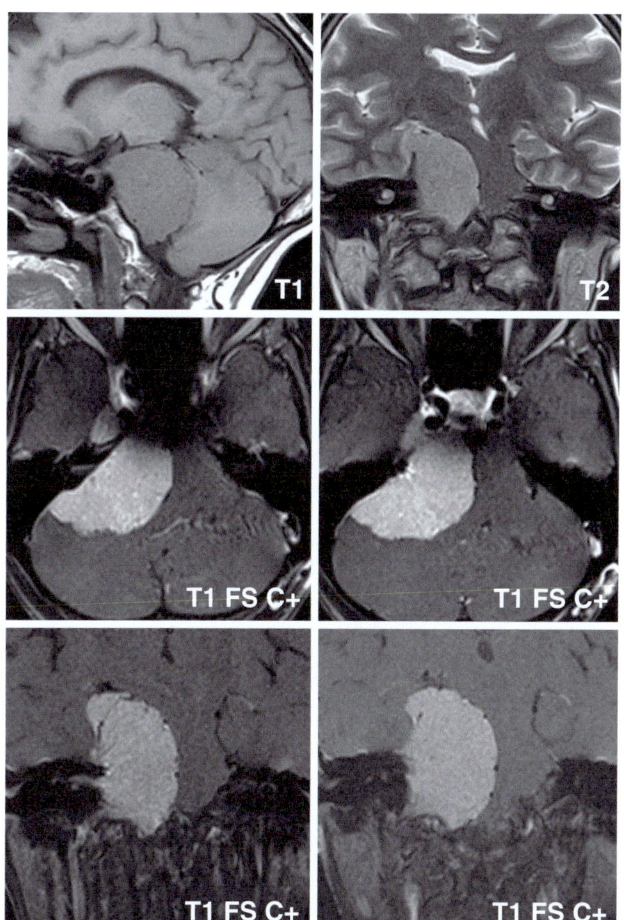

A. Haouimi et al., *Head and Neck Radiology Spot Diagnosis*,
https://doi.org/10.1007/978-3-032-14553-6_169

Findings

A right cerebellopontine angle (CPA) well-defined extraaxial lesion with a broad dural base along the petrous ridge. It appears isointense to the cortical grey matter on both T1 and T2, extending up to the ipsilateral Meckel's cave and internal auditory canal. Marked homogeneous enhancement with positive "dural tail sign." CSF cleft with signal voids separating the lesion and the brain: "CSF cleft sign." Positive "white matter buckling sign" better seen on T2. "Spoke wheel sign" better seen on postcontrast coronal view. Mass effect on adjacent trigeminal nerve, brainstem, middle cerebellar peduncle, and the fourth ventricle with a slight midline shift to the left.

Diagnosis

Cerebellopontine angle meningioma.

Discussion

CPA meningiomas account for up to 10% of all intracranial meningiomas. They arise from arachnoid cap cells in the meninges. The base of the lesions is usually along the cisternal face of the petrous bone. They are benign extraaxial tumors and the second most common slow-growing lesion in CPA in adults. In children, the diagnosis of NF type 2 should be considered.

The lesions may remain clinically silent and can be incidentally diagnosed. When symptomatic, hearing deficit, tinnitus, vertigo, and facial weakness are the major clinical issues. MRI is the investigation of choice but a characteristic CT finding (broad-based aligned with petrous ridge) can differentiate schwannoma from meningioma, especially in this location.

Common Differential Diagnosis

- Vestibular schwannoma: no dural tail, usually heterogeneous with cystic or hemorrhagic component, no dural base, negative "cleft sign".
- Metastasis: history of known cancer, rapid growth.
- Epidermoid cyst: restricted diffusion, no enhanced component.
- Arachnoid cyst: lesions of CSF signal with no restricted diffusion.

Management Options

Surgical excision if symptomatic. Adjunctive radiotherapy for incomplete excision.

References and Further Reading

1. Gao K, et al. Meningiomas of the cerebellopontine angle: radiological differences in tumors with internal auditory canal involvement and their influence on surgical outcome. PLoS One. 2015. https://pubmed.ncbi.nlm.nih.gov/25849220/. Accessed 15 July 2024.
2. Haouimi A. Meningioma - cerebellopontine angle. Radiopaedia.org. 2024. https://radiopaedia.org/cases/196950. Accessed 7 Dec 2024.

Case 170

170

Clinical History

A 50-year-old woman presented with a right-sided anosmia.

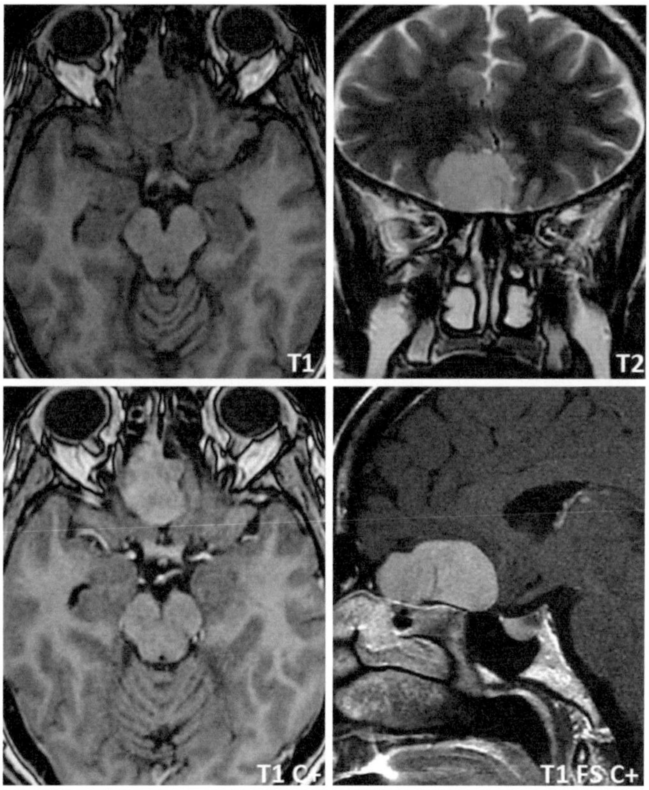

A. Haouimi et al., *Head and Neck Radiology Spot Diagnosis*,
https://doi.org/10.1007/978-3-032-14553-6_170

Findings

Anterior cranial fossa broad dural-based, well-defined, extraaxial lesion epicentered on the right cribriform plate. It is isointense to the cortical grey matter on T1 and slightly hyperintense on T2 with indentation on adjacent frontal lobe, revealing "white matter buckling sign." Marked homogeneous enhancement and positive "CSF cleft sign."

Diagnosis

Olfactory groove meningioma.

Discussion

Olfactory groove meningiomas are slow-growing tumors originating along the cribriform plate at the anterior cranial fossa, representing less than 10% of all meningiomas. Symptoms are of insidious onset. Anosmia can be explained by involvement and compression of olfactory nerve fibers. Frontal lobe compression may cause frontal lobe syndrome, including memory deficit. Visual disturbances may occur due to compression on the opto-chiasmatic pathway or parenchymal edema. Due to the slow-growing nature, delayed diagnosis is the rule rather than exception.

On MRI, the lesions appear as well-defined extraaxial masses, isointense to gray matter on T1 and iso/hyperintense on T2, showing intense enhancement. They can show a positive "dural tail sign" and "CSF cleft sign." Marked perilesional edema is often present. CT helps to define the bony relationship, including detecting hyperostosis or erosion and is thus helpful in planning the surgical approach, and to visualize intralesional calcifications.

Common Differential Diagnosis

- Esthesioneuroblastoma: both intra and extracranial components.
- Falx meningioma: lesion is based on the falx rather than the cribriform plate.
- Dural metastasis: history of known cancer, fast growth.

Management Options

The management of olfactory groove meningioma is most often surgical. Presurgical embolization may help to reduce intraoperative bleeding. For incomplete resection, adjuvant radiotherapy and/or radiosurgery may be used.

References and Further Reading

1. Haouimi A. Olfactory groove meningioma. Radiopaedia.org. https://radiopaedia.org/cases/195249. Accessed 25 Nov 2024.
2. Ikhuoriah T, et al. Olfactory groove meningioma: a case report with typical clinical and radiologic features in a 74-year-old Nigerian male. Radiol Case Rep. 2022. https://doi.org/10.1016/j.radcr.2022.08.077. Accessed 25 Nov 2024.

Case 171

171

Clinical History

A 45-year-old man presented with epilepsy.

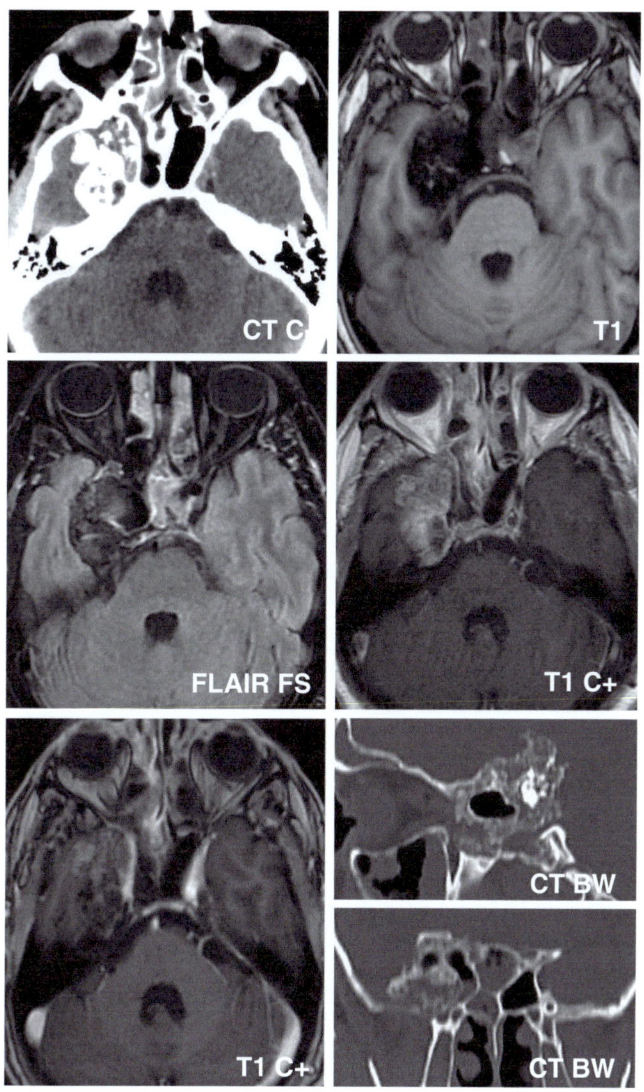

A. Haouimi et al., *Head and Neck Radiology Spot Diagnosis*,
https://doi.org/10.1007/978-3-032-14553-6_171

Findings

A heterogeneous extraaxial right off-midline intracranial lesion showing compression on the adjacent cavernous sinus and temporal lobe. No obvious perilesional edema. The lesion is heterogeneously isointense on all sequences with heterogeneous enhancement better seen on delayed scan. CT shows the aggressive lytic pattern of bone lesion epicentered on sphenoid wing with calcified "rings and arcs" suggesting chondroid matrix.

Diagnosis

Sphenoid wing chondrosarcoma.

Discussion

Chondrosarcomas are slow-growing malignant mesenchymal tumors, representing approximately 20% of skeletal system cancers in young adults. Although they can affect any bone, involvement of the sphenoid wing is exceedingly uncommon. These tumors often appear multilobulated due to their hyaline cartilage content. Because treatment strategies differ, distinguishing the chondroid subtype from myxoid chondrosarcoma is essential.

Clinical manifestations are largely determined by tumor size and local invasion. Symptoms such as headache and signs of raised intracranial pressure are nonspecific. Extension into the orbit may lead to diplopia, ptosis, and restricted ocular movements, while invasion of the cavernous sinus can result in multiple cranial nerve deficits.

CT imaging is valuable for evaluating calcification patterns, with "rings and arcs" or "popcorn" calcifications being highly indicative of a chondroid tumor. MRI remains the preferred modality for assessing the extent of locoregional invasion.

Common Differential Diagnosis

- Chordoma: midline lesions, no "rings and arc" like calcification.
- Meningioma: often with dural tail, no locoregional invasion.
- Trigeminal schwannoma: no calcification, dumbbell, or linear configuration.

Management Options

The mainstay of treatment is surgery. Due to extensive locoregional invasion, complete resection is often difficult. A large debulking followed by both radiation and chemotherapy often provides the best result.

References and Further Reading

1. Battal B, Zamora C. Imaging of skull base tumors. Tomography. 2023. Accessed 12 July 2024. https://doi.org/10.3390/tomography9040097.
2. Gaillard F, et al. Chondrosarcoma of the skull base. Radiopaedia.org. 2025. Accessed 12 July 2024. https://doi.org/10.53347/rID-6229.
3. Haouimi A. Chondrosarcoma sphenoid wing. Radiopaedia.org. 2024. Accessed 25 Nov 2024. https://doi.org/10.53347/rID-187775.

Case 172

172

Clinical History

A 70-year-old man presented with severe sensorineural hearing loss for cochlear implant assessment.

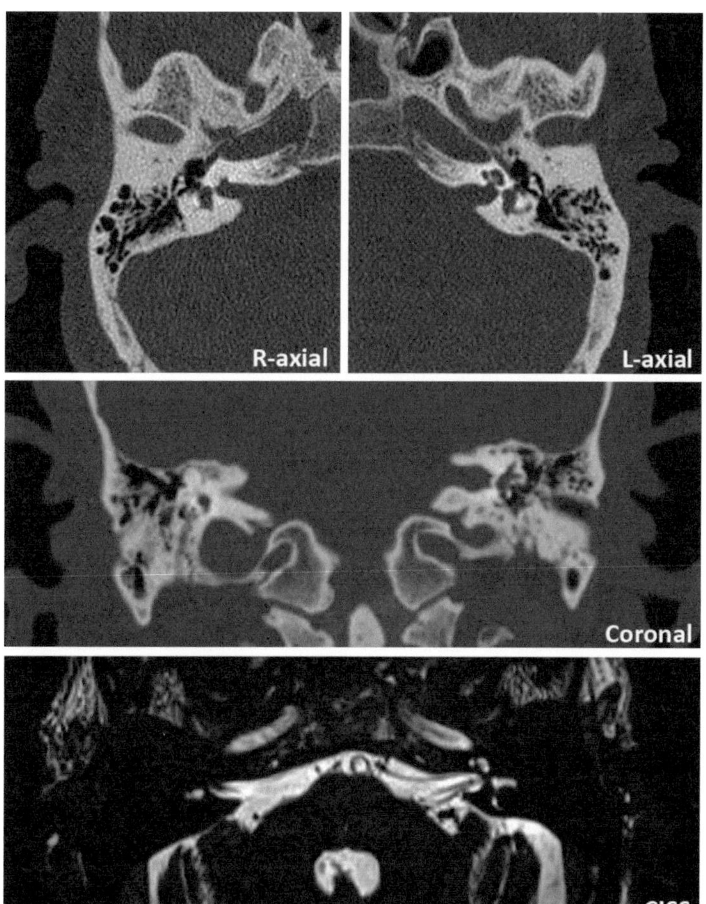

A. Haouimi et al., *Head and Neck Radiology Spot Diagnosis*,
https://doi.org/10.1007/978-3-032-14553-6_172

Findings

CT images show abnormal ossification/sclerosis of the right cochlea and semicircular canals. This is demonstrated on the axial CISS images as a complete loss of the normal high T2 signal of the membranous labyrinth.

Diagnosis

Labyrinthitis ossificans.

Discussion

Labyrinthitis ossificans refers to a process in which the structures of the membranous labyrinth of the inner ear undergo sclerosis and ossification in response to an insult. It is an acquired condition, and the main causes are infection (otologic or meningeal), autoimmune disorders, and trauma including iatrogenic injury. It can occur at all ages and is slightly more common in females.

The initial inflammation leads to endosteal cochlear damage, causing inflammatory exudate to fill the cochlear duct. Ultimately, the exudate is replaced by fibrous tissue, which undergoes ossification that interferes with hearing.

Labyrinthitis ossificans has been divided into four stages. The first serous and second purulent stages are considered as acute phases and patients can present with nonspecific symptoms such as dizziness, vertigo, vomiting, and hearing loss. The third fibrous and fourth osseous stages are the chronic irreversible phases leading to profound sensorineural hearing loss.

In the acute stages, CT may be normal while MRI may demonstrate enhancement of the labyrinthine structures, T2 hypointensity, and restricted diffusion. In the chronic stages, CT will show high-density bone deposition within the membranous labyrinth, while MRI shows loss of the normal fluid signal in the inner ear.

Common Differential Diagnosis

- Cochlear aplasia: no anatomic cochlear structure, possible association of absent CN VIII.
- Labyrinthine aplasia: congenital absence of inner ear structures, absent/hypoplastic IAC.
- Otosclerosis: spares cochlear lumen, semicircular canals, pericochlear lucency +/−.

Management Options

Labyrinthitis ossificans can be treated with cochlear implants. Imaging plays an important role in staging and level of ossification to ensure adequate surgical planning and electrode selection.

References and Further Reading

1. Buch K, et al. Etiology-specific mineralization patterns in patients with labyrinthitis ossificans. Am J Neuroradiol. 2019. https://doi.org/10.3174/ajnr.A5985. Accessed 12 Apr 2024.
2. Taxak P, et al. Labyrinthitis and labyrinthitis ossificans -a case report and review of the literature. J Radiol Case Rep. 2020. https://doi.org/10.3941/jrcr.v14i5.3706. Accessed 12 Apr 2024.

Clinical History

A 5-year-old boy presented with a history of fall from the first floor and otorrhea.

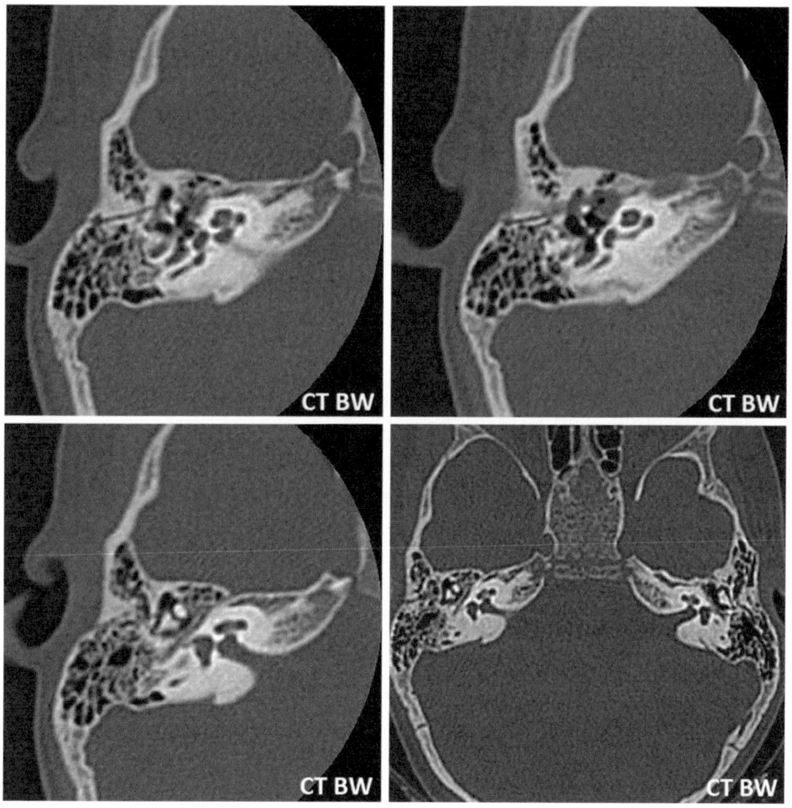

A. Haouimi et al., *Head and Neck Radiology Spot Diagnosis*,
https://doi.org/10.1007/978-3-032-14553-6_173

Findings

Longitudinal fracture of the right temporal bone extending into the middle ear with associated incudo-malleolar dislocation and widening of the joint space. Partial opacification of the epitympanic recess, suggesting hemotympanum. Normal left middle ear and both inner ears.

Diagnosis

Longitudinal temporal bone fracture with incudo-malleolar dislocation.

Discussion

The temporal bones comprise the thickest and densest components of the skull base. A minimum impact force of 6000–8000 Newton is necessary to fracture this bone. External impact can be anteroposterior or lateral. Temporal fractures are usually unilateral and 20% of all skull fractures will have a temporal bone fracture. Only 2.5% of fractures involve the otic capsule and 10% of the cases involve facial nerve injury, mostly at the geniculate ganglion.

The longitudinal fracture accounts for about 80% of all temporal bone fractures and is due to lateral impact. The fracture line runs parallel to the long axis of petrous bone. The structures at risk include the bony ossicles and mastoid air cells. Injuries may be associated with ossicular disruption and hemotympanum, causing conductive hearing loss.

The remaining 20% of fractures are transverse fractures where the fracture line runs perpendicular to the long axis and are associated with risk of damage to internal ear. The impact is usually anteroposterior. Fracture propagation through the otic capsule or damage to the round or oval windows can lead to perilymphatic fistula, causing sensorineural hearing loss with or without vertigo. There is also risk of facial and vestibulocochlear nerve damage in temporal bone fracture. CT is the investigation of choice. MRI is indicated for evaluation of internal ear.

Common Differential Diagnosis

- Diagnosis is straightforward in an appropriate clinical context.

Management Options

Management options are conservative with antibiotics and steroids. Surgical intervention for ossicular reconstruction, closure of persistent fistula, and repair of facial nerve, etc.

References and Further Reading

1. Haouimi A. Longitudinal temporal bone fracture with incudo-malleolar dislocation. Radiopaedia.org. 2021. https://doi.org/10.53347/rID-96042. Accessed on 7 Dec 2024.
2. Patel A, Lofgren DH, Varacallo M. Temporal fracture. Stat Pearls Publishing; 2024. https://www.ncbi.nlm.nih.gov/books/NBK535391/. Accessed 7 Dec 2024.

Case 174

174

Clinical History

A 30-year-old man presented with a history of chronic headache.

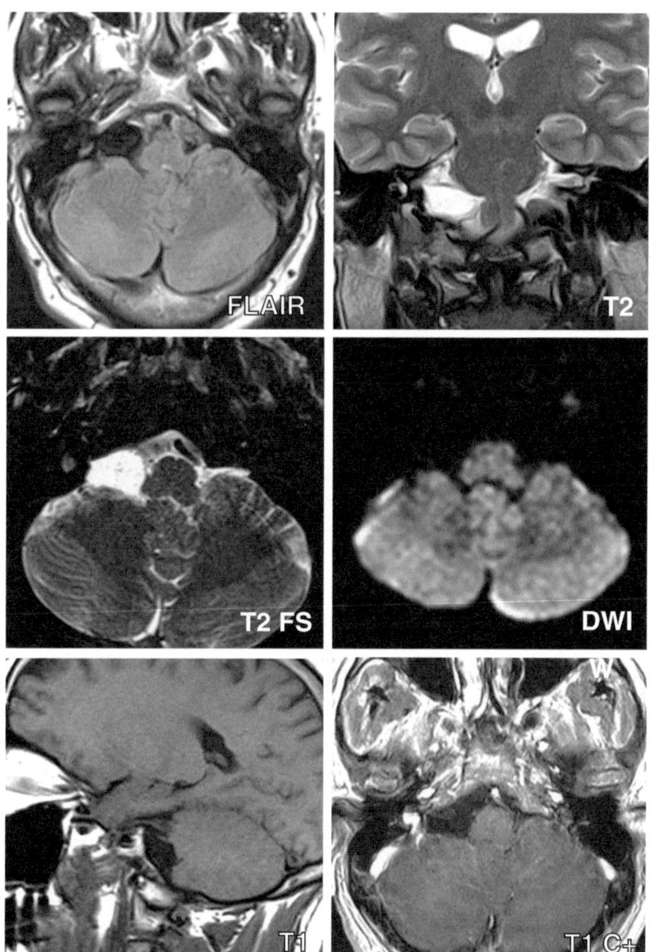

A. Haouimi et al., *Head and Neck Radiology Spot Diagnosis*,
https://doi.org/10.1007/978-3-032-14553-6_174

Findings

Small extraaxial cystic lesion at the right cerebellopontine angle of CSF signal on all sequences with no enhancement or restricted diffusion.

Diagnosis

Cerebellopontine arachnoid cyst.

Discussion

Primary arachnoid cysts are rare, benign developmental arachnoid duplication anomalies that arise during the early weeks of gestation. They cause CSF collection within the arachnoid membranes and are present at birth. Secondary arachnoid cysts develop because of head injury, meningitis, tumors, or as a complication of brain surgery.

Most lesions are asymptomatic and discovered incidentally. Occasionally, they can become symptomatic due to compression effect, involvement of cranial nerves, and obstruction of CSF. Headache, nausea, vomiting, vertigo, hearing, and visual impairment are common symptoms. Rarely can they have a valve mechanism leading to progressive enlargement.

CT scan is usually not helpful due to posterior fossa artifacts. On MRI, the lesions are isointense to CSF on all sequences with no sign of restricted diffusion or enhancement. They do not extend into the internal auditory meatus, nor do they demonstrate a "dural tail" sign.

Common Differential Diagnosis

- Epidermoid cyst: usually heterogeneous, insinuating the adjacent brain parenchyma with scalloped contour and restricted diffusion.
- Meningioma: usually shows "dural tail sign" with enhancement and restricted diffusion.
- Vestibular schwannoma: involvement of acoustico-facial bundle.

Management Options

Most arachnoid cysts are considered "do not touch" lesions and do not need any special attention. Open or endoscopic surgery is reserved only for bigger and symptomatic cases.

References and Further Reading

1. Gaillard F, et al. Arachnoid cyst. Radiopaedia.org. 2025. https://doi.org/10.53347/rID-929. Accessed 13 Aug 2024.
2. Haouimi A. Arachnoid cyst – cerebellopontine angle. Radiopaedia.org. 2024. https://doi.org/10.53347/rID-185870. Accessed 7 Dec 2024.
3. White ML, Das JM. Arachnoid cysts. Stat Pearls Publishing; 2024. https://www.ncbi.nlm.nih.gov/books/NBK563272/. Accessed 7 Dec 2024.

Case 175

175

Clinical History

A 16-year-old boy presented with a painful left ophthalmoplegia.

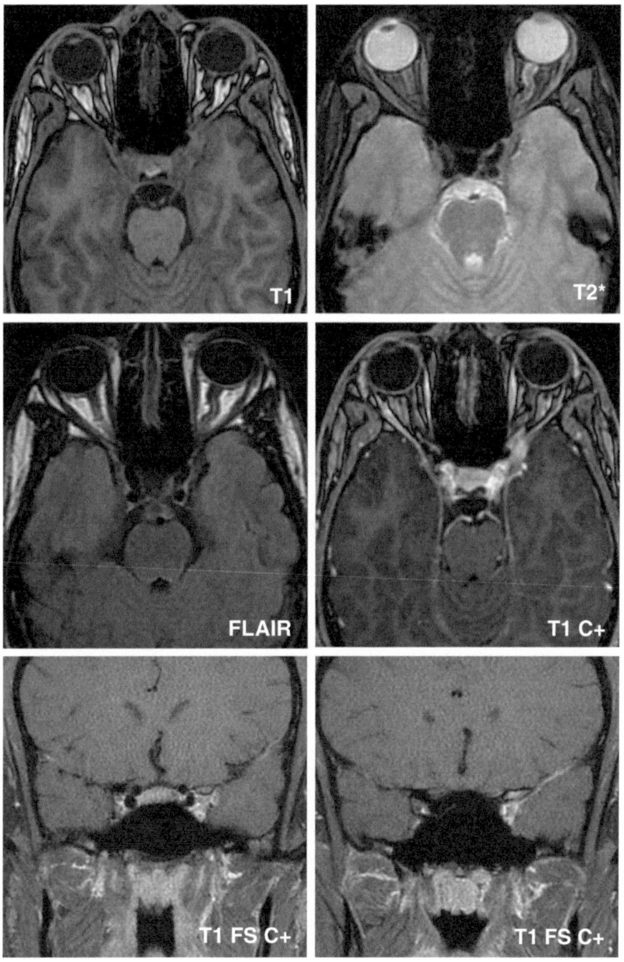

A. Haouimi et al., *Head and Neck Radiology Spot Diagnosis*,
https://doi.org/10.1007/978-3-032-14553-6_175

Findings

Enlargement of left anterior cavernous sinus compared to its counterpart by a soft-tissue lesion extending to the superior orbital fissure and orbital apex. The lesion appears isointense to muscle on T1, minimally hyperintense on T2 with marked enhancement.

Diagnosis

Tolosa–Hunt syndrome.

Discussion

Tolosa–Hunt syndrome represents the inflammation of the septae and wall of the cavernous sinus extending to the superior orbital fissure and orbital apex. It is usually seen in patients around their 40s. Possible etiologies are autoimmune and viral. The pathology is described as fibroblastic proliferation, lymphocytic, and plasmocytic infiltration.

The patients often present with severe unilateral orbital pain and ophthalmoplegia. The compression from intracavernous pathological changes along with dural thickening can explain the severe pain. Other symptoms are due to involvement of cranial nerves. Diplopia and ptosis may develop. Spontaneous recovery is possible but it tends to relapse and remit.

The diagnosis is clinical and by exclusion of other common conditions such as infection, tumor, and vascular aneurysm. The role of MRI is to rule out any other cause of painful ophthalmoplegia. On MRI, an intracavernous isointense soft-tissue mass is seen on both T1 and T2 with anterior extension into orbital apex. There is always an intense contrast enhancement.

Common Differential Diagnosis

- Pachymeningitis: generally, not as focal, positive CSF.
- Sarcoidosis: systemic involvement.
- Meningioma: broad dural base, hyperostosis.

Management Options

Corticosteroids are the treatment of choice and pain disappears within a couple of days. Ophthalmoplegia usually requires weeks to months to recover. Treatment with azathioprine, methotrexate, or even radiation therapy may be considered for refractory cases.

References and Further Reading

1. Haouimi A. Tolosa-Hunt syndrome. Case study. Radiopaedia.org. https://doi.org/10.53347/rID-176796. Accessed 7 Dec 2024.
2. Amrutkar CV, Burton EV. Tolosa-Hunt syndrome. In: Stat Pearls [Internet]. Treasure Island (FL): Stat Pearls Publishing; 2023. Available from: https://www.ncbi.nlm.nih.gov/books/NBK459225/.

Case 176

176

Clinical History

A 75-year-old woman presented with a unilateral left proptosis and pulsatile exophthalmos with subconjunctival hemorrhage.

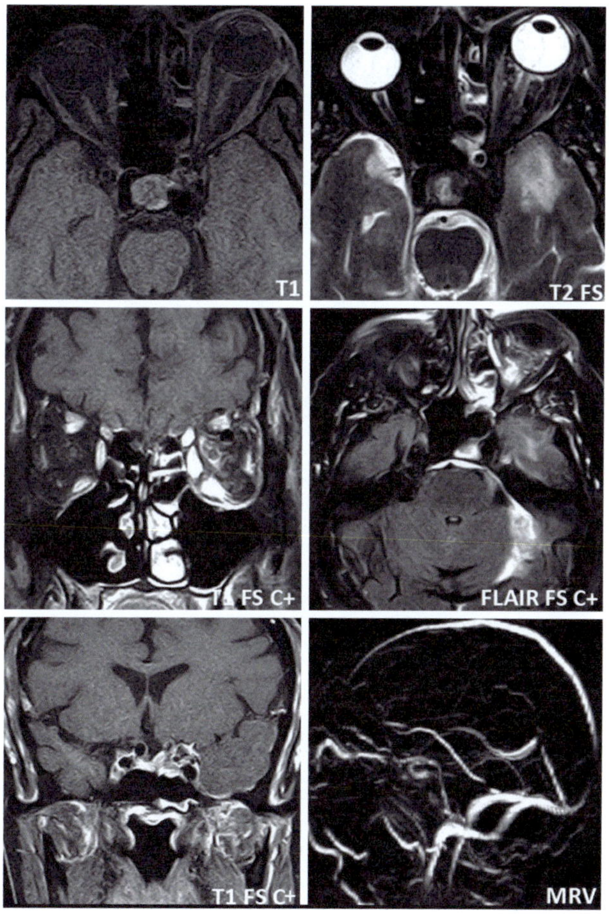

A. Haouimi et al., *Head and Neck Radiology Spot Diagnosis*,
https://doi.org/10.1007/978-3-032-14553-6_176

Findings

Left-sided proptosis with clouding of retrobulbar fat plane and swelling of the extraocular muscles. Markedly enlarged left cavernous sinus compared to its counterpart. Arterialization of superior ophthalmic vein and high velocity signal void. Marked dural thickening and enhancement mostly along the tentorium cerebelli.

Diagnosis

Carotid-cavernous fistula.

Discussion

Carotid-cavernous fistulas (CCFs) often disrupt the normal flow pattern and lead to increased pressure within the cavernous sinus and draining venous structures. The etiology can be spontaneous, associated with Ehlers–Danlos syndrome, atherosclerosis, hypertension, etc., or post-traumatic from skull fracture and penetrating injury. Based on hemodynamic factors, the CCF can be of high- and low-flow type, and finally, based on anatomy, the lesions can be either direct (communication between carotid artery and cavernous sinus) or indirect (dural arteriovenous fistula).

The onset of symptoms is usually sudden. Direct CCFs are characterized by a clinical triad of pulsatile proptosis, chemosis, and intracranial whistling. The patients can also present with diplopia. Optic nerve compression can lead to retinal ischemia and blindness.

Color Doppler may show arterialized, enlarged ophthalmic veins. CT and MRI can reveal enlarged cavernous sinus, arterialization of ophthalmic vein, and abnormal flow patterns.

Common Differential Diagnosis

- Dural arteriovenous fistula: slow flow.
- Cavernous sinus thrombosis: fever, neighboring infectious source, no bruit.
- Superior ophthalmic vein thrombosis: no pulsatile proptosis, high venous signal.

Management Options

The risk of visual loss and the severity must be evaluated to determine the timing of intervention. Reflux into cortical veins can lead to the risk of subarachnoid hemorrhage. Endovascular management is the mainstay of treatment.

References and Further Reading

1. Haouimi A. Caroticocavernous fistula. Radiopaedia.org. https://doi.org/10.53347/rID-174025. Accessed 14 Apr 2024.
2. Mittal M. Oronasal bleed: a rare case of carotid cavernous sinus fistula. Int J Head Neck Surg. 2014. https://doi.org/10.5005/jp-journals-10001-1187.
3. Nosko MG. Carotid-cavernous fistula: practice essentials, prognosis [Internet]. Medscape. 2021 [cited 2025 Oct 15]. Available from: https://emedicine.medscape.com/article/250591-overview.

Case 177

177

Clinical History

A 40-year-old woman presented with paroxysmal attacks of intense, sharp, electric shock-like unilateral facial pain along the distribution of the left trigeminal nerve.

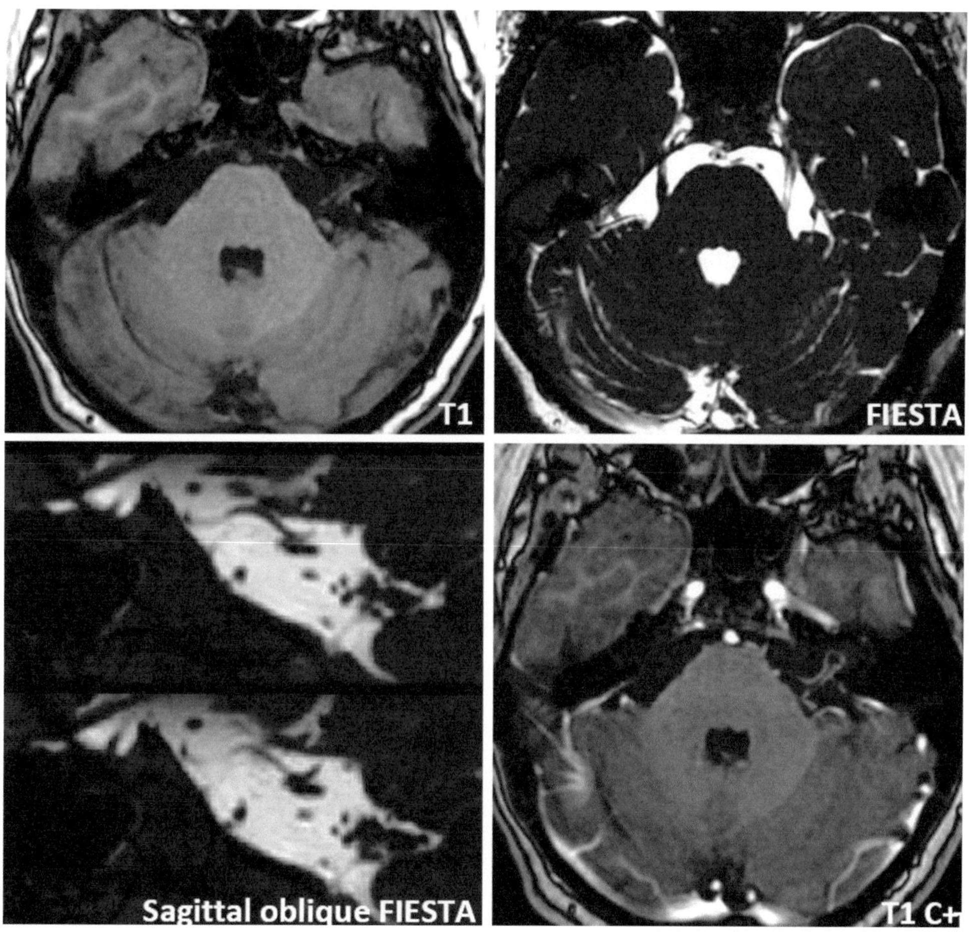

A. Haouimi et al., *Head and Neck Radiology Spot Diagnosis*,
https://doi.org/10.1007/978-3-032-14553-6_177

Findings

Neurovascular conflict involving the left superior cerebellar artery and adjacent cisternal segment of the trigeminal nerve. The conflict is at the superior aspect of the nerve at the transitional zone, approximately 3 mm from the "root entry zone." Focal high signal on axial FIESTA from the transitional zone of the left trigeminal nerve, suggesting neuritis.

Diagnosis

Neurovascular compression syndrome.

Discussion

Neurovascular compression syndrome (NVC) is a group of disorders resulting from compression and distortion of cisternal cranial nerves from adjacent redundant or aberrant vascular structures.

Trigeminal neuralgia, hemifacial spasm, glossopharyngeal neuralgia, and vestibular paroxysmia are by far the common clinical presentations. The symptoms depend on the nerve involved. Sudden intense episodic electric shock-like pain is seen in trigeminal neuralgia often triggered by simple touch, chewing, or even speaking. Involuntary muscular contraction and hemifacial twitching are the predominant symptoms in hemifacial spasm. Hemifacial spasm is due to compression of the facial nerve from AICA. Severe throat pain triggered by swallowing is seen in glossopharyngeal neuralgia and is due to neurovascular conflict arising from posterior inferior cerebellar artery (PICA) and the glossopharyngeal nerve. Brief episodes of vertigo with tinnitus and nausea can be seen in vestibular paroxysmia.

Common Differential Diagnosis

- Trigeminal neuralgia: superior cerebellar artery and trigeminal nerve conflict.
- Multiple sclerosis: no neurovascular conflict. Typical brain parenchymal changes.
- Cluster headache: autonomic symptoms, no neurovascular conflict.

Management Options

Most cases are managed by medical treatment. Carbamazepine is useful in trigeminal and glossopharyngeal neuralgia. Botulinum toxin injections are recommended in hemifacial spasm. Extreme and rare cases may be addressed by microvascular decompression procedure.

References and Further Reading

1. Haouimi A. Neurovascular compression syndrome – trigeminal nerve. Radiopaedia.org. 2021. https://doi.org/10.53347/rID-89835. Accessed 7 Dec 2024.
2. Weerakkody Y, et al. Neurovascular compression syndromes. Radiopaedia.org. 2025. https://doi.org/10.53347/rID-61146. Accessed 2 Aug 2025.

Case 178

178

Clinical History

A 30-year-old woman presented with a right trigeminal neuralgia.

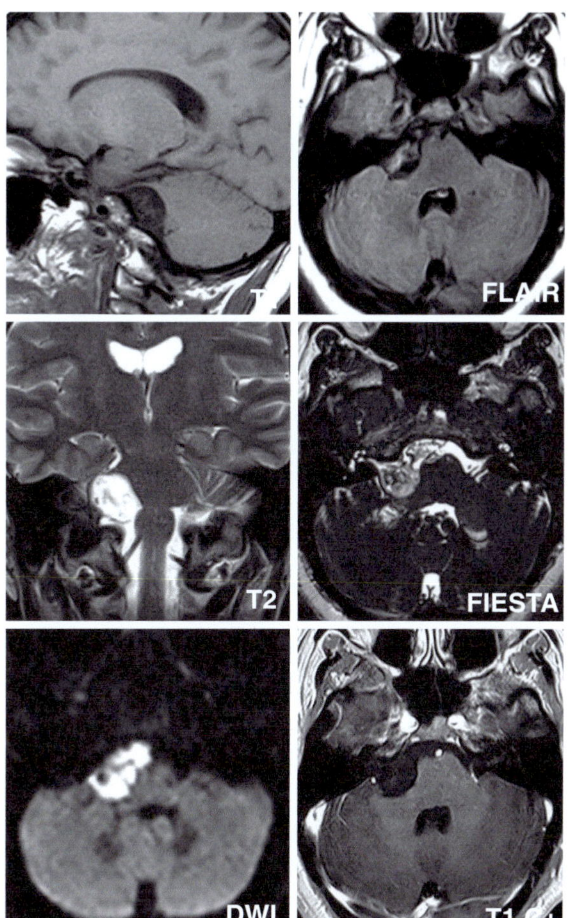

A. Haouimi et al., *Head and Neck Radiology Spot Diagnosis*,
https://doi.org/10.1007/978-3-032-14553-6_178

Findings

Right cerebellopontine angle extraaxial lesion, extending into the ipsilateral internal auditory canal, encasing the facial/vestibulocochlear nerves, and compressing the cisternal portion of the ipsilateral trigeminal nerve. It shows a low signal on T1, a heterogeneous signal on FLAIR, and a high signal on T2 with restricted diffusion and no enhancement. Minimal mass effect on adjacent brain parenchyma.

Diagnosis

Cerebellopontine angle (CPA) epidermoid cyst.

Discussion

CPA epidermoid cysts are the third most common congenital lesion of the cerebellopontine angle. They are benign, slow-growing lesions arising from ectodermal inclusions during neural tube closure in embryogenesis (third to fifth weeks). Cysts contain crystalline cholesterol and keratin debris lined by stratified squamous epithelium. Macroscopically, these "cauliflower"-like," well-defined, avascular, glistening lesions have a "mother-of-pearl" appearance. The shape of the lesion conforms to adjacent structures and has the tendency to encase the neighboring neurovascular bundle. Rare degenerative malignant transformation to squamous cell carcinoma has been reported.

The lesions are mostly clinically silent, or patients can complain of headache. Larger lesions can lead to obstructive hydrocephalus.

On MRI, the lesions are isointense to CSF on both T1 and T2 with restricted diffusion. Diffusion MRI helps to distinguish the lesions from arachnoid cysts. There is no enhancement except for minimal peripheral enhancement. Enhancing lesions may suggest malignant transformation.

Common Differential Diagnosis

- Arachnoid cyst: CSF-like signal on all sequences without restricted diffusion.
- Acoustic neuroma: "ice cream cone" lesion, intracanalar extension, enhancement.
- CPA meningioma: "CSF cleft sign," "dural tail sign," enhancement.

Management Options

The treatment is usually surgical resection.

References and Further Reading

1. Haouimi A. Epidermoid cyst – cerebellopontine angle. Radiopaedia.org. https://doi.org/10.53347/rID-161917. Accessed 7 Dec 2024.
2. Sirin S, et al. Imaging of posterior fossa epidermoid tumors. Clin Neurol Neurosurg. 2004. https://doi.org/10.1016/j.clineuro.2004.11.007. Accessed 7 Dec 2024.

Case 179

179

Clinical History

A 30-year-old man presented with signs of increased intracranial pressure. History of episodic gelastic seizures.

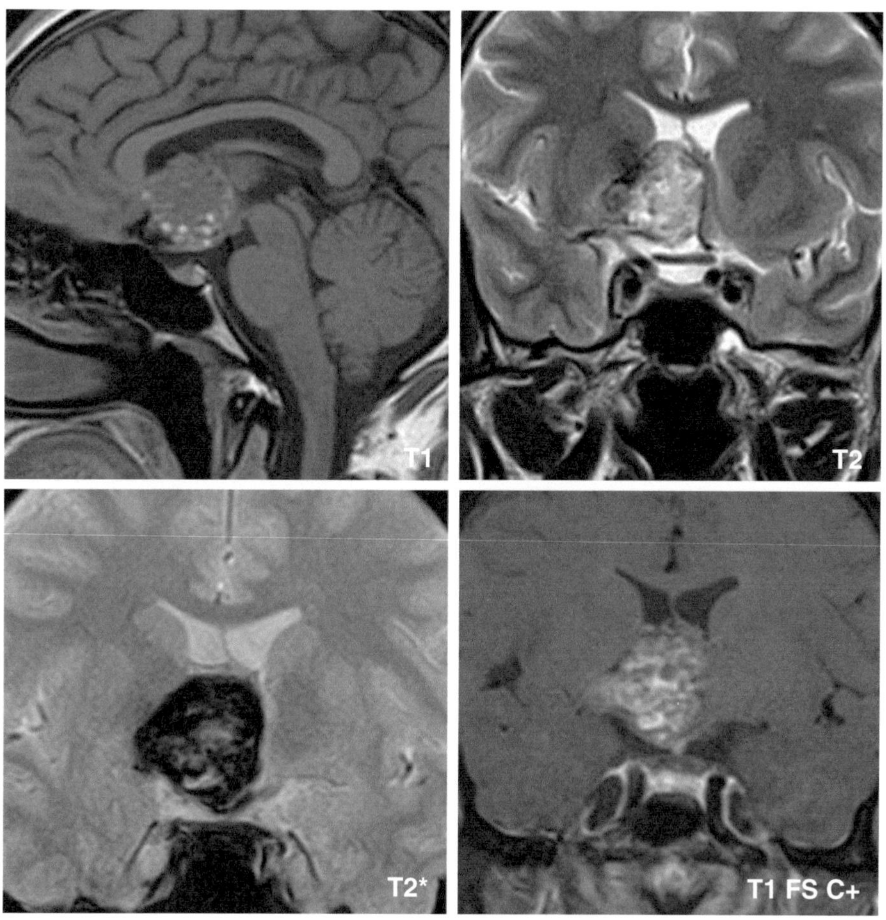

A. Haouimi et al., *Head and Neck Radiology Spot Diagnosis*,
https://doi.org/10.1007/978-3-032-14553-6_179

Findings

Both T1 and T2 images show a well-defined hypothalamic mixed-signal intensity lesion with prominent blooming on T2* and moderate heterogeneous enhancement. Mass effect on the optic chiasma and third ventricle with mild lateral ventricular dilatation.

Diagnosis

Hypothalamic cavernoma.

Discussion

Cavernomas are slow-flow vascular malformations, composed of a cluster of endothelial-lined dilated sinusoids (caverns). These represent up to 20% of all vascular malformations of the central nervous system. These angiographically occult lesions are the third most common cerebral vascular malformation after developmental venous anomaly and capillary telangiectasia. Macroscopically, they resemble "blackberry" or "raspberry" like lesions filled with blood, ranging from a few millimeters to a few centimeters. The hypothalamus is anatomically adjacent to the mammillary bodies and borders the thalamus, basal ganglia, and internal capsule. Cavernomas are predisposed to episodic hemorrhage and may exert mass effect on adjacent eloquent structures.

The unique clinical presentations given the location of this mass include endocrinopathies, visual disturbances, gelastic seizures, memory difficulty, and gait disturbance.

MRI is the investigation of choice. These lesions show a characteristic "popcorn" like appearance with a peripheral rim of low signal (hemosiderin). The internal signals depend on the contents of blood products of different amounts and ages. Recent bleeding can result in perilesional edema. Susceptibility-weighted sequences show a prominent blooming artifact and enhancement is unlikely.

Common Differential Diagnosis

- Tuber cinereum hamartoma: isosignal on all sequences, no enhancement, no calcification.
- Hypothalamic lipoma: high signal on both T1 and T2 with signal suppression on fat sat.

Management Options

Hypothalamic cavernomas are considered by some to be a "do not touch" lesion. Most patients are managed conservatively. Complete resection is curative for symptomatic cases.

References and Further Reading

1. Haouimi A. Cavernoma-hypothalamus. Radiopaedia.org. 2024. https://radiopaedia.org/cases/197912. Accessed 7 Dec 2024.
2. Khahera AS, Li Y, Steinberg GK. Cavernous malformations of the hypothalamus. J Neurosurg. 2021. https://doi.org/10.3171/2020.10.JNS201419. Accessed 18 Apr 2023.

Case 180

180

Clinical History

A 60-year-old woman presented with headache and decreased tongue mobility.

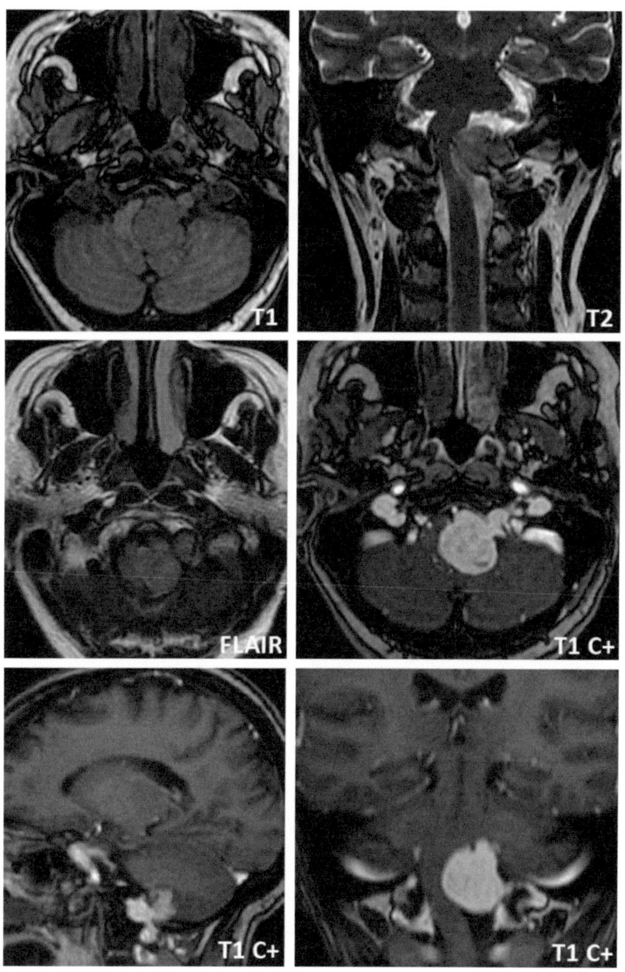

A. Haouimi et al., *Head and Neck Radiology Spot Diagnosis*,
https://doi.org/10.1007/978-3-032-14553-6_180

Findings

A lobulated left off-midline extraaxial well-circumscribed isointense mass at the foramen magnum, extending to the ipsilateral hypoglossal canal on all sequences (T1, T2, and FLAIR). The postcontrast sequences demonstrate vivid enhancement. The medulla oblongata is compressed and displaced to the right. No significant dilatation of the ventricular system.

Diagnosis

Foramen magnum hemangiopericytoma.

Discussion

Hemangiopericytomas, also known as solitary fibrous tumors, account for less than 1% of all central nervous system tumors. These tumors arise from pericytes of Zimmerman (contractile cells found along capillary walls). Posterior fossa hemangiopericytomas tend to occur near foramen magnum. Adults between 30 and 50 are mostly affected by these highly vascular tumors with equal male and female distribution. Only 10% are seen in children.

Immunohistochemical markers like STAT6, CD34, and vimentin are very useful in the diagnosis of hemangiopericytomas.

Unlike meningiomas, hemangiopericytomas do not show hyperostosis or calcification on CT. However, the lesions enhance very strongly. On MRI, the lesions are isointense on both T1 and T2 and may show "dural tail sign" (especially grade II type). The presence of flow voids and edema is the sign in favor of hemangiopericytoma rather than meningioma.

Common Differential Diagnosis

- Hypoglossal schwannoma: elongated, linear, without dural base.
- Meningioma: slow growing, no perilesional edema, "spoke wheel" appearance.

Management Options

Total surgical excision is recommended with prior embolization. Radiotherapy may be recommended to prevent recurrence.

References and Further Reading

1. D'Souza D, et al. Meningeal haemangiopericytoma (historical). Radiopaedia.org. 2024. https://doi.org/10.53347/rID-1437. Accessed 16 Dec 2024.
2. Haouimi A. Haemangiopericytoma – foramen magnum. Radiopaedia.org. 2022. https://doi.org/10.53347/rID-96085. Accessed 7 Dec 2024.
3. Kumar R, et al. Unusual tumors of the posterior fossa skull base. Skull Base. 2006. https://doi.org/10.1055/s-2006-934103. PMID: 17077871; PMCID: PMC1502038. Accessed 7 Dec 2024.

Case 181

181

Clinical History

A 68-year-old woman presented with low-grade fever, localized soft-tissue swelling with pain and tenderness in the right mandibular base and loosening of a few adjacent teeth.

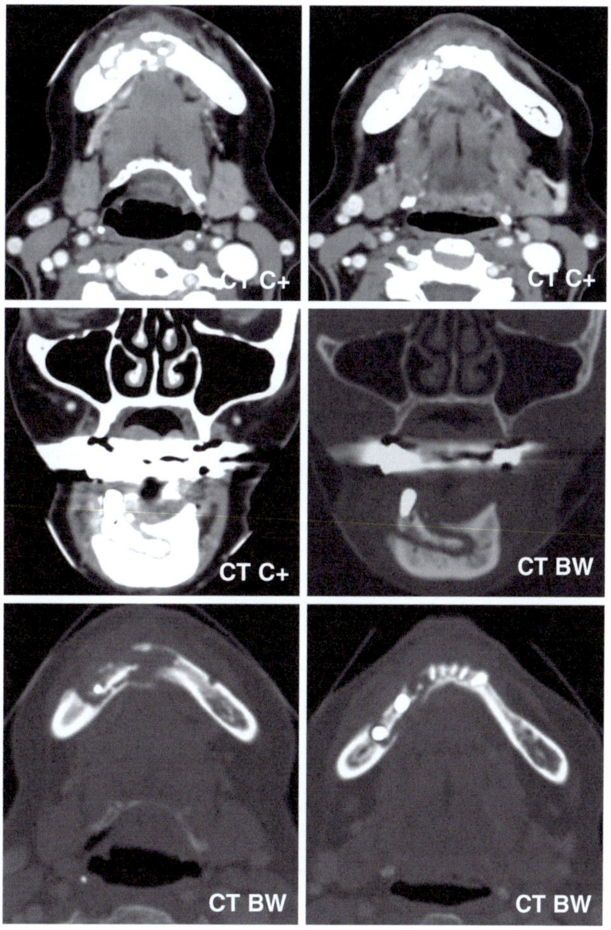

A. Haouimi et al., *Head and Neck Radiology Spot Diagnosis*,
https://doi.org/10.1007/978-3-032-14553-6_181

Findings

Right hemi-mandibular arch shows segmental osteolytic changes. The lesion shows a central detached sequestrum containing the prosthetic dental implants. Induration of perimandibular soft tissues without any abscess formation.

Diagnosis

Chronic mandibular osteomyelitis.

Discussion

Mandibular osteomyelitis is caused by bacterial infection. The predisposing factors include trauma, periapical abscesses, and inadequately treated periodontal disease. *Staphylococcus aureus* is the primary pathogen involved. Fungal osteomyelitis is uncommon and typically occurs in immunocompromised individuals.

Chronic mandibular osteomyelitis arises from unresolved acute infection and often presents with persistent swelling, draining sinus tracts, and sequestrum formation. Besides the discharging sinus, complications may include local spread to adjacent facial bones and pathological fractures. Chronic sclerotic forms of osteomyelitis can cause osteocondensation.

Laboratory findings often show elevated inflammatory markers such as CRP, ESR, and WBC count. Plain radiographs can reveal lytic lesions with periosteal reaction and sequestra in chronic cases. CT imaging is useful to delineate the extent of the lesion, while MRI provides superior visualization of soft-tissue involvement and bone marrow edema.

Common Differential Diagnosis

- Fibrous dysplasia: frosty ground glass swelling, cortical thinning, no sequestrum.
- Ossifying fibroma: radiolucent to radiopaque, no sequestrum, thin lucent fibrous capsule/periphery.
- Langerhans cell histiocytosis: punched-out lytic lesion, systemic, younger age.

Management Options

Multidisciplinary approach involves stomatologists, dentists, and infectious disease specialists. Prolonged antibiotherapy guided by microbiological findings. Surgical procedures include abscess drainage, sequestrectomy, and bone graft in severe cases.

References and Further Reading

1. Lucidarme Q, et al. Chronic osteomyelitis of the jaw: pivotal role of microbiological investigation and multidisciplinary management. Antibiotics. 2022. https://doi.org/10.3390/antibiotics11050568. Accessed 30 May 2024.
2. Mehra H. Chronic suppurative osteomyelitis of mandible. Craniomaxillofac Trauma Reconstr. 2013. https://doi.org/10.1055/s-0033-1343781. Epub 2013 May 31. PMID: 24436759; PMCID: PMC3773067. Accessed 31 May 2024.

Case 182

182

Clinical History

A 68-year-old man presented with stridor.

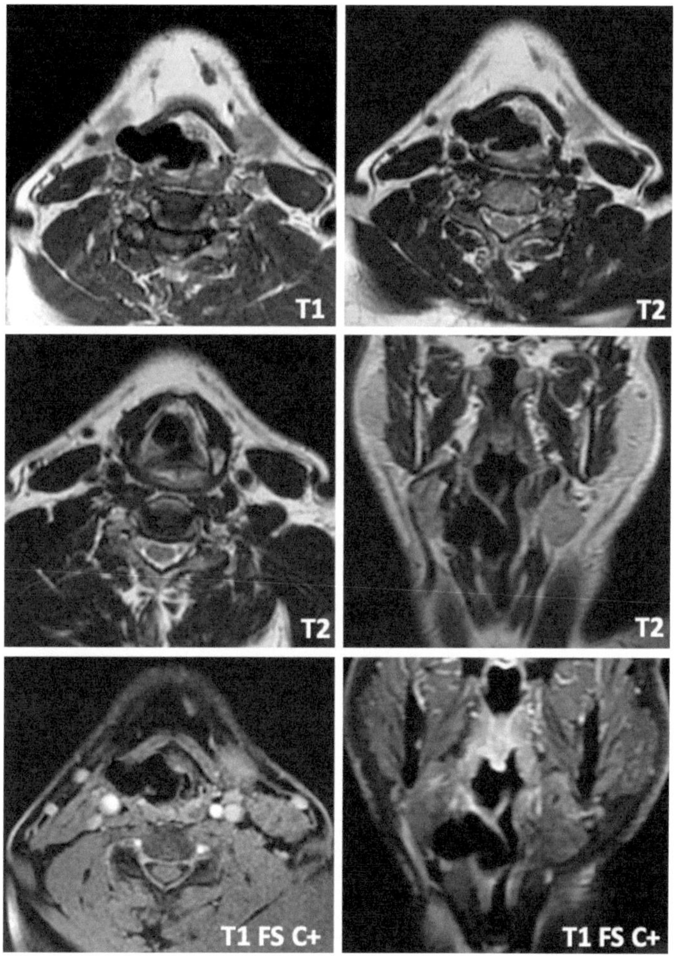

A. Haouimi et al., *Head and Neck Radiology Spot Diagnosis*,
https://doi.org/10.1007/978-3-032-14553-6_182

Findings

A small outpouching of the laryngeal lumen continuous with a narrowed endoluminal air column through the right thyrohyoid membrane. The extraluminal component is in contact with the inferomedial aspect of the right submandibular gland. No enhancement, no endoluminal lesion, nor any cervical adenopathy.

Diagnosis

Right lateral mixed laryngocele.

Discussion

Laryngoceles are benign dilatation of saccule of laryngeal ventricle, resulting in an outpouching of laryngeal mucosa through the thyrohyoid membrane. Most laryngoceles are acquired. Chronically raised intraglottic pressure in chronic coughers, professional wind blowers, musicians, and constipated patients predisposes to this condition. A prompt search for any underlying obstructive neoplastic lesion in the laryngeal ventricle needs to be ruled out in case of secondary laryngoceles.

Clinically, patients can present with a change of voice, hoarseness, stridor, dysphagia, as well as the sensation of a cervical lump which increases with straining and coughing.

Plain X-ray can show an outpouching of the air column in the upper cervical para-laryngeal soft tissues. CT shows a thin-walled air or fluid-filled cystic lesion. MRI may be useful for soft tissue differentiation and tumor detection in cases of secondary laryngocele.

Common Differential Diagnosis

- Thyroglossal duct cyst: embedded at strap muscles, no laryngeal luminal communication.
- Branchial cleft cyst: at mandibular angle, no laryngeal luminal communication.
- Lateral hypopharyngeal pouch: arising from lateral hypopharyngeal wall, not from larynx.

Management Options

Infected laryngoceles are managed with antibiotics. However, microlaryngoscopic excision, CO_2 laser resection, and open surgical excision are considered on a case-by-case basis.

References and Further Reading

1. Elfeky M, et al. Laryngocele. Radiopaedia.org. 2025. https://doi.org/10.53347/rID-1568. Accessed 22 July 2025.
2. Lu P. Laryngocele. Radiopaedia.org. 2025. https://doi.org/10.53347/rID-163116. Accessed 22 July 2025.

Case 183

183

Clinical History

A 60-year-old man presented with a right submandibular mass and difficulty in swallowing. History of smoking for the last 40 years.

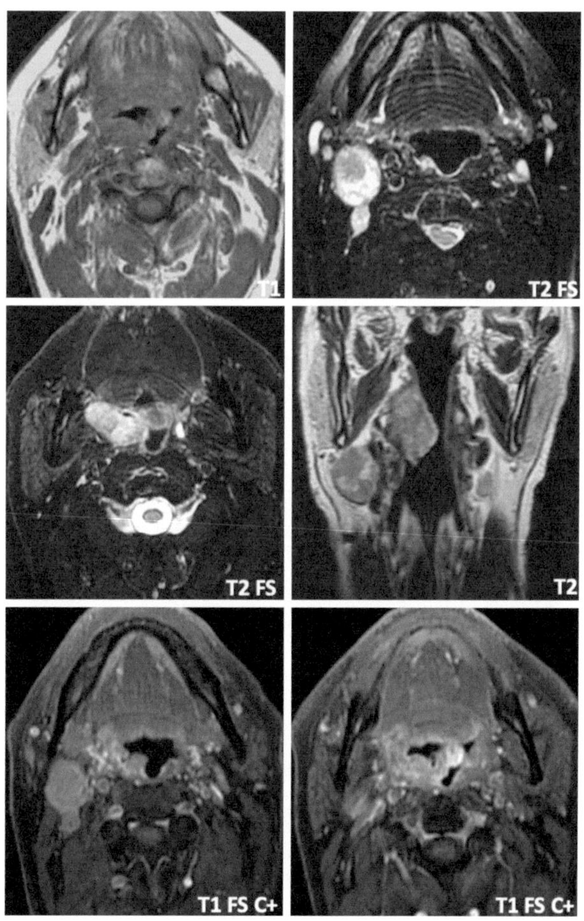

A. Haouimi et al., *Head and Neck Radiology Spot Diagnosis*,
https://doi.org/10.1007/978-3-032-14553-6_183

Findings

An irregular nonhomogeneous soft tissue lesion showing intermediate signal on T1 and high signal on T2 with marked heterogeneous enhancement involving the right palatine tonsil. Anterolateral extension to the pterygomandibular raphe. Locoregional extension into the right glossotonsillar sulcus. A partially necrotic ipsilateral level II lymph node with heterogeneous enhancement.

Diagnosis

Right palatine tonsil carcinoma with metastatic lymphadenopathy.

Discussion

Palatine tonsil cancers are a subset of oropharyngeal cancer originating from tonsillar tissue. Squamous cell carcinomas are by far the most common type with a male predominance.

Clinically, patients present with persistent sore throat, odynophagia, trismus, and retroauricular pain. Ipsilateral level II lymphadenopathy can occasionally be the only symptom.

Tobacco, alcohol, and HPV infection are predisposing factors. Imaging helps in the initial evaluation, staging, and management. Both enhanced CT and MRI show the lesion as an enlarged, exophytic, irregular, ill-defined mass along the lateral oropharyngeal wall with luminal narrowing. The lesions are epicentered in the tonsillar fossa and may show an invasive deep margin. Enlarged cervical lymph nodes can be necrotic and cystic and advanced cases can show bony involvement. MRI can better assess the invasion of the tongue base, as well as adjacent parapharyngeal and neurovascular involvement. As a rule of thumb, unilateral cervical level II lesions in an adult should be considered neoplastic until proven otherwise.

Common Differential Diagnosis

- Tonsillar lymphoid hyperplasia: bilateral, symmetric, no locoregional invasion.
- Tonsillar abscess: acute, febrile, retropharyngeal nodes, smooth, regular ring enhancement.
- Benign mixed tumor: marked T2 hyperintensity, well defined, calcification +/−.

Management Options

Treatment may include surgery, radiation, or chemotherapy.

References and Further Reading

1. Di Muzio B. Palatine tonsil squamous cell carcinoma. Radiopaedia.org. 2015. https://doi.org/10.53347/rID-37909. Accessed 22 Jan 2025.
2. Williamson AJ, Mullangi S, Gajra A. Tonsil cancer. Stat Pearls Publishing; 2023. https://www.ncbi.nlm.nih.gov/books/NBK537238. Accessed 22 Jan 2025.

Case 184

184

Clinical History

A 65-year-old man presented with a sensation of fullness in the right ear with hearing loss, positional vertigo, tinnitus, and foul-smelling otorrhea. Positive Hennbert sign.

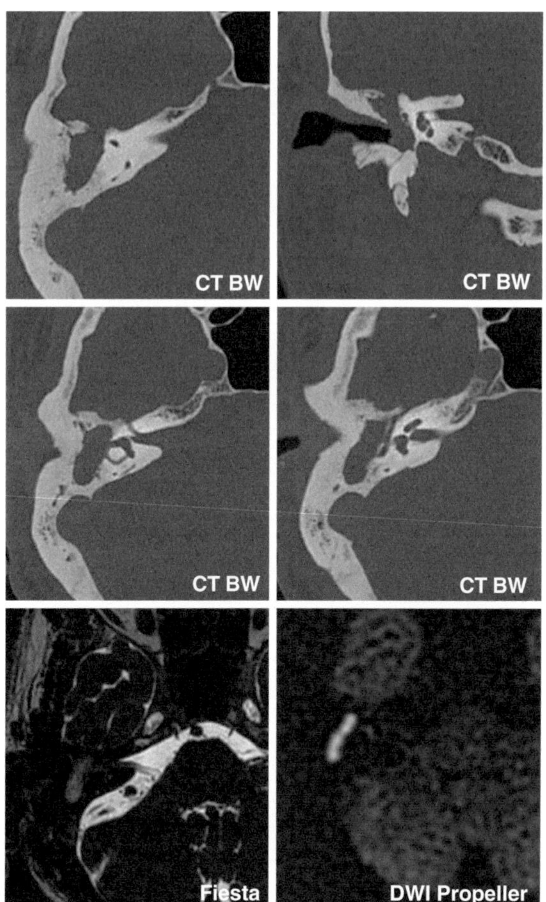

A. Haouimi et al., *Head and Neck Radiology Spot Diagnosis*,
https://doi.org/10.1007/978-3-032-14553-6_184

Findings

Complete soft-tissue opacity of the right middle ear with destruction of the ossicular chain. Lysis of anterior wall of the attic, tegmen tympani, as well as the bony wall of the lateral semicircular canal and the bony margins of the tympanic portion of the facial nerve. Restricted diffusion is noted involving the mass.

Diagnosis

Cholesteatoma with labyrinthine fistula.

Discussion

Cholesteatomas can be both acquired and congenital (epidermoid), mostly seen in children without history of chronic infection. Acquired cholesteatomas arise due to Eustachian tube dysfunction, chronic infection, and trauma. The lesions are benign with locally destructive features. The bony erosion is the result of the accumulation of a collection of abnormal keratinized squamous epithelium and waxy debris within the pneumatized temporal bone and middle ear, as well as from the production of collagenases.

Clinically, patients present with hearing deficit, foul-smelling otorrhea, and tinnitus. Bony erosion of the labyrinth and facial nerve canal can lead to facial numbness/paralysis.

High-resolution CT reveals nonenhancing soft-tissue mass with bony erosion often originating from Prussak's space and associated erosion of the scutum. The restricted diffusion on MRI is characteristic. MRI helps to rule out soft-tissue extension, including intracranial involvement.

Common Differential Diagnosis

- Chronic otitis media: No restricted diffusion, no bony erosion.
- Glomic tumor: hypervascularized lesion with typical "salt and pepper" appearance.
- Cholesterol granuloma: high signal T1, no restricted diffusion, mostly at petrous apex.

Management Options

Surgical resection. Interval monitoring for signs of recurrence.

References and Further Reading

1. Castle JT. Cholesteatoma pearls: practical points and update. Head Neck Pathol. 2018. https://doi.org/10.1007/s12105-018-0915-5. Epub 2018 Aug 1. PMID: 30069838; PMCID: PMC6081285. Accessed 30 Sept 2025.
2. Gaillard F, et al. Cholesteatoma. Radiopaedia.org. 2024. https://doi.org/10.53347/rID-1116. Accessed 25 Jan 2025.

Case 185

185

Clinical History

A 45-year-old woman known for left chronic otitis media. Suspicion of cholesteatoma on ENT exam.

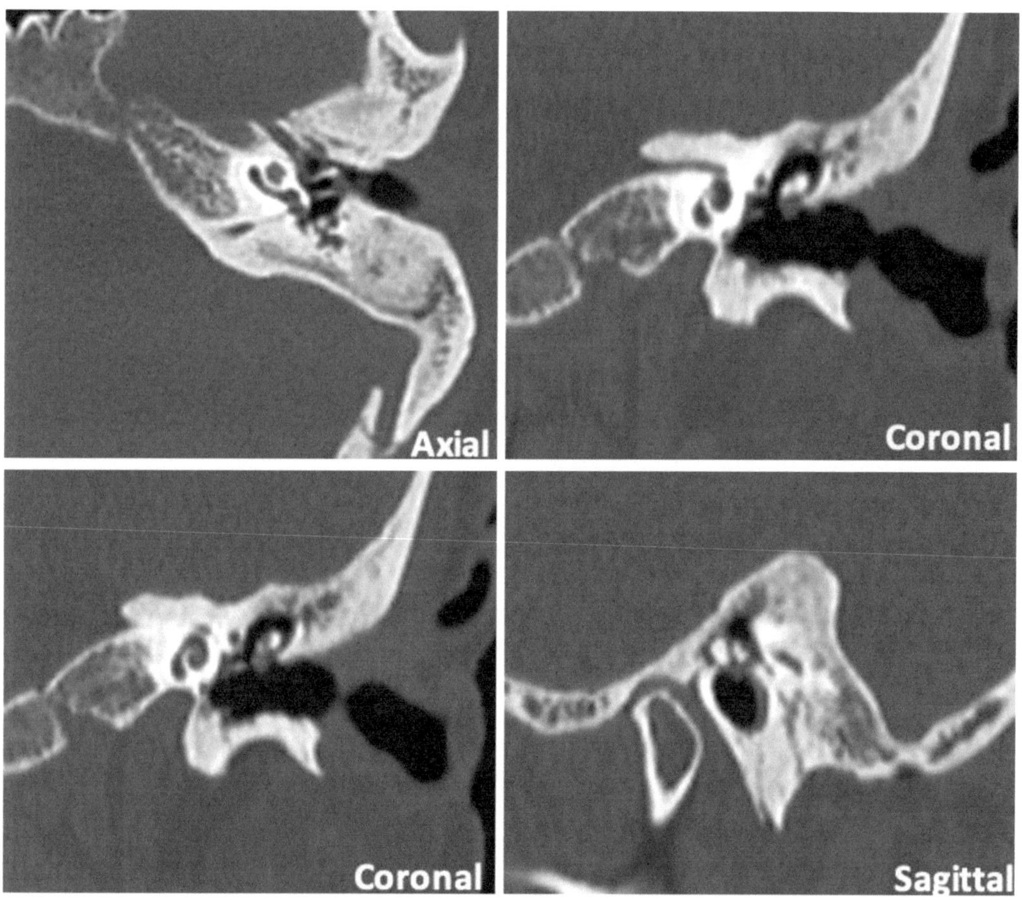

A. Haouimi et al., *Head and Neck Radiology Spot Diagnosis*,
https://doi.org/10.1007/978-3-032-14553-6_185

Findings

Stigmata of left tympanoplasty. A round epitympanic inflammatory soft-tissue opacity between the promontory and the posterior wall of the external acoustic meatus. Slight displacement of long process of incus. Erosion of scutum and bony ossicles.

Diagnosis

Pearl cholesteatoma.

Discussion

Cholesteatomas are benign but locally aggressive collections of keratinized squamous epithelium in an abnormal location. If left untreated, it can cause adjacent bony erosion including the ossicles, cochlea, and semicircular canals. It can cause locoregional invasion to the adjacent mastoid and in advanced cases, intracranial involvement. Macroscopically, they are soft-tissue waxy lesions with a pearly white appearance.

Most cholesteatomas are acquired and result of abnormal Eustachian tube function, which can lead to negative middle ear pressure. This in turn can cause a retraction of the tympanic membrane (often of the thinner pars flaccida portion), which leads to the migration of squamous epithelium and keratin debris into the middle ear.

Clinically, patients present with hearing loss. Vertigo and facial weakness can arise if there is associated labyrinthine fistula and erosion of facial nerve canal, respectively.

High-resolution CT in bone algorithm provides excellent anatomical detail for surgical planning. MRI shows restricted diffusion and can identify the soft-tissue involvement and rule out intracranial extension.

Common Differential Diagnosis

- CSOM: no bony erosion, effusion, or restricted diffusion.
- Glomus tumor: vascular-enhancing lesion.
- Cholesterol granuloma: clinical, retrotympanic “blue” mass.

Management Options

Surgery.

References and Further Reading

1. Baráth K, et al. Neuroradiology of cholesteatomas. Am J Neuroradiol. 2011. https://doi.org/10.3174/ajnr.A2052. Accessed 30 Apr 2024.
2. Castle JT. Cholesteatoma pearls: practical points and update. Head Neck Pathol. 2018. https://doi.org/10.1007/s12105-018-0915-5. Epub 2018 Aug 1. PMID: 30069838; PMCID: PMC6081285. Accessed 30 Apr 2024.
3. Gaillard F, et al. Cholesteatoma. Radiopaedia.org. 2024. https://doi.org/10.53347/rID-1116. Accessed 25 Jan 2025.

Case 186

186

Clinical History

A 70-year-old man presented with a history of mixed type of hearing loss on the left side, autophony, disequilibrium, and sound-induced vertigo.

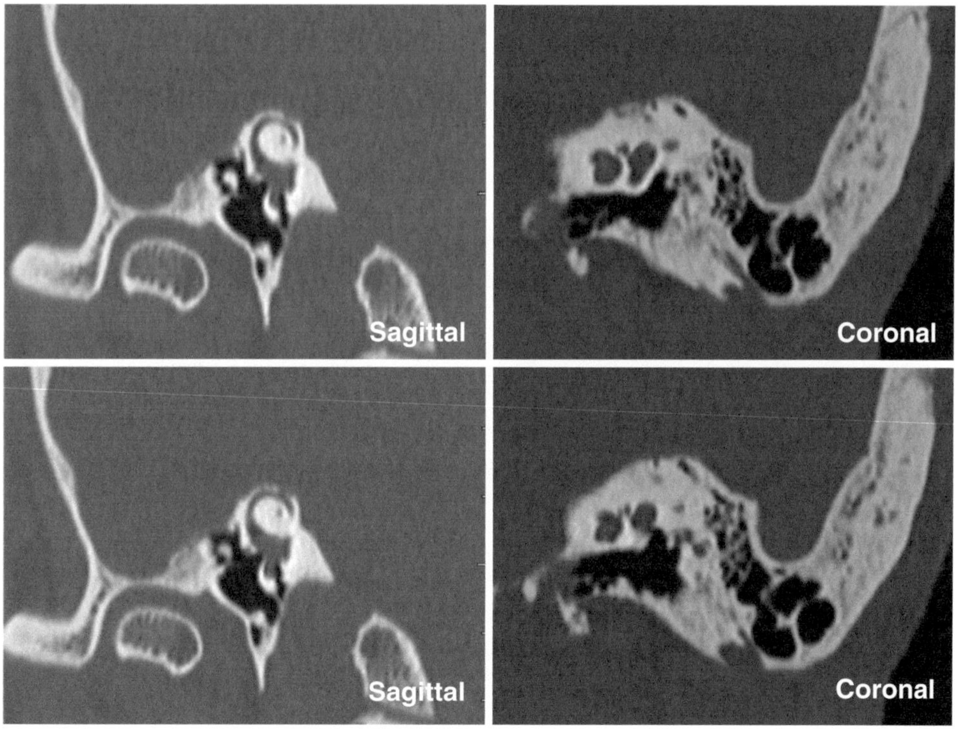

A. Haouimi et al., *Head and Neck Radiology Spot Diagnosis*,
https://doi.org/10.1007/978-3-032-14553-6_186

Findings

Defect at the bony roof of the superior semicircular canal.

Diagnosis

Dehiscent superior semicircular canal.

Discussion

Dehiscence of the superior semicircular canal refers to the presence of a bony defect at the roof of the superior semicircular canal. It can significantly affect the quality of life. This abnormal "third window" creates an additional pathway for pressure and sound transmission, causing abnormal stimulation of the vestibular system and direct communication of inner ear and cranial cavity. Dehiscent semicircular canal can be either congenital due to incomplete ossification of bony labyrinth or acquired from chronic increased intracranial pressure, barotrauma, or as a complication of cholesteatoma. Conditions such as osteogenesis imperfecta and Paget disease can predispose to this condition.

Clinically, the patient may present with Tullio phenomenon (sound-induced vertigo) with positive Hennebert sign (pressure-induced vertigo), oscillopsia, and autophony. Nonspecific symptoms like vertigo, tinnitus, disequilibrium, fullness of the ear, and hearing loss often coexist.

High-resolution CT in bone algorithm is the gold standard in diagnosing the defect at the roof of superior semicircular canal (up to <5 mm dehiscence). The MRI can show the fluid signal continuity through the defect and is mainly indicated to rule out conditions such as perilymphatic fistula and vestibular schwannoma.

Common Differential Diagnosis

- Normal variation: clinically silent.
- Large vestibular aqueduct syndrome: enlarged endolymphatic sac and duct, no Tullio phenomenon.
- Meniere's disease: hydrops +/−, episodic vertigo, intact semicircular canal.

Management Options

Mild cases are managed conservatively (avoiding the triggers). Surgery is reserved for severe, debilitating cases to stabilize hearing and to improve vestibular symptoms.

References and Further Reading

1. Campos A, et al. Superior semicircular canal dehiscence syndrome. Radiopaedia.org. 2025. https://doi.org/10.53347/rID-12317. Accessed 20 July 2025.
2. Thibodeau R. Superior semicircular canal dehiscence. Radiopaedia.org. 2023. https://doi.org/10.53347/rID-166543. Accessed on 25 Jan 2025.

Case 187

187

Clinical History

A 2-year-old girl with left-sided leukocoria.

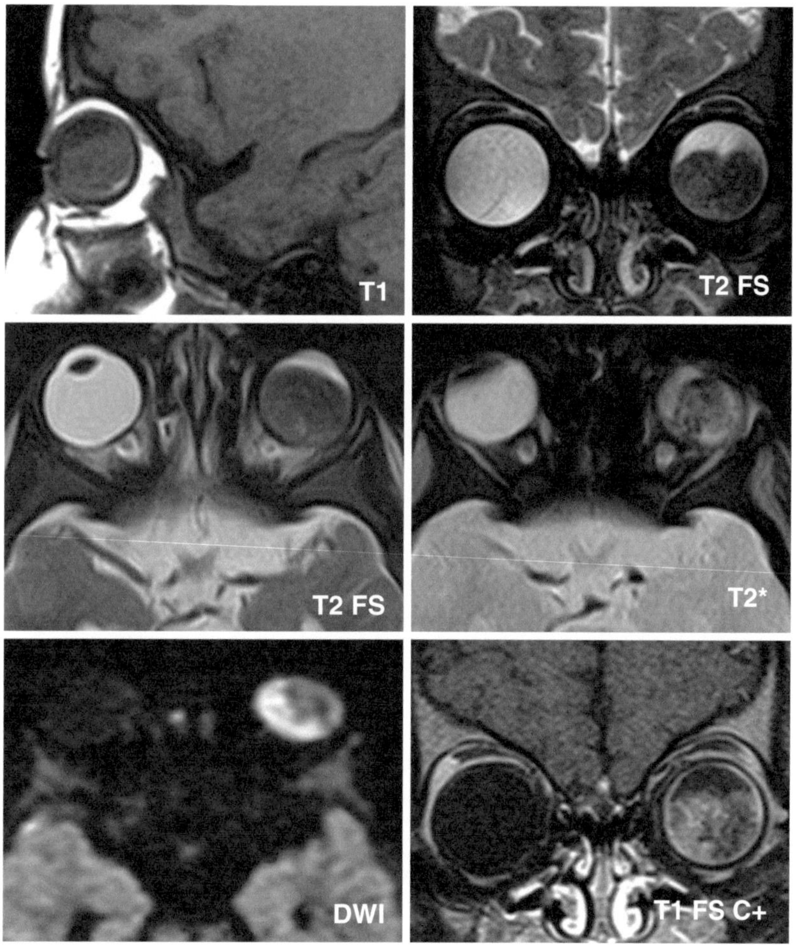

A. Haouimi et al., *Head and Neck Radiology Spot Diagnosis*,
https://doi.org/10.1007/978-3-032-14553-6_187

Findings

A well-defined left intraocular soft-tissue mass showing intermediate signal on T1 and homogeneously low signal on T2. Intralesional speckled hypointensities on T2* representing calcifications and showing restricted diffusion on DWI. Moderate heterogeneous enhancement without any cystic component. Linear enhancement beyond the margins of the lesion, suggesting possible choroidal involvement.

Diagnosis

Retinoblastoma.

Discussion

Retinoblastomas are the most common intraocular malignant tumor of childhood. The lesions arise from neuroectodermal cells of the retina and most of the tumors show both endophytic and exophytic growth into the vitreous chamber and the subretinal space, respectively. The infiltrative growth along the retina can cause retinal detachment as well as vitreous and subretinal tumor seeding.

Most children with retinoblastoma seem well, but the parents often notice a white glow in the center of their eye (leukocoria) and squinting (strabismus). They can also complain of "cat's eye" reflecting light.

Calcification is a key diagnostic feature. Though CT can better detect calcification, due to exposure to ionizing radiation, ultrasound has replaced CT. MRI is the modality of choice. The lesion is slightly hyperintense on T1 and hypointense on T2. Intralesional calcifications may show as a signal void on T2*. The lesions show restricted diffusion and heterogeneous enhancement; the necrotic components do not enhance.

Common Differential Diagnosis

- Coat disease: no calcification, retinal detachment, high signal on both T1 and T2.
- Retinopathy of prematurity: small, hyperintense, often bilateral, calcification ++.
- Coloboma: vitreous herniation through posterior defect.

Management Options

Intravenous chemotherapy remains the standard care for bilateral cases. Advanced unilateral cases are treated intraarterially by experienced neuroradiologists.

References and Further Reading

1. Haouimi A. Retinoblastoma. Radiopaedia.org. 2020. https://doi.org/10.53347/rID-78680. Accessed 1 Sept 2022.
2. Silvera VM, et al. Retinoblastoma. AJNR Am J Neuroradiol. 2021. https://doi.org/10.3174/ajnr.A6949. Epub 2021 Jan 28. PMID: 33509920; PMCID. Accessed 15 Apr 2023.

Case 188

188

Clinical History

A 40-year-old normotensive woman presented with a right earache, pulsatile tinnitus, and aural filling for the last 8 months.

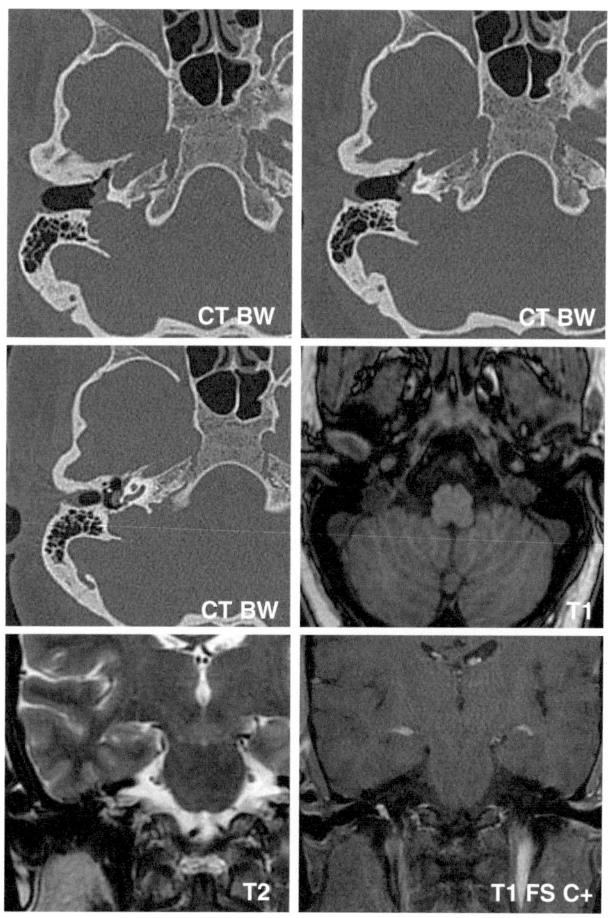

A. Haouimi et al., *Head and Neck Radiology Spot Diagnosis*,
https://doi.org/10.1007/978-3-032-14553-6_188

Findings

A lobulated soft tissue hypodense lesion of the right middle ear with mild ossicular erosion. Intact floor of the middle ear and bony wall of jugular foramen. On MRI, the lesion appears hypointense on T1, occupying both the epi- and mesotympanic regions, and isosignal on T2, neighboring the cochlear promontory. The lesion appears hypervascular with intense enhancement without extension toward jugular vein.

Diagnosis

Tympanic paraganglioma.

Discussion

Tympanic paragangliomas are the most common middle ear tumors. They are a distinct entity from glomus jugulare paragangliomas and are characterized by their smaller size and are confined to the middle ear. These indolent benign neuroendocrine tumors arise from tympanic cavity paraganglia neighboring Jacobson nerve and the cochlear promontory. They can rarely develop malignant potential.

Clinically, patients may be asymptomatic or present with unilateral otalgia, pulsatile tinnitus, and conductive hearing loss.

An intensely enhancing vascular mass neighboring the cochlear promontory with preservation of adjacent bony structures, including the floor of the middle ear in the appropriate clinical context is highly suggestive of tympanic paraganglioma.

Common Differential Diagnosis

- Glomus jugular: involve jugular bulb, permeative destruction of floor of middle ear.
- Facial schwannoma: pedunculated and connected to facial nerve, not hypervascular.
- Cholesterol granuloma: hyperdense, no enhancement.

Management Options

Surgery for symptomatic patients often after presurgical embolization. Radiotherapy is reserved only for inoperable cases or after recurrence.

References and Further Reading

1. Neto ME, et al. Tympanic paragangliomas: case reports. Braz J Otorhinolaryngol. 2005. https://doi.org/10.1016/s1808-8694(15)31293-3. Epub 2006 Jan 2. PMID: 16446900; PMCID: PMC9443525. Accessed 15 Jan 2025.
2. Sweeney AD, Carlson ML. Tympanic paraganglioma. In: Wanna G, Carlson M, Netterville J, editors. Contemporary management of jugular paraganglioma. Cham: Springer; 2018. https://doi.org/10.1007/978-3-319-60955-3_11. Accessed 15 Jan 2025.

Case 189

Clinical History

A 40-year-old man presented with an indolent lateral neck mass.

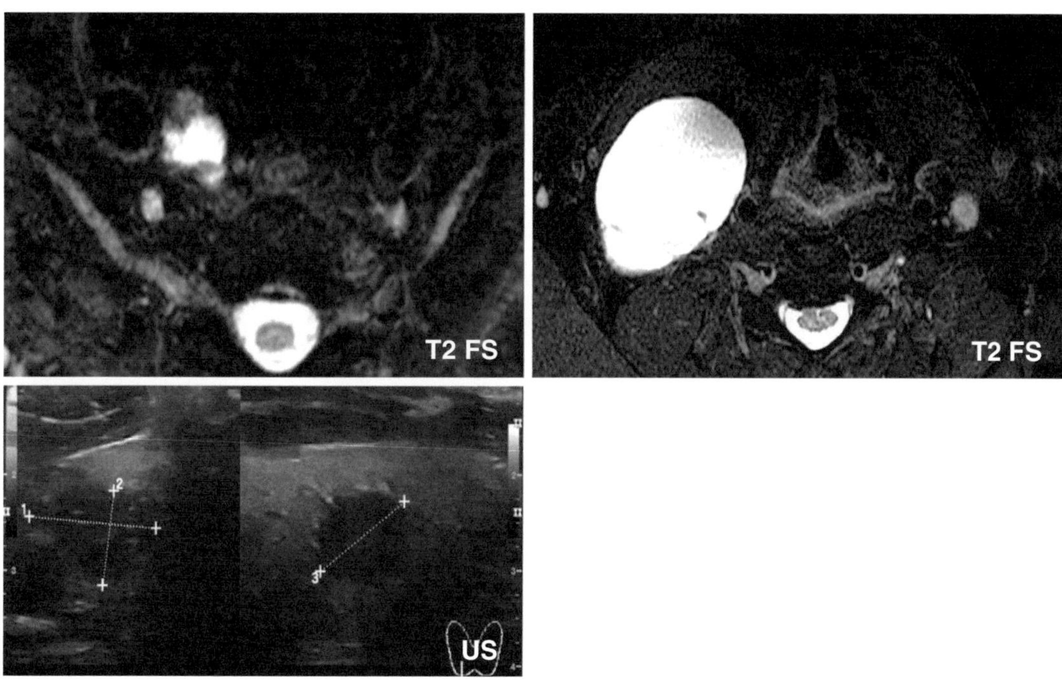

A. Haouimi et al., *Head and Neck Radiology Spot Diagnosis*,
https://doi.org/10.1007/978-3-032-14553-6_189

Findings

MRI shows multiple T2 high-signal cystic lymph nodes along the right jugular chain. They are extended from level II (A) to the mediastinum, with paratracheal and perithyroidal involvement. Ultrasound reveals an ill-defined hypoechoic thyroid nodule with intrinsic punctate echogenic foci.

Diagnosis

Papillary thyroid cancer.

Discussion

Papillary carcinoma of thyroid is the most prevalent type of thyroid cancer, representing approximately 80% of all thyroid malignancies. These tumors are slow growing and can remain limited to the thyroid tissue for extended periods. The highest incidence occurs around 40 years of age, with a higher frequency in females. Lymph node metastasis develops more rapidly in the papillary subtype compared to the follicular variant, yet long-term mortality remains low even in the presence of nodal involvement. In adults, any newly found cystic mass in the lateral neck should prompt suspicion for metastatic thyroid or tonsillar carcinoma, as cystic lymph node metastases may appear before the primary tumor is detected.

Ultrasound is the imaging modality of choice for detecting and evaluating thyroid nodules, proving superior to CT and MRI. The Thyroid Imaging Reporting and Data System (TI-RADS) score aids in determining appropriate management based on sonographic features. CT and MRI are useful for assessing tracheal invasion and for staging purposes.

Common Differential Diagnosis

- Branchial cleft cyst: single cystic neck mass, diagnosis of exclusion in adults.
- Thyroglossal duct cyst: typically, midline, no calcification, moves with swallowing.
- Cystic metastas3is of thyroid: known cancer, microcalcification, mural nodule, septations.

Management Options

Radioiodine nuclear medicine studies, including I-131 and I-123-MIBG, are effective for imaging and treatment of different thyroid cancer subtypes. Depending on subtype and staging, options range from active surveillance to total thyroidectomy.

References and Further Reading

1. King AD. Imaging for staging and management of thyroid cancer. Cancer Imaging. 2008. https://doi.org/10.1102/1470-7330.2008.0007. PMID: 18390389; PMCID: PMC2324369. Accessed 15 Apr 2025.
2. Tessler FN, et al. ACR thyroid imaging, reporting and data system (TI-RADS): white paper of the ACR TI-RADS Committee. J Am Coll Radiol. 2017. https://doi.org/10.1016/j.jacr.2017.01.046. Epub 2017 Apr 2. PMID: 28372962. Accessed 15 Apr 2025.

Case 190

190

Clinical History

A 19-year-old man presented with periorbital swelling and a bumpy protrusion from the right forehead.

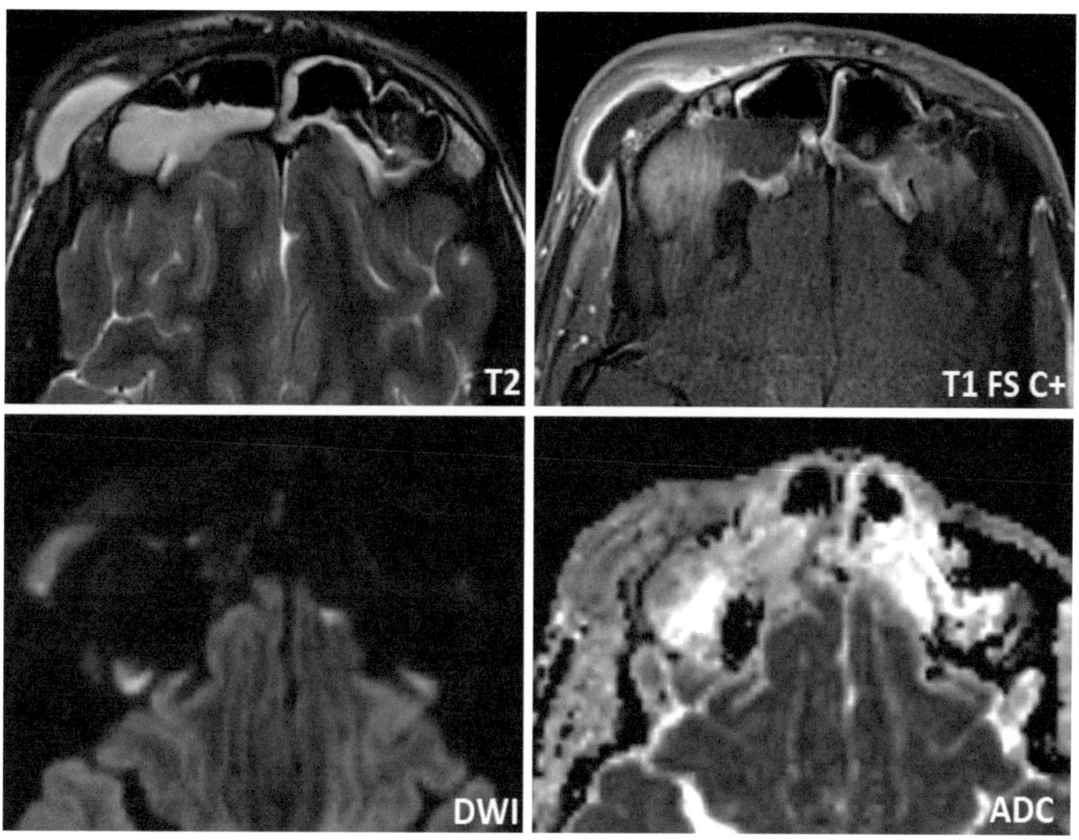

A. Haouimi et al., *Head and Neck Radiology Spot Diagnosis*,
https://doi.org/10.1007/978-3-032-14553-6_190

Findings

Right frontal sinusitis with an air-fluid level on MRI. Extension of the lesion across the external table into the subgaleal soft tissues, showing a collection in the right forehead. The collection shows peripheral rim enhancement and central restricted diffusion.

Diagnosis

Pott's puffy tumor.

Discussion

Pott's puffy tumor is a non-neoplastic pathology and hence a misnomer. It is a complication of acute sinusitis. Very rarely, it can also be a complication of mastoiditis. With the advent of antibiotics, its incidence has drastically reduced.

The lesion is characterized by extension of frontal sinusitis through the anterior table of the frontal bone into the subgaleal and subperiosteal soft tissues. The spread is either through venous drainage channels or direct extension through the bone. Its posterior intracranial extension can lead to complications such as subdural empyema, meningitis, and brain abscess.

Clinically, patients are often febrile and present with indolent, fluctuant, reddish forehead swelling with tenderness. Mental confusion, seizures, and the signs of meningeal irritation suggest intracranial extension. The forehead collection often evolves into an abscess with associated osteomyelitis.

CT scan often shows the signs of frontal sinusitis with stranding and swelling of the overlying scalp. The anterior wall defect of the frontal sinus can also be documented on CT scan. Postcontrast CT delineates abscess formation. Enhanced MRI is the investigation of choice to rule out intracranial complications including cerebritis, empyema, and cerebral abscess.

Common Differential Diagnosis

- Scalp hematoma: known clinical history.
- Soft tissue abscess: no sinusitis.
- Frontal sinus mucocele: nontender, nonfebrile.

Management Options

Antibiotics and emergency surgical drainage are required. Secondary obliteration of the sinus with adipose tissue is the mainstay to prevent recurrence.

References and Further Reading

1. Gaillard F, et al. Pott puffy tumour. Radiopaedia.org. 2010. https://doi.org/10.53347/rID-4895. Accessed 6 Mar 2025.
2. Masterson L, Leong P. Pott's puffy tumour: a forgotten complication of frontal sinus disease. Oral Maxillofac Surg. 2009. https://doi.org/10.1007/s10006-009-0155-7. PMID: 19352731. Accessed 6 Mar 2025.

191

Clinical History

A 40-year-old man presented with tinnitus. Pure tone audiogram revealed right-sided sensorineural hearing loss.

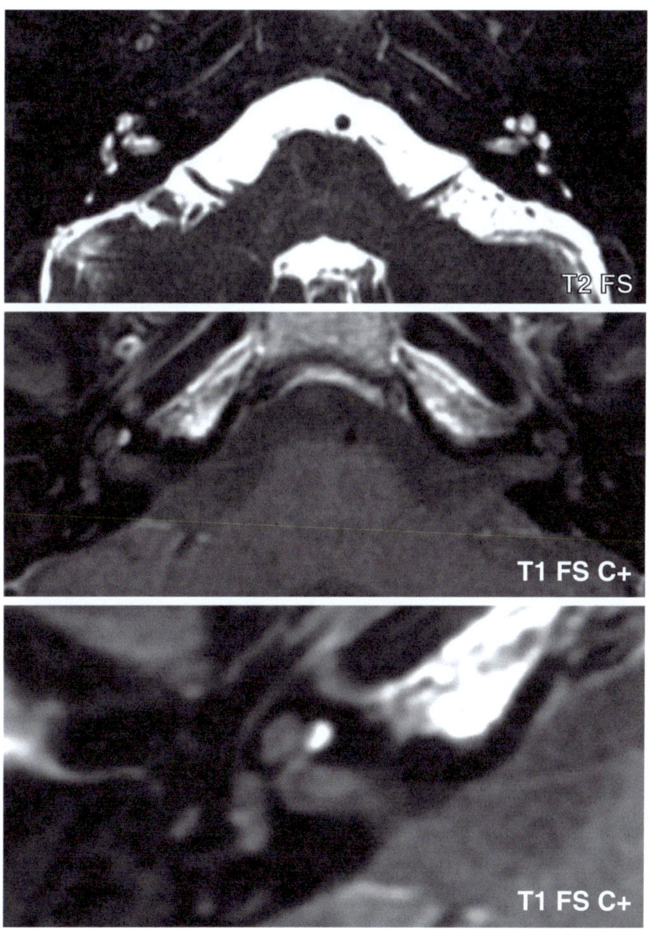

A. Haouimi et al., *Head and Neck Radiology Spot Diagnosis*,
https://doi.org/10.1007/978-3-032-14553-6_191

Findings

High-resolution MRI shows a focal T2 low signal at the anterior aspect of the basal turn of the right cochlea on a fat-suppression sequence. Intense postcontrast enhancement of the lesion.

Diagnosis

Intracochlear schwannoma.

Discussion

Isolated intracochlear schwannomas are rare benign lesions arising from cochlear Schwann cells. These are a subtype of intralabyrinthine schwannomas, often involving the modiolus or scalae, sparing the vestibular nerve with no malignant potential. They represent <1% of all internal ear tumors. Pathologically, they are identical to other schwannomas with Antoni A and B regions and S-100 protein positivity.

Most patients are clinically silent and discovered incidentally. Some patients may present with gradual sensorineural hearing loss. Rarely, acute onset hearing loss can mimic acute labyrinthitis. Intracochlear schwannomas are often misdiagnosed as idiopathic hearing loss. MRI is the investigation of choice and can identify the lesion as a well-defined enhancing intracochlear mass. A diagnosis of intracochlear schwannoma must be considered in any case of labyrinthine enhancement and needs follow-up. The labyrinthine enhancement often disappears on follow-up examinations in acute labyrinthitis, whereas the enhancement in intracochlear schwannomas persists and may continue to grow. Erosion and enlargement of the cochlear scalae on high-resolution CT are indirect signs. Audiometry often confirms sensorineural hearing loss.

Common Differential Diagnosis

- Acute labyrinthitis: no filling defect of endo/perilymph on high-resolution T2 (e.g., SPACE/FIESTA).
- Intralabyrinthine lipoma: hyperintense signal on T1.
- Intralabyrinthine hemorrhage: clinical history, signal depends on the age of blood products.

Management Options

Treatment options for intracochlear schwannomas include surgery or stereotactic radiosurgery, depending on size and growth.

References and Further Reading

1. Salzman KL, et al. Intralabyrinthine schwannomas: imaging diagnosis and classification. AJNR Am J Neuroradiol. 2012. https://doi.org/10.3174/ajnr.A2712. Epub 2011 Dec 8. PMID: 22158921; PMCID: PMC7966166. Accessed 12 Aug 2025.
2. Weerakkody Y, et al. Intracochlear schwannoma. Radiopaedia.org. 2023. https://doi.org/10.53347/rID-98098. Accessed 6 Mar 2025.

Case 192

192

Clinical History

A 70-year-old man presented with general malaise, fatigue, headaches, and sinus infections. CT images are from another 50-year-old man with similar complaints in the late stage.

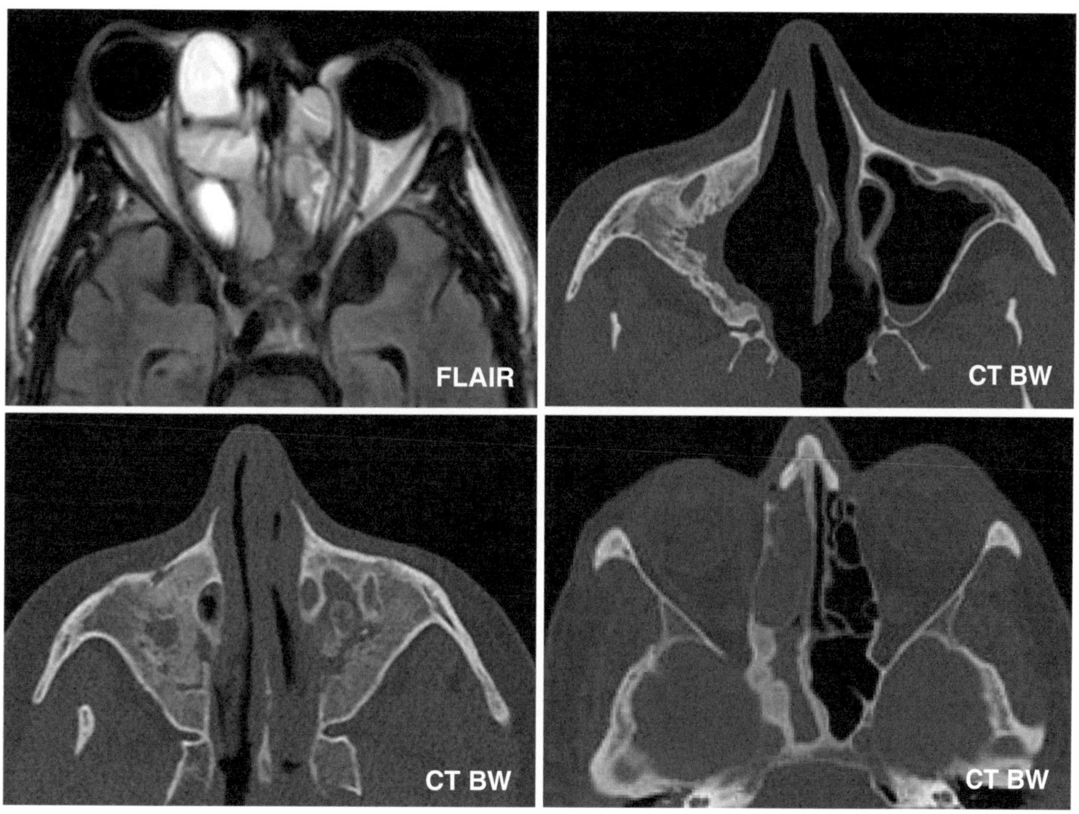

A. Haouimi et al., *Head and Neck Radiology Spot Diagnosis*,
https://doi.org/10.1007/978-3-032-14553-6_192

Findings

Multiple mucoceles in the paranasal sinuses secondary to sinonasal mucosal thickening with right proptosis (early stage). Sclerotic bone thickening with bone destruction of the paranasal sinuses in advanced stage on CT in the other patient (advanced stage).

Diagnosis

Granulomatosis with polyangiitis (GPA).

Discussion

GPA is a multisystem c-ANCA-positive vasculitis affecting the medium- and small-sized vessels. The hallmark features include noncaseating necrotizing granulomas and pauci-immune vasculitis, most commonly affecting the upper respiratory tract, lungs, and kidneys. The typical clinical triad includes respiratory tract inflammation (sinusitis, lung nodules, diffuse alveolar hemorrhage), systemic vasculitis, and glomerulonephritis.

In the early stages of GPA, the patients often present with upper respiratory tract involvement and are often mistaken for sinusitis. On CT, this can be seen as diffuse or nodular mucosal thickening with bony involvement progressing to inflammatory sclerotic bone thickening. Later, the findings become more destructive and include loss of the turbinates, septal perforation, and "saddle nose" deformity. On MRI, edema and granulomatous tissue are evidenced in the early stage with intense enhancement. In later stages, due to the presence of fibrosis, the soft tissue appears hypointense on T2. The granulomas with central necrosis may mimic malignancy.

Common Differential Diagnosis

- Early stages: acute or chronic sinusitis, fungal sinusitis, polyposis.
- Later stages: nasal septum perforation due to other inflammatory conditions such as syphilis or sarcoidosis, cocaine abuse, or destruction due to malignant disease.

Management Options

Corticosteroids and immunosuppressives to prevent relapses and antibiotics for secondary infections.

References and Further Reading

1. Gaillard F, et al. Granulomatosis with polyangiitis. Radiopaedia.org. 2024. https://doi.org/10.53347/rID-2285. Accessed 6 Mar 2025.
2. Guzman-Soto MI, et al. From head to toe: granulomatosis with polyangiitis. Radiographics. 2021. https://doi.org/10.1148/rg.2021210132. Epub 2021 Oct 15. PMID: 34652975. Accessed 9 June 2024.
3. Rout P, Garlapati P, Qurie A. Granulomatosis with polyangiitis. Stat Pearls Publishing; 2024. https://www.ncbi.nlm.nih.gov/books/NBK557827/. Accessed 6 Mar 2024.

Case 193

193

Clinical History

A 74-year-old man undergoing evaluation for TIA.

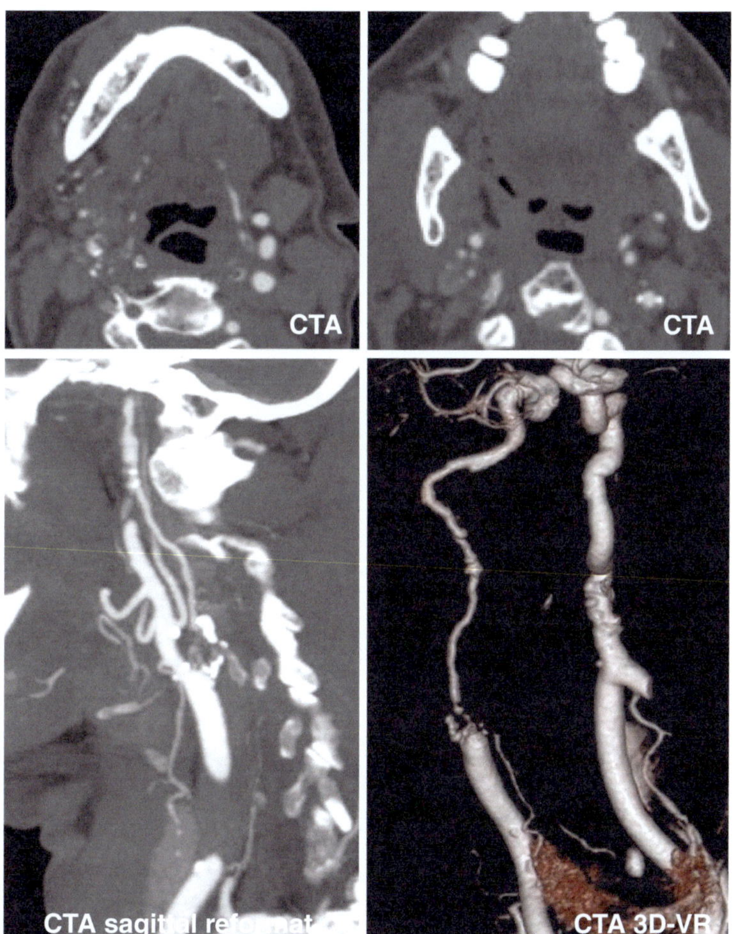

A. Haouimi et al., *Head and Neck Radiology Spot Diagnosis*,
https://doi.org/10.1007/978-3-032-14553-6_193

Findings

Near-complete vessel occlusion due to atherosclerotic plaque at the origin of the right ICA on CTA. The vessel lumen is collapsed distal to the plaque. MIP and VRT reformats further illustrate the ICA narrowing and poststenotic collapse.

Diagnosis

Carotid stenosis.

Discussion

Carotid stenosis is mostly caused by atherosclerosis, typically affecting the carotid bulb and/or the proximal segment of the ICA. Severe stenosis is referred to as "near-occlusion" when the post-stenotic arterial lumen is collapsed due to significantly reduced blood flow. The degree of stenosis is assessed by using the North American Symptomatic Carotid Endarterectomy Trial (NASCET) or European Carotid Surgery Trial (ECST) criteria.

Clinically, patients may remain asymptomatic if the compromised blood supply is compensated for by collateral circulation via the circle of Willis. Some patients may complain of TIA. The limb shaking and crescendo TIAs, as well as RIND, are considered as "red flags" in patients with carotid stenosis.

The stenosis may lead to stroke via atherothrombembolism. Major risk factors include hypertension, a higher degree of stenosis, and vulnerable plaque morphology. Irregular or ulcerated plaques increase the risk of stroke by initiating thrombotic cascades, while features such as a lipid core, intraplaque hemorrhage, thin fibrous cap, or ulceration increase the risk of plaque rupture. The vulnerable plaque features can be characterized by US and MRI.

Common Differential Diagnosis

- Carotid dissection: "string sign," no calcified plaque, "flame-shaped" narrowing and/or double lumen on CTA, T1 high-signal mural hematoma on MRI.
- Carotid web: no plaque, shelf-like filling defect at carotid bulb on MRA and DSA.

Management Options

Mild to moderate carotid stenosis can be managed medically, while severe stenosis combined with a history of TIA or stroke requires either endovascular angioplasty, stenting, or endarterectomy.

References and Further Reading

1. David E, et al. Imaging of carotid stenosis: where are we standing? Comparison of multiparametric ultrasound, CT angiography, and MRI angiography, with recent developments. Diagnostics. 2024. https://doi.org/10.3390/diagnostics14161708. Accessed 12 July 2024.
2. Kassem M, et al. Magnetic resonance imaging of carotid plaques: current status and clinical perspectives. Ann Transl Med. 2020. https://doi.org/10.21037/atm-2020-cass-16. PMID: 33178798; PMCID: PMC7607136. Accessed 12 July 2024.

Case 194

194

Clinical History

A 41-year-old man presented with left-sided neck pain following chiropractic manipulation.

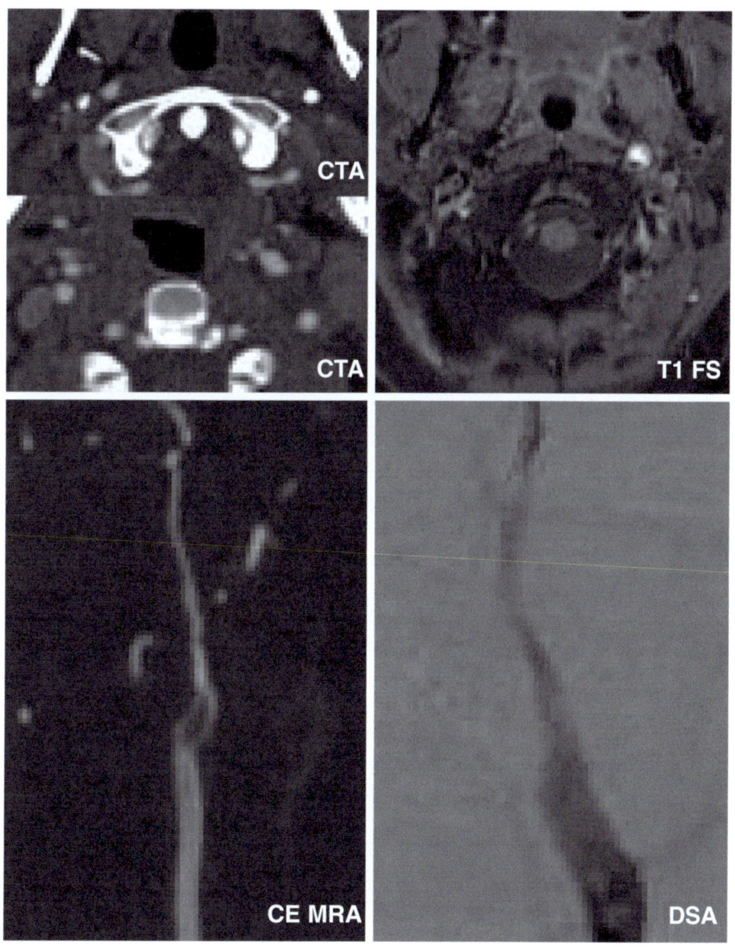

A. Haouimi et al., *Head and Neck Radiology Spot Diagnosis*,
https://doi.org/10.1007/978-3-032-14553-6_194

Findings

Narrowing of the left ICA distal to the bifurcation. A crescentic, mural T1 high signal focus suggesting hematoma. Reformatted MRI correlated with DSA findings. The initial "flame-shaped" tapering is followed by a long-segment "string sign." A small pseudoaneurysm is seen in the cervical ICA below the skull base.

Diagnosis

Carotid dissection.

Discussion

Dissection is an intimal tear allowing the blood to enter the vessel wall, creating a false lumen with luminal narrowing. Thrombosis, embolism, and vessel occlusion secondary to dissection are responsible for TIA or even ischemic stroke. Carotid dissection is a significant cause of stroke in younger patients. Risk factors include hypertension, connective tissue disorders, and cervical trauma. The patients commonly present with local neck pain, headache, or Horner syndrome.

A long tapering arterial stenosis with a "flame-shaped" configuration is the typical appearance responsible for "string-sign" on DSA and reformatted CTA. On MRI, the mural hematoma appears as a T1 high signal crescentic focus from day 3, due to the presence of methemoglobin. Any sudden narrowing or tapering of the carotid lumen should raise the suspicion of dissection. Unlike aortic dissection, intimal flaps or "double lumen" appearances are rarely seen in cervical arteries.

Common Differential Diagnosis

- Atherosclerosis: plaque deposition, irregular narrowing, high PSV with turbulence on ultrasound.
- Fibromuscular dysplasia: "strings of beads" appearance involves mid to distal carotid.

Management Options

The dissection itself is generally managed by anticoagulants or antiplatelet therapy. For severe stenosis or expanding dissecting aneurysm, endovascular or surgical intervention is considered.

References and Further Reading

1. Debette S, et al. ESO guideline for the management of extracranial and intracranial artery dissection. Eur Stroke J. 2021. https://doi.org/10.1177/23969873211046475. Epub 2021 Oct 13. Accessed 11 May 2025.
2. Leira EC. Dedicated guidelines for arterial dissections: more specific amid uncertainty. Stroke. 2022. https://doi.org/10.1161/STROKEAHA.121.037324. Epub 2021 Dec 23. PMID: 34937422. Accessed 11 May 2025.

Case 195

195

Clinical History

A 61-year-old man presented with episodic spells of dizziness and hearing loss.

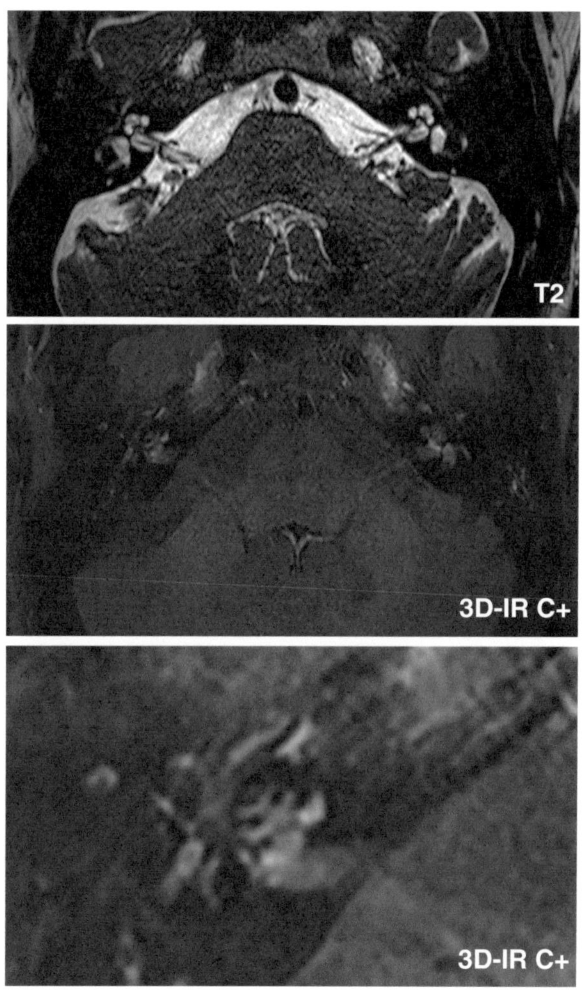

A. Haouimi et al., *Head and Neck Radiology Spot Diagnosis*,
https://doi.org/10.1007/978-3-032-14553-6_195

Findings

Normal bilateral cochlea and vestibule on T2 high-resolution MRI. The 3D real inversion recovery sequence acquired 4 h after contrast reveals endolymphatic hydrops of the cochlea and vestibule on the right side.

Diagnosis

Ménière disease.

Discussion

Ménière disease, also known as endolymphatic hydrops, is an inner ear disorder presenting with recurrent episodes of vertigo, fluctuating sensorineural hearing loss, tinnitus, and a sensation of aural fullness or pressure. The presence of at least two spontaneous vertigo attacks lasting 20 min or longer is required to establish a clinical diagnosis. The condition slowly progresses over time and patients have a substantial impact on daily life and social functioning. The etiology is multifactorial, involving interaction between genetic, environmental, and physiological factors. Clinical symptoms are associated with labyrinthine fluid imbalance. The abnormal build-up of endolymph disrupts the normal balance and hearing.

MRI is the modality of choice to confirm the diagnosis. Delayed postcontrast 3D inversion recovery performed after 4 h helps to differentiate the enhancement patterns within the inner ear structures. The nonenhancing endolymphatic space displaces the contrast-filled perilymphatic space, creating a characteristic striped or layered cochlear appearance. Distension of the endolymphatic structures in the vestibular region, specifically in the utricle and saccule, produces a filling-defect pattern. A proposed grading system can categorize the severity of Ménière disease based on imaging findings seen during visual assessment.

Common Differential Diagnosis

- None apart from false positives.

Management Options

Mild forms of Ménière disease are typically managed medically, which can be escalated to middle ear injections for improved resorption. Surgery is considered for severe vertigo attacks.

References and Further Reading

1. Baráth K, et al. Detection and grading of endolymphatic hydrops in Menière disease using MR imaging. AJNR Am J Neuroradiol. 2014. https://doi.org/10.3174/ajnr.A3856. Epub 2014 Feb 13. PMID: 24524921; PMCID: PMC7966587. Accessed 21 June 2025.
2. Koenen L, Andaloro C. Meniere disease. Stat Pearls Publishing; 2025. https://www.ncbi.nlm.nih.gov/books/NBK536955/. Accessed 21 June 2025.

Case 196

196

Clinical History

A 49-year-old man on immunosuppressive therapy presented to the hospital in septic shock.

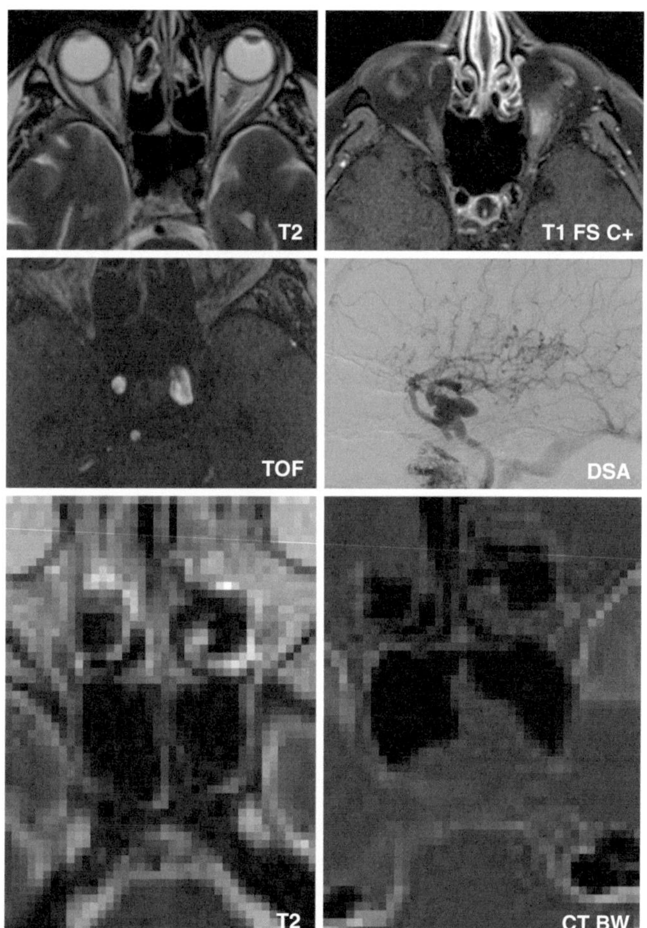

A. Haouimi et al., *Head and Neck Radiology Spot Diagnosis*,
https://doi.org/10.1007/978-3-032-14553-6_196

Findings

A T2-marked low-intensity lesion at posterolateral aspect of left sphenoid sinus showing contrast enhancement of the adjacent left ICA. TOF-angiography demonstrates the formation of an aneurysm of the ICA. DSA performed 3 weeks later shows rapid progression of the mycotic aneurysm.

Diagnosis

Invasive fungal sinusitis.

Discussion

Fungal sinusitis is broadly categorized into invasive and noninvasive forms. Among these, the invasive variant represents the most virulent and rapidly progressive type, frequently associated with substantial morbidity and mortality. It predominantly occurs in immunocompromised individuals, including patients with diabetes mellitus (particularly those experiencing diabetic ketoacidosis), neutropenia, or AIDS. The disease often extends beyond the paranasal sinuses, infiltrating adjacent structures such as the orbits and intracranial compartment. Histopathologically, the causative fungi exhibit an angiocentric pattern of spread, resulting in vascular invasion, ischemia, and tissue necrosis.

Radiologically, unilateral involvement of the ethmoid and sphenoid sinuses, bony destruction, and fat stranding within the orbits or perisinus fat are characteristic findings that raise suspicion for invasive fungal sinusitis. On T2-weighted MRI, the fungal elements typically demonstrate intermediate- to low-signal intensity, which may simulate the appearance of air. Additionally, the absence of mucosal enhancement following contrast administration often reflects underlying tissue necrosis.

Common Differential Diagnosis

- Chronic invasive fungal sinusitis: hyperdense on CT and sclerotic bony changes.
- Sinonasal carcinoma: soft tissue involvement ++, T2 hyperintensity, perineural spread.

Management Options

Invasive fungal sinusitis requires medical and often surgical management to contain the infection. The underlying neutropenia should be corrected.

References and Further Reading

1. Akhondi H, Woldemariam B, Rajasurya V. Fungal sinusitis. Stat Pearls Publishing; 2025. https://www.ncbi.nlm.nih.gov/books/NBK551496/.
2. Aribandi M, et al. Imaging features of invasive and noninvasive fungal sinusitis: a review. Radiographics. 2007. https://doi.org/10.1148/rg.275065189. PMID: 17848691. Accessed 14 June 2025.
3. Fadda GL, et al. Definition and management of invasive fungal rhinosinusitis: a single-centre retrospective study. Acta Otorhinolaryngol Ital. 2021. https://doi.org/10.14639/0392-100X-N0848. Accessed 14 June 2025.

Case 197

197

Clinical History

An 81-year-old man presented with cervicalgia, fever, and dysphagia.

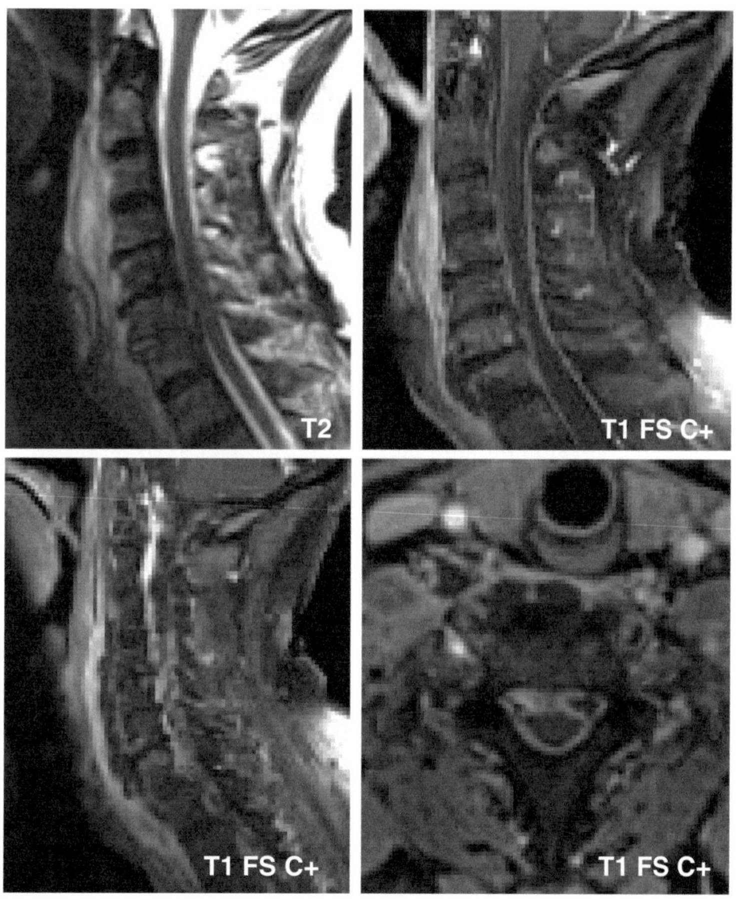

A. Haouimi et al., *Head and Neck Radiology Spot Diagnosis*,
https://doi.org/10.1007/978-3-032-14553-6_197

Findings

Markedly thickened prevertebral soft tissue causing midline bulge at posterior esophagopharyngeal juncture. An elongated fluid collection with peripheral enhancement involving both longus colli anteriorly and epidural tissue posteriorly at C6/C7 level. Associated C6/C7 discitis/osteomyelitis.

Diagnosis

Prevertebral abscess.

Discussion

The prevertebral space is the space between the prevertebral fascia and vertebral bodies and deep cervical musculature extending the entire length of the vertebral column from clivus to the coccyx. The fibrous attachments between the prevertebral fascia and deep cervical muscles tend to contain longitudinal prevertebral infections. In the cervical region, the prevertebral and retropharyngeal spaces are separated by the alar fascia and are indistinguishable in a healthy patient.

The primary site of infection determines which space will be predominantly involved. Infectious processes from the spinal column, such as discitis/osteomyelitis, primarily involve the prevertebral space and prevertebral muscles. In contrast, infectious processes originating from the visceral space of the neck predominantly affect the retropharyngeal space. The alar fascia extends from the clivus to the C7 level, where the two potential spaces merge. Narrowing of the aerodigestive tract and extension of infection into the mediastinum are life-threatening complications.

Common Differential Diagnosis

- Retropharyngeal abscess: no vertebral or epidural involvement, mediastinal extension +/−.
- Longus colli calcific tendinitis: clinical, amorphous calcification, no restricted diffusion.

Management Options

Emergency surgical drainage and antibiotic treatment.

References and Further Reading

1. Hoang JK, et al. Multiplanar CT and MRI of collections in the retropharyngeal space: is it an abscess? AJR Am J Roentgenol. 2011. https://doi.org/10.2214/AJR.10.5116. PMID: 21427307. Accessed 11 Aug 2024.
2. Jalisi S, et al. Features of prevertebral disease in patients presenting to a head and neck surgery clinic with neck pain. Ann Maxillofac Surg. 2017. https://doi.org/10.4103/ams.ams_54_17. PMID: 29264290; PMCID: PMC5717899. Accessed 11 Aug 2024.

Case 198

198

Clinical History

An 18-year-old girl presented with a profound hearing loss. CT for preoperative assessment.

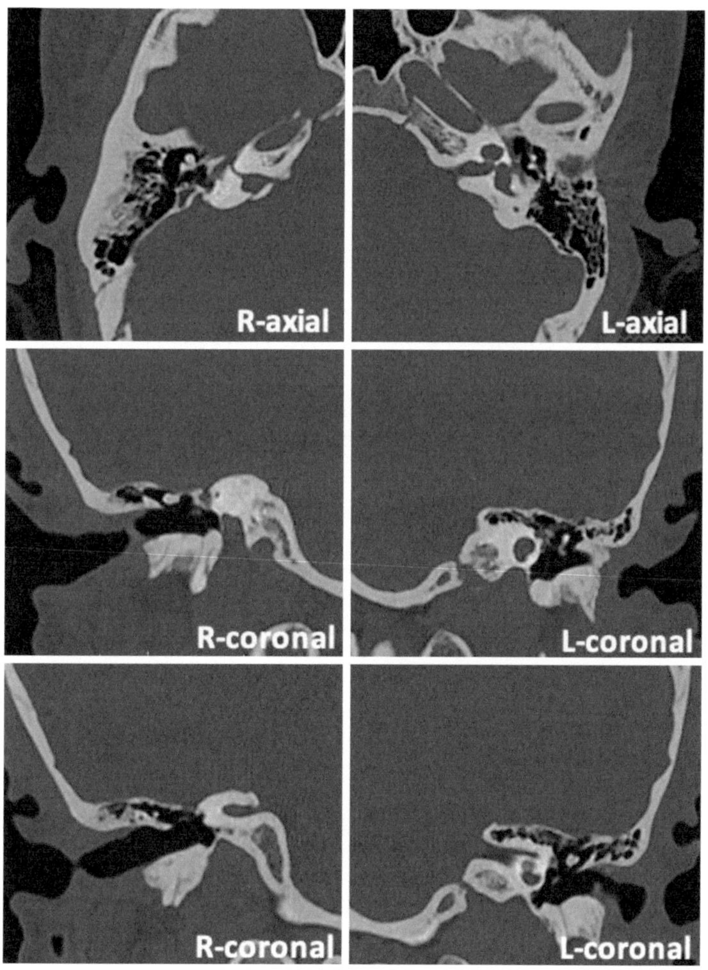

A. Haouimi et al., *Head and Neck Radiology Spot Diagnosis*,
https://doi.org/10.1007/978-3-032-14553-6_198

Findings

Complete absence of the right labyrinth and narrowing of the right internal auditory canal. Absent modiolus and interscalar septum giving a hypodense cystic appearance to the left inner ear. Dilated and globular left vestibule. Normal left internal auditory canal indirectly suggesting normal vestibulocochlear nerve (needs to be confirmed by MRI).

Diagnosis

Right "Michel aplasia" and type 1 left partial cochlear partition.

Discussion

Cochlear malformations are congenital abnormalities. Cochlear aplasia, also known as "Michel aplasia," is the complete absence of cochlea due to developmental arrest during the third week of gestation from failure of otic placode differentiation. Michel aplasia is extremely rare, accounting for less than 1% of all inner ear malformations. On imaging, no cochlear structure is identified.

The cochlear malformation is an umbrella term to describe cochlear abnormalities ranging from mild hypoplasia to severe abnormalities such as a partial partition in Mondini dysplasia. Cochlear aplasia is the most severe form of cochlear malformation. The developmental arrest during the fourth gestational week is responsible for a common cavity appearance, arrest at the sixth week causes cochlear hypoplasia, and Mondini malformation occurs when the arrest occurs at the seventh week.

Clinically, patients with cochlear malformations suffer from profound uni- or bilateral hearing loss often detected by newborn hearing screening. Vestibular dysfunction may lead to delayed milestones (sitting and walking). Cochlear malformation can be isolated or syndromic.

Common Differential Diagnosis

- Labyrinthine ossificans: progressive acquired hearing loss, history of infection/trauma.
- CHARGE syndrome: associated coloboma, nasal atresia, cardiac and genital abnormality.
- Goldenhar syndrome: associated hemifacial abnormality, spinal abnormality.

Management Options

Multidisciplinary approach for hearing and vestibular rehabilitation. Cochlear implantation can be considered for Mondini dysplasia but not for Michel aplasia.

References and Further Reading

1. Brotto D, et al. Genetics of inner ear malformations: a review. Audiol Res. 2021. https://doi.org/10.3390/audiolres11040047. PMID: 34698066; PMCID: PMC8544219. Accessed 15 June 2024.
2. Ibrahim D, et al. Cochlear aplasia. Radiopaedia.org. https://doi.org/10.53347/rID-47542. Accessed 2 Feb 2025.

Case 199

199

Clinical History

A 44-year-old man presented with a recent history of stroke for investigation.

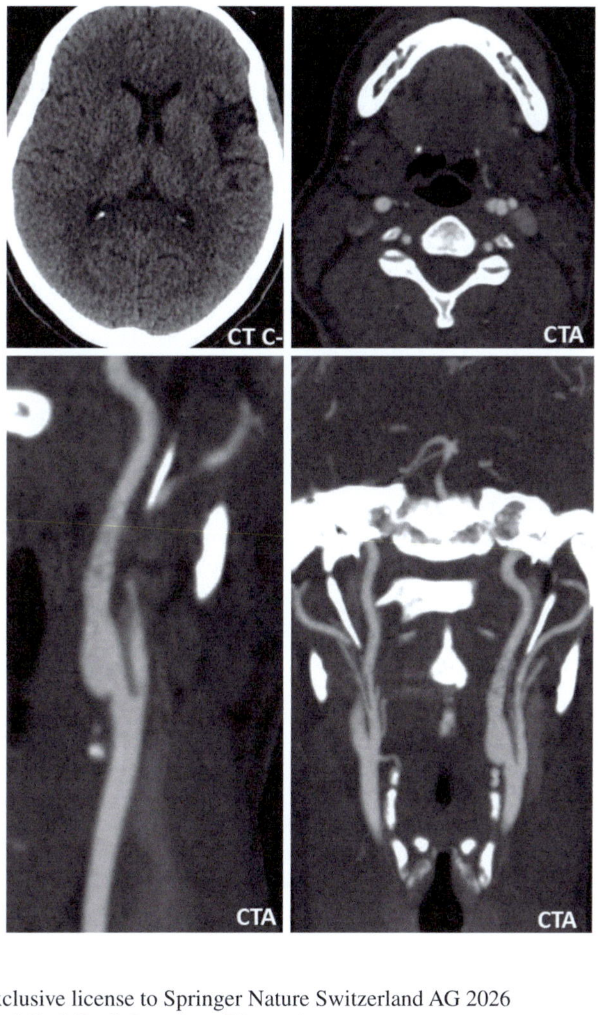

A. Haouimi et al., *Head and Neck Radiology Spot Diagnosis*,
https://doi.org/10.1007/978-3-032-14553-6_199

Findings

Left insular and superior temporal gyrus old infarct seen on CT. CTA shows a small, thin, smooth eccentric filling defect at posterior wall of left ICA origin with no stenosis or occlusion.

Diagnosis

Carotid web.

Discussion

Carotid web is a variant of intimal fibromuscular dysplasia and an underrecognized nonatherosclerotic cause of cryptogenic stroke in young patients without any obvious risk factors. It is a fibrous shelf-like intimal flap arising typically from the wall of the carotid bulb and projecting into the lumen. The shelf creates turbulent blood flow and facilitates thrombus formation, which causes embolic strokes. Unlike atherosclerosis, there is no significant luminal narrowing.

Stroke in young patients without risk factors is the typical clinical presentation. CTA is a reasonable initial test, though DSA is the gold standard. Other imaging modalities, such as US and MRA, are less reliable. The diagnosis can be missed on US due to its non-atherosclerotic nature, but a high-velocity flow jet at the carotid bulb can be seen on color Doppler.

Common Differential Diagnosis

- Internal carotid artery dissection flap: usually more distal, irregular borders.
- ICA atherosclerotic plaque: associated calcifications, more distal, irregular borders.
- Carotid aneurysm: focal outpouching.

Management Options

Treatment options are both medical and endovascular. A single antiplatelet drug is insufficient due to the high rates of recurrent stroke. Symptomatic patients are usually given dual anti-thrombotic or anticoagulation medication. For patients with multiple strokes, revascularization has been proposed via carotid stenting or carotid endarterectomy in stenotic cases.

References and Further Reading

1. Chen H, et al. Carotid webs: a review of pathophysiology, diagnostic findings, and treatment options. J Neurointerv Surg. 2024. https://doi.org/10.1136/jnis-2023-021243. Accessed 1 Dec 2024.
2. Liang S, et al. The carotid web: current research status and imaging features. Front Neurosci. 2023. https://doi.org/10.3389/fnins.2023.1104212. Accessed 1 Dec 2024.
3. Madaelil TP, et al. Multimodality imaging in carotid web. Front Neurol. 2019. https://doi.org/10.3389/fneur.2019.00220. Accessed 1 Dec 2024.

Case 200

200

Clinical History

A 54-year-old man presented to the ENT clinic with a slow-growing left neck mass.

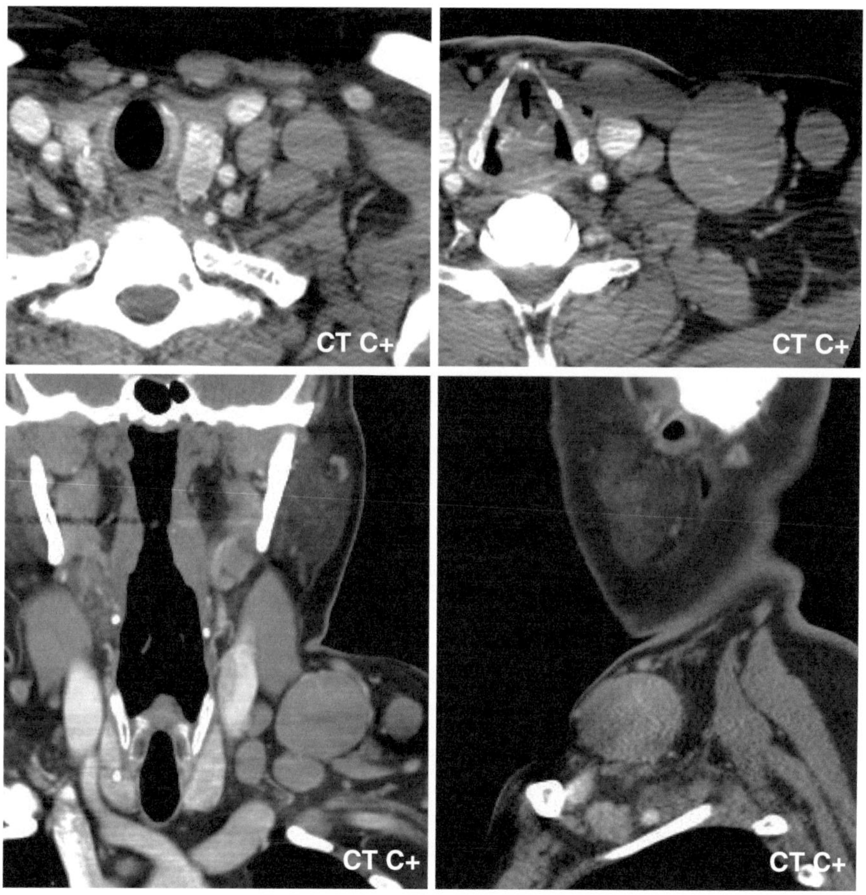

A. Haouimi et al., *Head and Neck Radiology Spot Diagnosis*,
https://doi.org/10.1007/978-3-032-14553-6_200

Findings

Homogenously enhancing non-necrotic nodal masses of variable sizes involving the left lower neck. No calcification or perinodal fat infiltration. No mediastinal masses.

Diagnosis

Castleman disease.

Discussion

Castleman disease (CD) is a rare hematologic disorder of unknown etiology involving B-cell proliferation. Lymph node involvement can be both uni- and multicentric.

Most unicentric CD is asymptomatic apart from localized painless swelling and compression on adjacent structure. They are thought to be linked to immune system dysfunction. Multicentric CD affects lymph nodes throughout the body and may or may not be associated with HHV-8. The commonest site of multicentric involvement is the chest and neck, followed by the abdomen. Negative HHV cases are considered idiopathic.

Unicentric CD demonstrates the presence of well-defined hypervascular non-necrotic enlarged lymph nodes with prolonged enhancement on delayed CT and MRI. Occasionally, perinodal infiltration, calcifications, and hypertrophied vasculature can be seen. Multicentric type is usually associated with hepatosplenomegaly. On MRI, the nodes are typically iso- to hyperintense to muscle on T1, hyper- or isointense on T2, with homogeneous contrast enhancement. Diagnostic certitude however requires core or excisional biopsy.

Common Differential Diagnosis

- Lymphoma: extranodal involvement, high FDG (SUV > 10) on PET CT.
- Kimura disease: subcutaneous nodule, eosinophilia, enlarged nodes with fatty hilum.
- Metastatic cancer: known primary.

Management Options

Complete surgical excision for symptomatic unicentric cases with excellent prognosis. When surgery is not feasible, radiation, embolization, or monoclonal antibodies are considered. Multicentric cases are treated with monoclonal antibodies and steroids, followed by chemotherapy.

References and Further Reading

1. Din F, et al. Radiology of Castleman disease: the pivotal role of imaging in diagnosis, staging, and response assessment of this rare entity. Clin Radiol. 2022. https://doi.org/10.1016/j.crad.2022.01.045. Accessed 11 Aug 2025.
2. Lang E, Van Rhee F. Idiopathic multicentric Castleman disease: an update in diagnosis and treatment advances. Blood Rev. 2023. https://doi.org/10.1016/j.blre.2023.101161. Accessed 11 Aug 2025. CC.

Blurb

Head and neck radiology is an exciting field that requires a deep understanding of the complex anatomy, pathology, and imaging techniques involved. This is a region that is at the crossroads between several medical specialties, including otolaryngology, ophthalmology, skull-base neurosurgery, dental surgery, radiation, and medical oncology. It is tough to diagnose, and endoscopy provides only a limited view. Hence, cross-sectional imaging and standard x-rays are vital in the assessment of patients.

This book aims to bridge the gap between theory and practice by presenting key topics in a visually appealing and interactive format. Cases are designed to engage readers through self-assessment. Each case starts with high-quality images and a clinical history, prompting the reader to evaluate the findings and propose a diagnosis or differential. Concise explanatory notes follow, explaining the imaging features, pathophysiology, and clinical relevance of each condition. Differential considerations are highlighted concisely to train the reader in systematic diagnostic reasoning. A short description accompanies every case, including management options, distilling essential information without overwhelming details.

This approach ensures clarity while covering the wide range of head and neck disorders. Emphasis is placed on correlation with clinical scenarios, helping readers understand the broader context of imaging findings. The interactive design promotes self-paced learning, making it ideal for radiologists, residents, fellows, and other healthcare professionals involved in treating the diseases of the head and neck. By blending visual learning with concise explanations, this book provides an engaging resource to enhance diagnostic accuracy. This companion book aims to promote an intuitive understanding of anatomy, pathology, and imaging nuances across all major modalities, including CT, MRI, and ultrasound. The case-based pedagogy allows readers to test their diagnostic skills before revealing guided interpretations, fostering an interactive and self-directed learning experience. The interactive format not only reinforces key imaging patterns but also encourages self-assessment, making it an ideal companion for board preparation, clinical rotations, or daily practice. This book aims to inspire confidence, curiosity, and a deeper understanding of this complex and fascinating area of radiology.

Features

- Randomly arranged 200 head and neck cases for self-evaluation.
- More than 1000 high-quality MRI, CT, and Ultrasound images.
- Description of findings to identify typical radiologic signs.
- Tips to narrow down the diagnostic spectrum.
- Brief notion of choice of treatment and management.
- Guidance for further reading and references.

A. Haouimi et al., *Head and Neck Radiology Spot Diagnosis*,
https://doi.org/10.1007/978-3-032-14553-6

Index

A. Haouimi et al., *Head and Neck Radiology Spot Diagnosis*,
https://doi.org/10.1007/978-3-032-14553-6

MIX
Papier aus verantwortungsvollen Quellen
Paper from responsible sources
FSC® C105338

If you have any concerns about our products,
you can contact us on
ProductSafety@springernature.com

In case Publisher is established outside the EU,
the EU authorized representative is:
Springer Nature Customer Service Center GmbH
Europaplatz 3, 69115 Heidelberg, Germany

Printed by Libri Plureos GmbH
in Hamburg, Germany